Atlas of Graft-versus-Host Disease

Jonathan A. Cotliar
Editor

Atlas of Graft-versus-Host Disease

Approaches to Diagnosis and Treatment

Springer

Editor
Jonathan A. Cotliar
Division of Dermatology
City of Hope National Medical Center
Division of Dermatology
Duarte, California
USA

ISBN 978-3-319-46950-8 ISBN 978-3-319-46952-2 (eBook)
DOI 10.1007/978-3-319-46952-2

Library of Congress Control Number: 2016963253

Printed on acid-free paper

This Springer imprint is published by Springer Nature
The registered company is Springer International Publishing AG
The registered company address is Gewerbestrasse 11, 6330 Cham, Switzerland

To the University of Kentucky College of Medicine for taking a chance on me; Dr. Victor Newcomer, whose enthusiasm and teaching was the inspiration for my career; Dr. Amy Paller, whose support and guidance I will never forget; Dr. Ronald Cotliar, whose energy and compassion I admire and try to emulate daily; my mother Ellen for your endless supply of love and support; my wife Sumie and children Zoe and Zach, whom I love more than anything. A special recognition to the patients and their families that have entrusted me with their care, a privilege that I never take for granted.

Foreword

Allogeneic hematopoietic cell transplantation was developed as a therapy in the early 1970s as a treatment for inherited and acquired diseases of the blood and immune system. Although initially utilized predominantly for patients with severe aplastic anemia or advanced acute leukemia who had a matched sibling donor, the therapy has evolved to be a potential treatment for all diseases of the hematopoietic and immune system, including inherited diseases such as sickle cell disease, acquired diseases involving all of hematologic malignancies, and numerous rare disorders where the underlying cause of the disease is in the hematopoietic stem cell. Among the major early complications are those related to treatment regimens that were usually total body irradiation– or high-dose chemotherapy–based and infections during the early phase of transplant. The other major challenge to patients is the development of the acute and chronic graft-versus-host reaction that occurs despite molecular matching between donor and recipient, both in the family and through international registries. All patients undergoing allogeneic transplant require some degree of either systemic graft-versus-host disease (GVHD) prevention therapy or graft manipulation to reduce this complication and to induce a state of tolerance where the donor's immune system protects the patient and a functioning hematopoietic and immune system organ functions for the life of the patient. Although considered the most challenging of transplant complications, graft-versus-host reaction is associated with a reduced chance for relapse of the original disease, which is an important consideration in those patients undergoing transplant for treatment of hematologic malignancy where prevention of relapse is the reason for this treatment.

Over the years, numerous treatments have evolved for preventing and treating graft-versus-host reaction. The field has evolved to understand at the cellular and molecular level the basis for this reaction, which is donor derived, but results from interactions with the residual hematopoietic system of the recipient as well, of course, with target antigens on nonhematopoietic tissue. Strategies have been explored to try to achieve the ultimate goal of the transplant, which is to engraft the patient with cells that will cure the disease but not cause complications.

In addition to changes in conditioning regimens and GVHD prevention and treatment strategies, there has also been a change in the patient population who are undergoing transplantation. In the early decades, allogeneic transplant was restricted predominantly to patients who had a matched sibling donor and who were under the age of 45–50. However, with the development of newer and safer approaches that consistently facilitate donor stem-cell engraftment and rely heavily on the donor immune system to control the malignancy, older patients have been transplanted. It is common now to see patients undergoing transplant for treatment of hematologic malignancy in their 60s and 70s. Thus, the spectrum of manifestations of graft-versus-host reaction is also evolving thanks to the type of transplant (sibling, matched unrelated, cord blood, haploidentical) that is used as the age diversity increases.

This Atlas, as edited by Dr. Jonathan Cotliar at the City of Hope Comprehensive Cancer Center, is focused on manifestations of both acute and chronic graft-versus-host reaction in its various forms but, in particular, the dermatologic and mucosal manifestations. This book provides the reader with an initial introduction to hematopoietic stem cell transplantation, reflecting the evolution of the treatment over the past four decades, and provides both text and images reflecting the various aspects of the GVHD, including the clinical presentations of cutaneous and mucosal GVHD and the pathologic manifestations derived from biopsy material of patients who have this syndrome. One of the observations that was made with the development of a reduced-intensity transplant has been the changing manifestations of graft-versus-host reaction and its timing, and this book is useful in understanding this change in the clinical presentation that is no longer simply acute GVHD in the first 100 days and chronic GVHD and its manifestations after that time. Dr. Cotliar and his collaborators in this project provide practical and scientific information for both the diagnosis and treatment of these GVHD manifestations, which can be so challenging for patients and physicians. The chapters emphasize how early recognition and early intervention can sometimes blunt the evolving manifestations that affect quality of life for patients and result in long-term immunosuppression and a full recovery. To their credit, he has included chapters on wound care in the management of chronic GVHD.

Although numerous books have chapters on graft-versus-host reaction, this Atlas provides both visual and text to aid physicians and other health care personnel in helping to both recognize and manage patients with graft-versus-host reaction so that the overall goal of the procedure, namely cure of the underlying hematopoietic disorder, can be realized. This book, therefore, should have wide appeal for those who have been in the field for many years and for those who are entering it to make their own contributions to both research and care to help improve the outcome for patients undergoing transplant to cure their disease.

Duarte, CA, USA Stephen J. Forman

Preface

I am grateful to have received help from so many friends and colleagues in this undertaking. Individual dermatologists, oncologists, and pathologists from many of the leading clinical centers in the United States all contributed to this effort. As such, we were able to generate a text that I believe will provide valuable guidance for those medical students, residents, fellows, nurses, attending physicians, and other allied health professionals who take care of patients with graft-versus-host disease (GVHD). Our understanding about the intricacies of GVHD diagnosis and treatment are constantly developing as basic and translational science in the field evolves. As such, I believe this text is reflective of the best current evidence we have to date for clinicians treating patients with GVHD.

As a young physician taking care of patients suffering from GVHD, it would have been nice to have a resource handy that could have provided the type of comprehensive guidance required for a disease entity that has such a heterogeneous and complicated clinical presentation. The collaboration we sought in generating this text was based upon input from individuals with varied training backgrounds and current clinical practice, which I believe enabled us to capture the perspectives and nuances of GVHD diagnosis/management that can only result from the input of both oncologists and dermatologists. When combining the experiences of clinicians from these different backgrounds, it creates a more powerful and useful resource for readers.

I am hopeful that the efforts of the contributors to this textbook will be recognized in a way that ultimately benefits patients. If any of the photographs or pearls that lie within these pages can help clinicians better recognize GVHD at the bedside, gain better insight into the presentation of the disease, or provide a patient with a therapeutic option that otherwise would not have been considered, then the goals of constructing this atlas will have been met.

Duarte, CA, USA   Jonathan A. Cotliar, MD

Contents

Contributors

Timothy H. Almazan, MD Division of Dermatology, City of Hope Comprehensive Cancer Center, Duarte, CA, USA

Amin M. Alousi, MD Department of Stem Cell Transplantation and Cellular Therapies, University of Texas M. D. Anderson Cancer Center, Houston, TX, USA

Valerie Carlberg, MD Department of Dermatology, School of Medicine, Oregon Health and Science University, Portland, OR, USA

Christine M. Cornejo, MD Department of Dermatology, Perelman School of Medicine, University of Pennsylvania, Philadelphia, PA, USA

Edward W. Cowen, MD, MHSc Dermatology Branch, Center for Cancer Research, National Cancer Institute, National Institutes of Health, Bethesda, MD, USA

Lauren Curtis, MD Experimental Transplantation and Immunology Branch, National Cancer Institute, National Institutes of Health, Bethesda, MD, USA

Sophia Delano, MD Division of Dermatology, Department of Medicine, University of Massachusetts Medical School, Worcester, MA, USA

Jennifer T. Huang, MD Department of Dermatology, Harvard Medical School, Dermatology Program, Boston Children's Hospital, Boston, MA, USA

Sharon R. Hymes, MD Department of Dermatology, University of Texas M. D. Anderson Cancer Center, Houston, TX, USA

Samantha M. Jaglowski, MD, MPH Department of Internal Medicine, Division of Hematology, The Ohio State University Wexner Medical Center, Columbus, OH, USA

Jae Y. Jung, MD Division of Dermatology, City of Hope Comprehensive Cancer Center, Duarte, CA, USA

Benjamin H. Kaffenberger, MD Division of Dermatology, The Ohio State University Wexner Medical Center, Columbus, OH, USA

Rachel I. Kornik, MD Department of Dermatology, University of California, San Francisco, San Francisco, CA, USA

Jacqueline W. Mays Oral and Pharyngeal Cancer Branch, National Institute of Dental and Craniofacial Research, National Institutes of Health, Bethesda, MD, USA

Robert G. Micheletti, MD Department of Dermatology and Medicine, Perelman School of Medicine, University of Pennsylvania, Philadelphia, PA, USA

Anar Mikailov, MD Department of Dermatology, Brigham and Women's Hospital and Harvard Medical School, Boston, MA, USA

Daniel D. Miller, MD Department of Dermatology, University of Minnesota Medical Center, Minneapolis, MN, USA

Haley B. Naik, MD, MHSc Department of Dermatology, University of California, San Francisco, San Francisco, CA, USA

Ryotaro Nakamura, MD Division of Dermatology, City of Hope Comprehensive Cancer Center, Duarte, CA, USA

Cuong V. Nguyen, MD Department of Dermatology, University of Minnesota, Minneapolis, MN, USA

Dominique C. Pichard, MD Dermatology Branch, Center for Cancer Research, National Cancer Institute, National Institutes of Health, Bethesda, MD, USA

Sarah S. Pinney, MD Department of Dermatology, University of Texas Houston Medical School, Houston, TX, USA

Molly Elizabeth Plovanich, MD Department of Dermatology, Brigham and Women's Hospital and Harvard Medical School, Boston, MA, USA

Christiane Querfeld, MD Division of Dermatology, City of Hope Comprehensive Cancer Center, Duarte, CA, USA

Arturo P. Saavedra, MD Department of Dermatology, Massachusetts General Hospital and Harvard Medical School, Boston, MA, USA

Amandeep Salhotra, MD Hematology and Hematopoietic Cell Transplantation, City of Hope National Medical Center, Duarte, CA, USA

Emily A. Simons, MPH Dermatology Program, Boston Children's Hospital, Boston, MA, USA

1 Overview of Hematopoietic Cell Transplantation

Amandeep Salhotra and Ryotaro Nakamura

Allogeneic hematopoietic stem cell transplantation (HSCT) is a form of immune therapy used to treat a variety of malignant and nonmalignant diseases. The procedure involves transfusion of multipotent hematopoietic stem cells derived from bone marrow, peripheral blood, or umbilical cord blood from a donor, usually matched in human leukocyte antigens (HLA). Immediately prior to HSCT, patients receive conditioning chemoradiotherapy to eliminate underlying hematologic malignant cells, and to sufficiently suppress the host's immune functions for successful engraftment of donor hematopoietic cells. Following the conditioning regimen and HSCT, donor-derived hematopoietic recovery and immune reconstitution occur, during which patients require intensive supportive care, including prevention and treatment of complications such as infections and acute or chronic graft-versus-host disease (GVHD).

Currently, between 55,000 and 60,000 HSCTs are performed worldwide each year, including approximately 8000 in the United States alone [1]. With the use of alternative donor strategies, reduced intensity conditioning (RIC) regimens, and greater availability of donors, the application of this form of immunotherapy is set to increase in the coming years (Fig. 1.1). Although allogeneic HSCT is the most effective and intensive therapy for hematologic disorders, there are significant barriers towards improving outcomes of HSCT, including transplant-related morbidity and mortality associated with acute and chronic GVHD, infection or delayed immune reconstitution, and regimen-related organ toxicities. In addition, despite intensive conditioning regimens and potent graft-versus-leukemia (GVL) effects, post-transplant relapse remains a significant cause of treatment failure. Thus, ongoing efforts are focused on improving patient selection criteria, preventing and treating GVHD and infection, and devising methods to reduce post-HSCT relapse of the underlying disease.

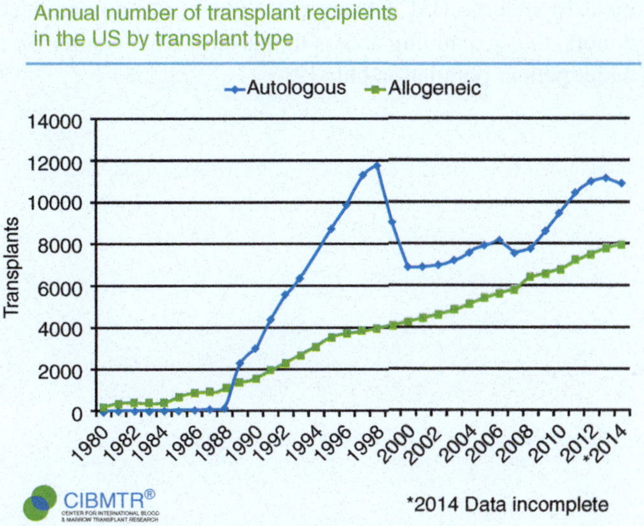

Fig. 1.1 Increasing numbers of patients are undergoing allogeneic hematopoietic stem cell transplantation (HSCT) every year (*Adapted from* Pasquini and Zhu [1]; *with permission*)

A. Salhotra (✉)
Hematology and Hematopoietic Cell Transplantation, City of Hope National Medical Center, 1500 East Duarte Road, Duarte, CA 91010, USA
e-mail: asalhotra@coh.org

R. Nakamura
Division of Dermatology, City of Hope Comprehensive Cancer Center, 1500 East Duarte Road, Duarte, CA 91010, USA
e-mail: rnakamura@coh.org

J.A. Cotliar (ed.), *Atlas of Graft-versus-Host Disease*, DOI 10.1007/978-3-319-46952-2_1

Historical Perspective

Pioneering experimentation by Jacobson in the 1940s showed that mice were protected from the deleterious effects of radiation if their spleens were shielded with lead foils [2]. The cellular basis of this protection was proved when infusion from marrow and spleen cells conferred a similar protective effect from radiation. Barnes et al. [3] were the first investigators to report treatment of murine leukemia with high-dose radiation followed by infusion of healthy marrow from littermates. The first group to publish results of long-term survival of patients with acute leukemia was from the Seattle group led by Dr. E.D. Thomas [4]. Patients received total body irradiation (TBI) and cyclophosphamide (Cy)–based conditioning and bone marrow grafts from HLA-matched sibling donors. Only 13 of the initial 100 enrolled patients in this trial eventually survived on long-term follow up, but this initial study gave an indication that this form of therapy could be curative in a proportion of leukemia patients. Similar results published by Blume and Beutler from City of Hope [5] confirmed the initial results from Seattle. Another advance in the field was the introduction of calcineurin inhibitors in combination with methotrexate for prevention of GVHD [6, 7]. This combination was associated with significantly lower risk of Grades II–IV aGVHD and improved disease-free survival. Other advancements in the field have been the development of alternative conditioning regimens to TBI/Cy [8], the introduction of prophylactic ganciclovir for cytomegalovirus (CMV) pulmonary infection [9], and the introduction of allele-level HLA typing as a result of improvement in molecular typing techniques, resulting in better-matched transplants [10]. Introduction of RIC regimens has allowed elderly patients and patients with comorbidities who cannot tolerate fully myeloablative regimens to undergo HSCT from matched sibling and unrelated donors, thus expanding access to this curative modality for a wider patient population [11, 12].

Indications for Allogeneic Hematopoietic Cell Transplantation

Allogeneic HSCT is often the only potentially curative treatment for hematologic malignancies in an advanced stage or for relapsed disease. For early-stage disease such as acute myeloid leukemia (AML) or acute lymphoblastic leukemia (ALL) in first complete remission (CR1), the risk of relapse can be significantly reduced by allogeneic HSCT, but the medical decision is complex and has to be carefully balanced against the risk of transplant-related mortality. In general, allogeneic HSCT is considered for acute leukemia in CR1 with intermediate-risk or high-risk features, or cases that are beyond CR1. In the United States, AML/ALL and myelodysplastic syndromes (MDS) account for 65 % of patients who undergo allogeneic HSCT based on the most recent data provided by the Center for International Blood and Marrow Transplant Research (CIBMTR) [13]. With the introduction of targeted therapy with tyrosine kinase inhibitors for chronic myeloid leukemia (CML), HSCT is reserved only for patients with refractory disease. Refractory non-Hodgkin's lymphoma, chronic lymphocytic leukemia (CLL), and nonmalignant diseases such as aplastic anemia, and paroxysmal nocturnal hemoglobinuria (PNH) comprise the remainder of indications for allogeneic HSCT.

The American Society of Blood and Marrow Transplantation (ASBMT) established a multiple-stakeholder taskforce to study role of HSCT in established disease states and identify emerging indications where HSCT may potentially be beneficial. This task force came out with a white paper in 2015 with clearly defined indications across disease states where HSCT has been shown to be of clinical benefit based on available clinical trial data. Published systematic evidence reviews or guidelines were used as the basis for recommendations to categorize indications for HSCT in pediatric and adult populations [13]; this comprehensive review of indications for HSCT based on currently available clinical evidence is highly recommended (Table 1.1) (Fig. 1.2) [14].

Table 1.1 Diseases for which allogeneic and autologous hematopoietic stem cell transplantation is used [13]

Malignant
Leukemia/preleukemia
Chronic myeloid leukemia
Myeloproliferative syndromes (other than chronic myeloid leukemia)
Acute myeloid leukemia
Acute lymphoblastic leukemia
Juvenile chronic myeloid leukemia
Myelodysplastic syndromes
Therapy-related myelodysplasia/leukemia
Kostmann's agranulocytosis
Chronic lymphocytic leukemia
Non-Hodgkin's and Hodgkin's lymphoma
Multiple myeloma
Solid tumors
Breast cancer
Neuroblastoma
Sarcomas
Ovarian cancer
Small cell lung cancer
Testicular cancer
Nonmalignant
Severe aplastic anemia
Paroxysmal nocturnal hemoglobinuria
Hemoglobinopathies
Thalassemia major
Sickle cell disease
Congenital disorders of hematopoiesis
Fanconi anemia
Diamond-Blackfan syndrome
Familial erythrophagocytic histiocytes
Dyskeratosis congenita
Schwachman-Diamond syndrome
Severe combined immune deficiency and related disorders
Wiskott-Aldrich syndrome
Inborn errors of metabolism
Acquired autoimmune diseases

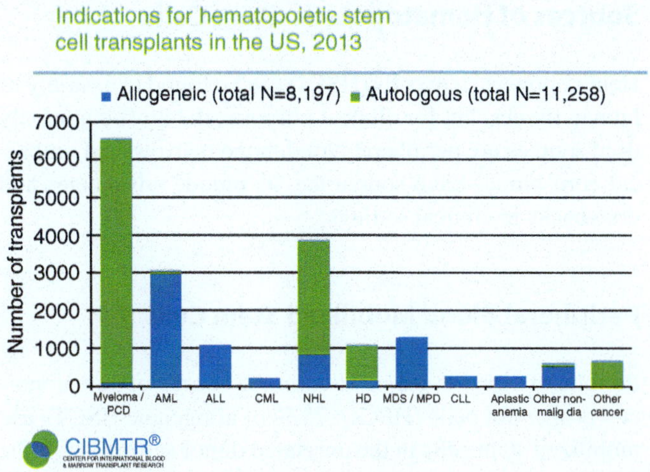

Fig. 1.2 Common indications for allogeneic and autologous HSCT (Adapted from Pasquini and Zhu [1]; *with permission*)

Sources of Hematopoietic Stem Cells

Hematopoietic stem cells (HSCs) can be found in a variety of human tissues, but for clinical purposes the most commonly used sources are peripheral blood, bone marrow, and umbilical cord blood. Each source has its unique advantages and drawbacks in clinical settings.

Peripheral Blood Mobilized Stem Cells

Peripheral blood is the most common source of hematopoietic progenitor cells (HPCs); 75 % of allogeneic HSCTs use mobilized stem cells in the unrelated donor setting [15]. The benefits of peripheral blood mobilized stem cells in the matched sibling setting are faster hematopoietic engraftment and fewer infectious complications due to higher numbers of CD34+ HSCs than in bone marrow grafts [16, 17]. Moreover, the procedure is less invasive than bone marrow harvest and more donor-friendly. In healthy donors, the concentration of CD34+ cells is 0.06 % in peripheral blood and 1.1 % in bone marrow [18]. This percentage can be readily augmented by growth factor priming and by chemotherapy in the setting of autologous stem cell transplantation. After four doses of granulocyte colony-stimulating factor (G-CSF) at 12 µg/kg per day, the mean peripheral blood CD34+ count increased from a baseline of 3.8×10^9/L to 61.9×10^9/L [19], allowing apheresis of CD34+ HPCs from the peripheral blood for infusion purposes. The peripheral blood stem cell (PBSC) graft has 10 times higher concentrations of T cells, monocytes, and NK cells compared with bone marrow graft, and the higher concentration of T cells in the PBSC grafts has been correlated with a higher incidence of acute and chronic GVHD in both related and unrelated HSCTs [15, 20]. The optimal CD34 dose is 2 to 5×10^6 cells/kg in the allogeneic HSCT setting; a CD34 dose exceeding 8×10^6 cells/kg has been associated with the development of chronic GVHD [21].

Bone Marrow Hematopoietic Stem Cells

Traditionally, bone marrow has been the source of HPCs used in the sibling and unrelated-donor settings. Five to 10 mL of bone marrow is typically obtained from healthy donors from the posterior iliac crest under general anesthesia, with a goal of 10–15 mL/kg of recipient weight, corresponding to a marrow volume of 700–1500 mL for an adult donor. The goal is to collect a minimum total nucleated cell dose of 2×10^8 cells/kg for successful engraftment. The bone marrow graft has lower numbers of T cells, correlated with a lower incidence of chronic GVHD in the unrelated-donor setting, although the graft failure rate is higher at 9 % [15].

Umbilical Cord Blood Stem Cells

Umbilical cord blood (UCB) contains high numbers of HPCs, and double cord stem cell transplants have been successfully used in adults for hematologic malignancies [22]. When mismatched UCB HSCT was compared with mismatched bone marrow HSCT for acute leukemia in the myeloablative setting, the transplant-related mortality, treatment failure, and overall mortality were similar [23], indicating that UCB is a viable source of HSCs for treatment of advanced hematologic malignancies. The major disadvantage to the use of UCB is the significant delay in neutrophil engraftment (average 27 days) and platelet engraftment (average 29 days) compared with bone marrow and PBSC graft sources. This delay in hematopoietic engraftment increases transfusion requirements and the risk of infectious complications. Graft failure is a major concern with UCB transplants (10 % in RIC and 20 % in myeloablative conditioning [24, 25]) because of the low numbers of passively transferred T cells.

In the HLA-matched sibling and unrelated-donor setting in adults, HSCT is most often performed using PBSCs as the source of stem cells (Fig. 1.3). In the pediatric population, bone marrow continues to be the preferred source of HSCs.

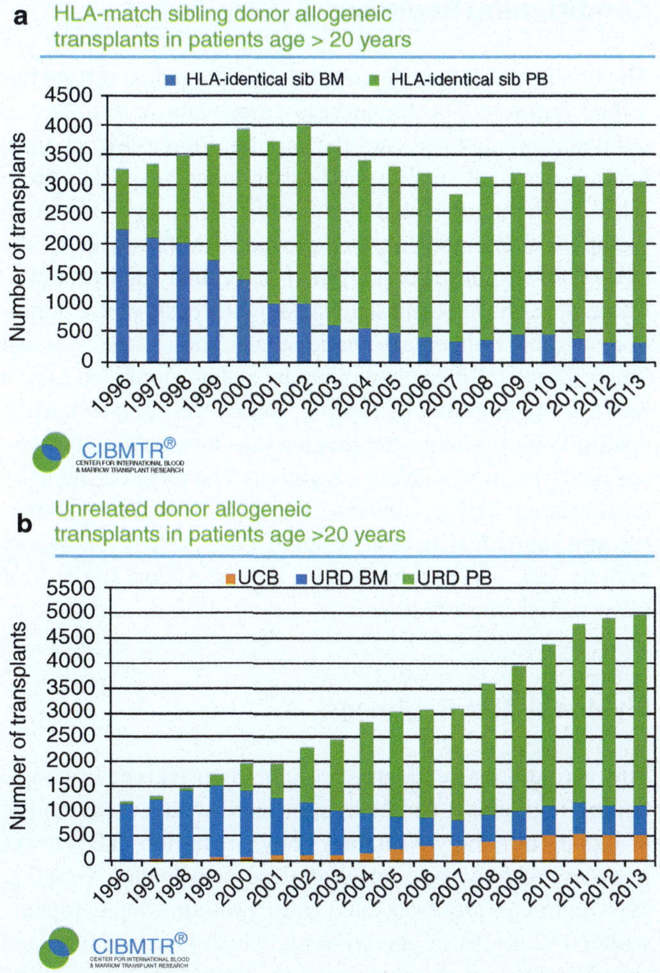

Fig. 1.3 (**a**, **b**) Increasing utilization of peripheral blood stem cells (PBSCs) as the source of hematopoietic stem cells in the sibling and unrelated donor settings in adults (*Adapted from* Pasquini and Zhu [1]; *with permission*)

Stem Cell Donors

Matched Related Donor

This type of allogeneic HSCT involves a donor who is an HLA-matched sibling of the recipient. The formula for calculating the chances of a particular person having an HLA-matched sibling is $1 - (0.75)^N$, where N denotes the number of potential sibling donors. In general, a patient with one sibling has a 25 % chance of having a match. The average American family size usually limits the success of finding a family donor to approximately 30 % of patients.

Matched Unrelated Donor

If the patient needs an allogeneic transplant and a donor cannot be found within the family, the identification of a matched unrelated donor (MUD) is accomplished by searching the computer files of the National Marrow Donor Program (NMDP) as well as other, international registries (Bone Marrow Donors Worldwide: BMDW). Through international connections, the NMDP searches more than 27.8 million potential donors worldwide as of 2016 (https://www.bmdw.org).

Haploidentical Stem Cell Donors

A recent source of hematopoietic stem cells that has emerged is from a haploidentical donor, which refers to complete half mismatch (4 of 8 HLA loci) from a related donor. This technique has greatly expanded the applicability of HSCT for patients with hematologic malignancies, as almost everyone will have a haploidentical donor (parent, child, or half sibling) who can potentially be used as an HSC donor source. The haploidentical donor is readily available and the cost of collection is lower than for MUD or UCB donors. Early attempts at haploidentical transplants were unsuccessful owing to severe GVHD in T-replete grafts and graft rejection in T-depleted grafts. The use of posttransplantation cyclophosphamide (Cytoxan), pioneered by a group at the Johns Hopkins Oncology Center [26], has allowed successful engraftment with low rates of acute and chronic GVHD. The risk of graft failure can be reduced by increasing the CD34+ stem cell dose, as shown by a group at the University of Perugia, Italy [27] (Fig. 1.4).

In 2006, MUD HSCTs exceeded the number of sibling transplants for the first time, and the gap continues to widen. From 2003 to 2011, UCB transplantation increased steadily in popularity, but owing to the rapid adoption of haploidentical donors with posttransplantation cyclophosphamide, the number of haploidentical HSCTs exceeded UCB transplants in 2014 and now accounts for 11 % of all allogeneic HSCT in the United States [1]. The survival data for MUD transplantation is similar to sibling HSCT outcomes in certain disease states [28].

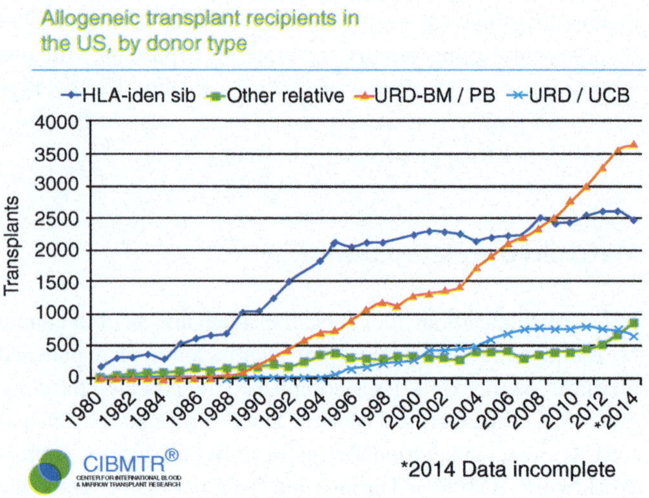

Fig. 1.4 Distribution of allogeneic HSCT based on various donor sources (*Adapted from* Pasquini and Zhu [1]; *with permission*)

Conditioning Regimens

The conditioning regimen used in the allogeneic setting has a dual purpose: The therapeutic component is designed to eliminate tumor cells, and the immunosuppressive component is intended to prevent host immune responses from rejecting the transplanted donor cells. The doses of radiation therapy and chemotherapy employed take advantage of the steep dose-response curve that exists for many malignancies. These doses have been established on the basis of the limitations of other nonhematopoietic organs, such as the liver and lungs. The combined chemotherapy agents employed have a nonoverlapping toxicity profile. Based on their intensity, conditioning regimens are divided into myeloablative (MA) regimens, nonmyeloablative regimens, and reduced-intensity conditioning (RIC) regimens. The type of regimen chosen for any individual patient depends on a variety of factors such as age, performance status, disease status, the risk of relapse, and comorbidities.

Myeloablative Regimens

This is traditionally the most commonly used type of conditioning regimen. It can be administered with a combination of radiation therapy with total body irradiation (TBI) doses in excess of 5 Gy or a busulfan dose greater than 8 mg/kg. MA regimens are associated with profound pancytopenia within 1–2 weeks of conditioning, which is irreversible and requires infusion of autologous or allogeneic stem cells to restore normal hematopoiesis. Busulfan-based regimens are most commonly used worldwide for allogeneic transplantation, but the oral administration of busulfan leads to unpredictable absorption, which has been correlated with relapse (low absorption) and increased toxicity (increased absorption). Studies with an intravenous formulation of the drug have shown much more predictable pharmacokinetics, less toxicity, and good survival when used in the transplant regimen. Studies have shown that when an intravenous formulation of busulfan is used, it is associated with a decreased incidence of hepatic venoocclusive disease and the 100-day survival is significantly higher [29]. The advent of therapeutic drug monitoring using pharmacokinetic dosing strategy can further help in achieving steady-state drug levels in the desired range, thereby improving HSCT outcomes [30].

Reduced-Intensity Conditioning

Reduced-intensity conditioning (RIC) uses lower doses of chemotherapy, with or without TBI, and relies on immunosuppression to facilitate engraftment of donor stem cells. These conditioning regimens are associated with significant lymphopenia, allowing successful engraftment of donor

HSCs in the recipient. The major therapeutic effect that results from this type of transplant is a graft-versus-tumor effect, because the nonmyeloablative regimen has limited long-term antitumor effect. Some disorders, such as CML, AML, and low-grade lymphoma, are particularly sensitive to this approach.

RIC transplantation is used primarily for patients who are older or who have comorbid conditions that might increase the risk of a fully ablative regimen. The most common regimens use fludarabine combined with either melphalan or busulfan or with a single fraction of TBI, followed by infusion of either donor bone marrow or peripheral blood–derived stem cells. All patients still require posttransplant immunosuppression similar to all other patients receiving non–T-cell–depleted transplants. For patients receiving either a matched sibling or fully matched unrelated transplant, the engraftment of donor cells after RIC is usually 100 % by day 30–60 after transplantation, and the immunosuppressive medications are tapered over a few months. Although the chemotherapy does have antitumor activity in this type of transplant, the major factor in eliminating the malignancy is the donor immune system. As in the fully ablative transplant setting, the presence or absence of GVHD influences the outcome.

Graft-Versus-Host Disease Prophylaxis and Treatment

GVHD can be broadly divided into acute and chronic, based on clinical manifestations rather than on the temporal relation to the time of transplantation. Acute GVHD includes classic acute GVHD (manifested by maculopapular rash, GI symptoms, or cholestatic hepatitis) and persistent, recurrent, or late-onset acute GVHD (occurring more than 100 days after HSCT). Chronic GVHD (cGVHD) comprises classic chronic GVHD, presenting with clinical manifestations attributable to GVHD alone, and overlap syndrome, which has diagnostic or distinctive cGVHD manifestations together with features typical of acute GVHD [31].

Prophylaxis

All patients who undergo non–T-cell–depleted transplantation require some form of GVHD prophylaxis. The most common regimens involve a combination of methotrexate (MTX) and a calcineurin inhibitor (cyclosporine or tacrolimus). In reduced-intensity HSCT, mycophenolate mofetil (MMF) plus a calcineurin inhibitor has also been used. The combination of tacrolimus and sirolimus has been studied and appears to be an effective approach for the prevention of GVHD. These medications, in the absence of GVHD, are tapered over 6– 12 months after HSCT. The regimens of sirolimus and tacrolimus are tapered in a similar manner. Adverse effects of tacrolimus and cyclosporine include renal toxicity, hypertension, magnesium wasting, seizures, and microangiopathy. Sirolimus, an oral agent, can cause hemolytic uremic syndrome in association with tacrolimus and requires careful monitoring of dosage and drug levels. It can also raise blood triglyceride levels. Newer approaches to prevent GVHD include the addition of maraviroc (CCR5 antagonist) [32], vorinostat (histone deacetylase inhibitor) [33], or bortezomib (proteasome inhibitor) [34] to the calcineurin inhibitor and MMF or MTX. Posttransplantation cyclophosphamide has also showed promising results in matched donor and haploidentical donor transplantation [35, 36].

Treatment of Acute GVHD

Despite prophylaxis, many allogeneic transplant recipients still develop some degree of GVHD and require increasing doses of prednisone (1–2 mg/kg per day). There is no single standard therapy for patients who do not respond to corticosteroids. Antithymocyte globulin (Atgam; 10 mg/kg per day for 5–10 days) has been used in this setting. More recent options include anti-CD25 monoclonal antibodies (basiliximab, daclizumab), pentostatin, anti-TNF agents (etanercept, infliximab), and MMF. There have been many efforts to improve upfront therapy beyond steroids, but a multicenter randomized trial comparing prednisone *versus* prednisone plus MMF for newly diagnosed acute GVHD did not show a benefit of additional MMF in this setting [37]. Active clinical trials are being done to study the role of inhibition of the JAK 1/2 pathway and complement pathway in the treatment of established GVHD. The ongoing BMT CTN 1301 trial is exploring the role of acute GVHD prophylaxis with CD34+ selected HSCs (T depletion) and posttransplantation cyclophosphamide versus standard tacrolimus and MTX-based prophylaxis. The HIV drug maraviroc has also shown activity in prevention of visceral GVHD by inhibition of the CCR5 pathway, which targets lymphocyte trafficking. The BMT CTN 1203 trial recently completed accrual; it tests three novel strategies for acute GVHD prophylaxis (tacrolimus/MTX with bortezomib or maraviroc and posttransplantation cyclophosphamide) in a multicenter phase 2 design to pick the most efficacious combination. Results from this trial are eagerly awaited.

Chronic GVHD

In patients surviving beyond 100 days after HSCT, cGVHD is the major cause of late mortality. Recent improvements in supportive care, GVHD regimens, and graft manipulation have not impacted the incidence of cGVHD or the mortality associated with it. GVHD is a chronic, multisystem, alloimmune disorder characterized by immune deregulation, impaired organ functioning, and increased mortality. Its clinical presentation has features resembling Sjögren syndrome, scleroderma, primary biliary cirrhosis, bronchiolitis obliterans, immune cytopenias, and chronic immunodeficiency. The pathogenesis of cGVHD is poorly understood, but the general consensus is that organ damage is secondary to organ toxicity caused by donor alloreactive T cells, cytokine dysregulation, and antibodies produced by donor-derived B cells. The reported incidence of cGVHD after allogeneic HSCT varies from 6 to 60 % based on cell source (PBSC *vs* bone marrow), donor type (sibling *vs* unrelated), conditioning regimen (MA *vs* non-MA), and graft manipulation (T-depleted or not). The variability in reported incidence of cGVHD is also due to lack to standard diagnostic guidelines in the past, interobserver variability in diagnosing cGVHD, differences in statistical methods of reporting, and limited follow-up of patients who are discharged from the transplant center.

Risk Factors Associated with Chronic GVHD

A number of risk factors are traditionally associated with the development of cGVHD:

- Prior development of acute GVHD
- HLA disparity or mismatched donor
- Intensity of conditioning regimen
- Female donor to male recipient
- Increasing recipient or donor age
- Use of PBSCs as HSC source [15]
- HSCT in CML, aplastic anemia, or other autoimmune conditions
- Alloimmunization of donor (*e.g.*, multiparous woman or multiple transfusions)
- Donor lymphocyte infusion [38, 39]

Most cases of cGVHD are diagnosed in the first year after transplantation, but 5–10 % of cases have delayed presentation beyond 1 year. Multisystem involvement occurs in 50 % of patients, requiring systemic immunosuppressive therapy for 2–3 years. A fraction of patients require immunosuppressive therapy lasting 5 years or more. The morbidity secondary to cGVHD is secondary to organ damage caused by the primary disease process and immune suppression caused by medications and GVHD [40]. The skin (75 %) is the most common site of involvement, followed by the mouth (51–63 %), liver (29–51 %), and eye (22–33 %). Less frequently involved sites are GI tract/weight loss (23–45 %), lung (4–19 %), esophagus (7 %), joints (6 %), and female genital tract (1 %).

Treatment of Chronic GVHD

Chronic GVHD is generally treated with prolonged courses of corticosteroids, cyclosporine/tacrolimus, and other medications, such as MMF, sirolimus, and pentostatin. Extracorporeal photopheresis has been used with varying response rates. Recently, the pathogenic role of B cells in cGVHD has been increasingly recognized, and rituximab has been successfully used in both therapy and prophylaxis. There are also promising results from phase 1 and 2 studies using low-dose IL-2, which increases the number of regulatory T cells (T_{reg}) in vivo. The prognosis for cGVHD (as for acute GVHD) is related to the extent of organ compromise and the response to treatment.

Causes of Treatment Failure

Despite major advances in conditioning regimens, posttransplantation maintenance strategies, and improved GVHD prophylactic regimens, a significant number of patients succumb either to disease relapse or to GVHD or infectious complications after HSCT. Based on data reported by the CIBMTR, the major causes of treatment failure after allogeneic HSCT from sibling and unrelated donors are relapse of primary disease (40–50 % of cases) and transplant-related morbidity secondary to GVHD and infectious complications (Fig. 1.5).

To prevent post-HSCT disease relapse, maintenance chemotherapy such as sorafenib in FLT3-ITD mutated AML or tyrosine kinase inhibitors in Ph-positive ALL can be employed to prevent relapse of the primary disease [41]. Minimal residual disease monitoring [42] is an emerging technique that is frequently employed in the posttransplant setting to detect early disease relapse. Multicolor flow cytometry, PCR-based assays, and chimerism analysis [43] can give an advance warning of impending relapse, allowing withdrawal of immunosuppression or donor lymphocyte infusion (DLI) [44] to potentially prevent full-blown disease relapse. DLI responses are not uniform across disease states; the best responses are noted in CML [45]. Responses are also noted in the setting of AML, MDS, and lymphoma, but responses are rare in the setting of ALL [46]. DLI infusions are typically followed by a flare of GVHD, so they should be restricted to patients who have relapse of primary disease without GVHD and who are partial donor chimeras. DLI typically works best when the disease burden is low, so it can be used in patients who are positive for minimal residual disease or after debulking with cytotoxic chemotherapy.

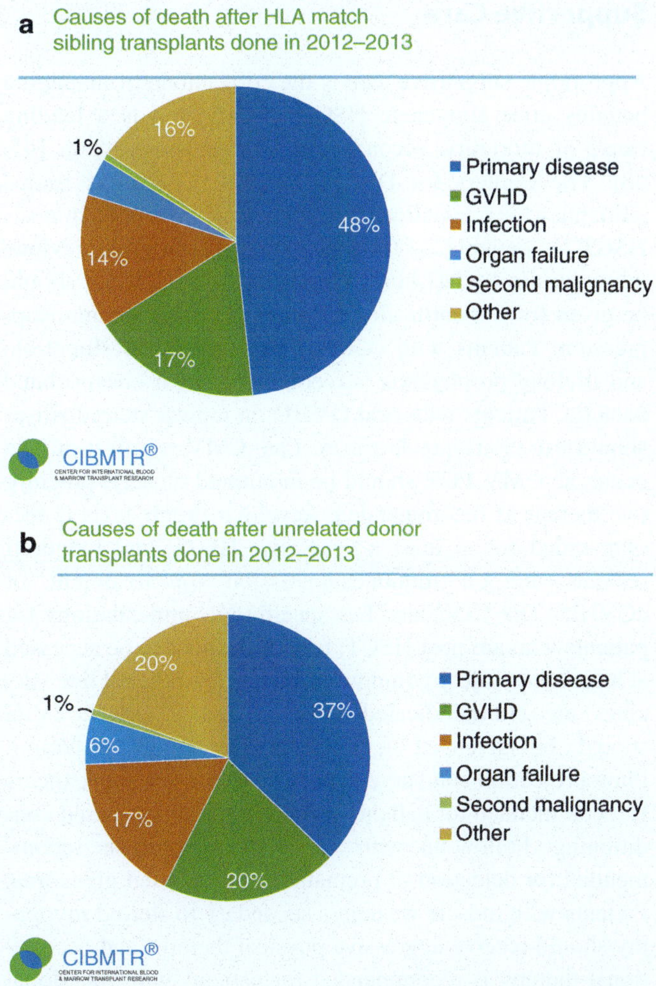

Fig. 1.5 Causes of mortality after allogeneic HSCT. (**a**) HLA-matched sibling transplants. (**b**) Unrelated donor transplants (*Adapted from* Pasquini and Zhu [1]; *with permission*)

Supportive Care

Appropriate supportive care is the cornerstone of managing patients after allogeneic HSCT, as infection is a leading cause of mortality, secondary to immunosuppression [47, 48]. The Centers for Disease Control (CDC) has issued guidelines for prevention of opportunistic infections in post-HSCT patients (http://www.cdc.gov/mmwr/preview/mmwrhtml/rr4910a1.htm). Prophylaxis of *P. jerovici* should be given for 6 months after discontinuation of immunosuppression. Patients with cGVHD have splenic dysfunction, and lifelong prophylaxis is recommended for encapsulated bacteria. Patients with oral GVHD on topical steroid rinses should use clotrimazole rinses. Late CMV reactivation can occur, so CMV PCR should be monitored closely; preemptive therapy is recommended. Acyclovir prophylaxis is recommended for at least a year after HSCT, and longer if patients are on immunosuppression for treatment of cGVHD. The CDC also has specific recommendations for patients who are post HSCT; further details can be accessed at http://www.cdc.gov/mmwr/pdf/rr/rr6207.pdf. All live vaccines are contraindicated after allogeneic HSCT. IVIG should be given if IgG levels are below $400/mm^3$. Photoprotection and surveillance for secondary skin cancers is recommended for patients exposed to radiation-based conditioning. Follow-up with an ophthalmologist is recommended for detection of premature cataracts and glaucoma. Patients with muscle weakness secondary to steroid myopathy should receive aggressive physical therapy, and occupational therapy is recommended for patients with functional disabilities due to neuropathy or skin sclerosis. Nuclear medicine dual-energy x-ray absorptiometry (DEXA) scans should be performed to detect osteopenia or osteoporosis, which should be aggressively treated with calcium, vitamin D, and bisphosphonates. Ancillary therapy and supportive care form critical components in long-term management after allogeneic HSCT, and a multidisciplinary approach with specialists is encouraged.

Conclusion

Use of allogeneic HSCT as a strategy to cure hematologic malignancies is increasing exponentially worldwide and is projected to continue to increase. Improvement in RIC and nonmyeloablative conditioning regimens, expansion of the worldwide unrelated donor registries, and adoption of alternative donor stem cell transplants (including cord blood and haploidentical HSCT) has made this immunotherapy more widely applicable. Significant obstacles still remain, such as posttransplantation relapse, transplant-related morbidity due to GVHD and infections, and impaired quality of life. With collaborative efforts of clinicians and emerging data from clinical trials, we hope to continue to improve patient outcomes with allogeneic HSCT [49].

References

1. Pasquini MC, Zhu X. Current uses and outcomes of hematopoietic stem cell transplantation: CIBMTR Summary Slides. 2015. Available at: http://www.cibmtr.org.
2. Jacobson LO, Marks EK, Gaston EO, et al. The role of the spleen in radiation injury. Proc Soc Exp Biol Med. 1949;70:740–2.
3. Barnes DW, Corp MJ, Loutit JF, Neal FE. Treatment of murine leukaemia with X rays and homologous bone marrow; preliminary communication. Br Med J. 1956;2(4993):626–7.
4. Thomas ED, Buckner CD, Banaji M, Clift RA, Fefer A, Flournoy N, et al. One hundred patients with acute leukemia treated by chemotherapy, total body irradiation, and allogeneic marrow transplantation. Blood. 1977;49:511–33.
5. Blume KG, Beutler E. Allogeneic bone marrow transplantation for acute leukemia. JAMA. 1979;241:1686.
6. Storb R, Deeg HJ, Whitehead J, Appelbaum F, Beatty P, Bensinger W, et al. Methotrexate and cyclosporine compared with cyclosporine alone for prophylaxis of acute graft versus host disease after marrow transplantation for leukemia. N Engl J Med. 1986;314:729–35.
7. Storb R, Deeg HJ, Pepe M, Appelbaum F, Anasetti C, Beatty P, et al. Methotrexate and cyclosporine versus cyclosporine alone for prophylaxis of graft-versus-host disease in patients given HLA-identical marrow grafts for leukemia: long-term follow-up of a controlled trial. Blood. 1989;73:1729–34.
8. Laport GG, Alvarnas JC, Palmer JM, Snyder DS, Slovak ML, Cherry AM, et al. Long-term remission of Philadelphia chromosome-positive acute lymphoblastic leukemia after allogeneic hematopoietic cell transplantation from matched sibling donors: a 20-year experience with the fractionated total body irradiation-etoposide regimen. Blood. 2008;112:903–9.
9. Schmidt GM, Horak DA, Niland JC, Duncan SR, Forman SJ, Zaia JA. A randomized, controlled trial of prophylactic ganciclovir for cytomegalovirus pulmonary infection in recipients of allogeneic bone marrow transplants; The City of Hope-Stanford-Syntex CMV Study Group. N Engl J Med. 1991;324:1005–11.
10. Petersdorf EW, Hansen JA, Martin PJ, Woolfrey A, Malkki M, Gooley T, et al. Major-histocompatibility-complex class I alleles and antigens in hematopoietic-cell transplantation. N Engl J Med. 2001;345:1794–800.
11. Storb R, Yu C, Wagner JL, Deeg HJ, Nash RA, Kiem HP, et al. Stable mixed hematopoietic chimerism in DLA-identical littermate dogs given sublethal total body irradiation before and pharmacological immunosuppression after marrow transplantation. Blood. 1997;89:3048–54.
12. Champlin R, Khouri I, Anderlini P, Gajewski J, Kornblau S, Molldrem J, et al. Nonmyeloablative preparative regimens for allogeneic hematopoietic transplantation. Bone Marrow Transplant. 2001;27(Suppl 2):S13–22.
13. Horowitz MM. Uses and growth of hematopoietic cell transplantation. In: Forman SJ, Negrin RS, Antin JH, Appelbaum FR, editors. Thomas' hematopoietic cell transplantation. 5th ed. Hoboken: Wiley; 2016. p. 8–17.
14. Majhail NS, Farnia SH, Carpenter PA, Champlin RE, Crawford S, Marks DI, et al. Indications for autologous and allogeneic hematopoietic cell transplantation: guidelines from the American Society for Blood and Marrow Transplantation. Biol Blood Marrow Transplant. 2015;21:1863–9.
15. Anasetti C, Logan BR, Lee SJ, Waller EK, Weisdorf DJ, Wingard JR, et al. Blood and Marrow Transplant Clinical Trials Network. Peripheral-blood stem cells versus bone marrow from unrelated donors. N Engl J Med. 2012;367:1487–96.
16. Blaise D, Kuentz M, Fortanier C, Bourhis JH, Milpied N, Sutton L, et al. Randomized trial of bone marrow versus lenograstim-primed blood cell allogeneic transplantation in patients with early-stage leukemia: a report from the Societe Francaise de Greffe de Moelle. J Clin Oncol. 2000;18:537–46.

17. Faucher C, Mohty M, Vey N, Gaugler B, Bilger K, Moziconnacci MJ, et al. Bone marrow as stem cell source for allogeneic HLA-identical sibling transplantation following reduced-intensity preparative regimen. Exp Hematol. 2003;31:873–80.
18. Korbling M, Anderlini P. Peripheral blood stem cell versus bone marrow allotransplantation: does the source of hematopoietic stem cells matter? Blood. 2001;98:2900–8.
19. Körbling M, Huh YO, Durett A, Mirza N, Miller P, Engel H, et al. Allogeneic blood stem cell transplantation: peripheralization and yield of donor-derived primitive hematopoietic progenitor cells (CD34+ Thy-1dim) and lymphoid subsets, and possible predictors of engraftment and graft-versus-host disease. Blood. 1995;86: 2842–8.
20. Schmitz N, Beksac M, Hasenclever D, Bacigalupo A, Ruutu T, Nagler A, et al. European Group for Blood and Marrow Transplantation. Transplantation of mobilized peripheral blood cells to HLA-identical siblings with standard-risk leukemia. Blood. 2002;100:761–7.
21. Zaucha JM, Gooley T, Bensinger WI, Heimfeld S, Chauncey TR, Zaucha R, et al. CD34 cell dose in granulocyte colony-stimulating factor-mobilized peripheral blood mononuclear cell grafts affects engraftment kinetics and development of extensive chronic graft-versus-host disease after human leukocyte antigen-identical sibling transplantation. Blood. 2001;98:3221–7.
22. Laughlin MJ, Barker J, Bambach B, Koc ON, Rizzieri DA, Wagner JE, et al. Hematopoietic engraftment and survival in adult recipients of umbilical-cord blood from unrelated donors. N Engl J Med. 2001;344:1815–22.
23. Laughlin MJ, Eapen M, Rubinstein P, Wagner JE, Zhang MJ, Champlin RE, et al. Outcomes after transplantation of cord blood or bone marrow from unrelated donors in adults with leukemia. N Engl J Med. 2004;351:2265–75.
24. Ballen KK, Spitzer TR, Yeap BY, McAfee S, Dey BR, Attar E, et al. Double unrelated reduced-intensity umbilical cord blood transplantation in adults. Biol Blood Marrow Transplant. 2007;13:82–9.
25. Rocha V, Labopin M, Sanz G, Arcese W, Schwerdtfeger R, Bosi A, et al. Transplants of umbilical-cord blood or bone marrow from unrelated donors in adults with acute leukemia. N Engl J Med. 2004;351:2276–85.
26. Luznik L, Jalla S, Engstrom LW, Iannone R, Fuchs EJ. Durable engraftment of major histocompatibility complex-incompatible cells after nonmyeloablative conditioning with fludarabine, low-dose total body irradiation, and posttransplantation cyclophosphamide. Blood. 2001;98:3456–64.
27. Aversa F, Terenzi A, Tabilio A, Falzetti F, Carotti A, Ballanti S, et al. Full haplotype-mismatched hematopoietic stem-cell transplantation: a phase II study in patients with acute leukemia at high risk of relapse. J Clin Oncol. 2005;23:3447–54.
28. Saber W, Opie S, Rizzo JD, Zhang MJ, Horowitz MM, Schriber J. Outcomes after matched unrelated donor versus identical sibling hematopoietic cell transplantation in adults with acute myelogenous leukemia. Blood. 2012;119:3908–16.
29. Kashyap A, Wingard J, Cagnoni P, Roy J, Tarantolo S, Hu W, et al. Intravenous versus oral busulfan as part of a busulfan/cyclophosphamide preparative regimen for allogeneic hematopoietic stem cell transplantation: decreased incidence of hepatic venoocclusive disease (HVOD), HVOD-related mortality, and overall 100-day mortality. Biol Blood Marrow Transplant. 2002;8:493–500.
30. Pidala J, Kim J, Anasetti C, Kharfan-Dabaja MA, Nishihori T, Field T, et al. Pharmacokinetic targeting of intravenous busulfan reduces conditioning regimen related toxicity following allogeneic hematopoietic cell transplantation for acute myelogenous leukemia. J Hematol Oncol. 2010;3:36.
31. Socie G, Ritz J. Current issues in chronic graft-versus-host disease. Blood. 2014;124:374–84.
32. Reshef R, Luger SM, Hexner EO, Loren AW, Frey NV, Nasta SD, et al. Blockade of lymphocyte chemotaxis in visceral graft-versus-host disease. N Engl J Med. 2012;367:135–45.
33. Reddy P, Maeda Y, Hotary K, Liu C, Reznikov LL, Dinarello CA, Ferrara JL. Histone deacetylase inhibitor suberoylanilide hydroxamic acid reduces acute graft-versus-host disease and preserves graft-versus-leukemia effect. Proc Natl Acad Sci U S A. 2004;101:3921–6.
34. Koreth J, Stevenson KE, Kim HT, McDonough SM, Bindra B, Armand P, et al. Bortezomib-based graft-versus-host disease prophylaxis in HLA-mismatched unrelated donor transplantation. J Clin Oncol. 2012;30:3202–8.
35. Robinson TM, O'Donnell PV, Fuchs EJ, Luznik L. Haploidentical bone marrow and stem cell transplantation: experience with post-transplantation cyclophosphamide. Semin Hematol. 2016;53: 90–7.
36. Kekre N, Antin JH. Cord blood versus haploidentical stem cell transplantation for hematological malignancies. Semin Hematol. 2016;53:98–102.
37. Bolaños-Meade J, Logan BR, Alousi AM, Antin JH, Barowski K, Carter SL, et al. Phase 3 clinical trial of steroids/mycophenolate mofetil vs steroids/placebo as therapy for acute GVHD: BMT CTN 0802. Blood 2014;124:3221–3227; quiz 3335.
38. Reinherz EL, Parkman R, Rappeport J, Rosen FS, Schlossman SF. Aberrations of suppressor T cells in human graft-versus-host disease. N Engl J Med. 1979;300:1061–8.
39. Storb R, Prentice RL, Sullivan KM, Shulman HM, Deeg HJ, Doney KC, et al. Predictive factors in chronic graft-versus-host disease in patients with aplastic anemia treated by marrow transplantation from HLA-identical siblings. Ann Intern Med. 1983;98:461–6.
40. Lee SJ, Flowers ME. Recognizing and managing chronic graft-versus-host disease. Hematology Am Soc Hematol Educ Program. 2008:134–41.
41. Nishiwaki S, Imai K, Mizuta S, Kanamori H, Ohashi K, Fukuda T, et al. Impact of MRD and TKI on allogeneic hematopoietic cell transplantation for Ph+ALL: a study from the adult ALL WG of the JSHCT. Bone Marrow Transplant. 2016;51:43–50.
42. van Dongen JJ, van der Velden VH, Bruggemann M, Orfao A. Minimal residual disease diagnostics in acute lymphoblastic leukemia: need for sensitive, fast, and standardized technologies. Blood. 2015;125:3996–4009.
43. Pérez-Simón JA, Caballero D, Diez-Campelo M, Lopez-Pérez R, Mateos G, Cañizo C, et al. Chimerism and minimal residual disease monitoring after reduced intensity conditioning (RIC) allogeneic transplantation. Leukemia. 2002;16:1423–31.
44. Deol A, Lum LG. Role of donor lymphocyte infusions in relapsed hematological malignancies after stem cell transplantation revisited. Cancer Treat Rev. 2010;36:528–38.
45. Kolb HJ, Schmid C, Barrett AJ, Schendel DJ. Graft-versus-leukemia reactions in allogeneic chimeras. Blood. 2004;103:767–76.
46. MacKinnon S. Who may benefit from donor leucocyte infusions after allogeneic stem cell transplantation? Br J Haematol. 2000;110:12–7.
47. Higman MA, Vogelsang GB. Chronic graft versus host disease. Br J Haematol. 2004;125:435–54.
48. Couriel D, Carpenter PA, Cutler C, Bolaños-Meade J, Treister NS, Gea-Banacloche J, et al. Ancillary therapy and supportive care of chronic graft-versus-host disease: national institutes of health consensus development project on criteria for clinical trials in chronic Graft-versus-host disease: V. Ancillary Therapy and Supportive Care Working Group Report. Biol Blood Marrow Transplant. 2006;12:375–96.
49. Gooley TA, Chien JW, Pergam SA, Hingorani S, Sorror ML, Boeckh M, et al. Reduced mortality after allogeneic hematopoietic-cell transplantation. N Engl J Med. 2010;363:2091–101.

Pathophysiology and Immunology of Chronic Graft-Versus-Host Disease

2

Amandeep Salhotra and Ryotaro Nakamura

Chronic graft-versus-host disease (cGVHD) is the leading cause of late morbidity and mortality in patients undergoing allogeneic hematopoietic stem cell transplant (HSCT) [1, 2]. Chronic GVHD and its associated complications result in increased resource utilization, poor quality of life parameters, and decreased overall survival in patients. Early detection and appropriate intervention will help in improving long-term outcomes of HCT patients. Detection of biomarkers in blood or involved tissue (skin, gut, etc.) may help in early diagnosis and risk-stratification of patients, thereby impacting the type and intensity of immunosuppressive therapy chosen. To date, early intervention and successful treatment of cGVHD patients has lagged due to difficulty in scoring organ involvement due to lack of uniform and objective scoring tools. Another major problem in the field is the absence of approved therapies in the steroid refractory setting, which is a result of the difficulties of clinical trials in this patient population due to poor standardization of scoring systems and evaluation of objective responses. There are other competing causes of death, including disease relapse and infectious complications that may confound survival data. Establishment of standardized cGVHD scoring systems has helped enormously in staging the disease and evaluating responses to new therapies, thereby helping to make objective response evaluations possible [3].

A. Salhotra (✉)
Hematology and Hematopoietic Cell Transplantation, City of Hope National Medical Center, Duarte, CA, USA
e-mail: asalhotra@coh.org

R. Nakamura
Division of Dermatology, City of Hope Comprehensive Cancer Center, Duarte, CA, USA
e-mail: rnakamura@coh.org

Basic Biology of cGVHD

The underlying pathophysiologic mechanisms of cGVHD are complex and are related to donor T-cells recognizing recipient as "non-self" based on a variety of factors. The most important of these is degree of human leukocyte antigen (HLA) disparity between the donor-recipient pair. cGVHD consists of an early initiating phase, followed by gradual evolution to the full-blown syndrome, which can involve multiple organs. The "prime targets" are skin, GI tract, and liver, all of which are organs that undergo tissue damage as part of prior chemotherapy and conditioning regimens. Other organs, such as lung, salivary and lacrimal glands, oral mucosa, skin, and subcutaneous tissues can also be involved and contribute to morbidity associated with cGVHD. During the initiation phase of cGVHD, recipient antigen presenting cells (rAPCs) engage Donor CD8+ T cells by presenting self-antigens in conjunction with MHC class I complex. Donor CD4+ T cells are activated by the MHC class II pathway, wherein shed donor proteins and apoptotic cells are processed by endosome and presented to donor CD4+ cells by rAPCs. After antigen presentation and appropriate co-stimulatory signaling, donor CD4+ and CD8+ undergo activation and expansion. In the evolution phase, donor APCs continue ongoing activation of donor-derived T cells by presenting recipient antigens via MHC class I and II peptides. The activated T cells cause tissue damage by release of inflammatory cytokines (TNF-α, IL-2 IFN-γ) and by direct tissue infiltration [4] causing manifestation of acute GVHD. Chronic GVHD is postulated to occur due to thymic damage during conditioning which leads to defective negative selection of T cells, deficiency of regulatory T cells (Tregs), auto antibody production by aberrant B cells, and formation of fibrotic lesions.

J.A. Cotliar (ed.), *Atlas of Graft-versus-Host Disease*, DOI 10.1007/978-3-319-46952-2_2

cGVHD Biomarker

The properties of an ideal biomarker as defined by Schultz et al. [5] include its ability to (1) predict response to therapy; (2) measure disease activity and distinguish irreversible damage from continued disease activity; (3) predict the risk of developing chronic GVHD; (4) diagnose chronic GVHD; (5) predict the prognosis of chronic GVHD; (6) evaluate the balance between GVHD and graft-versus-leukemia (GVT) effects; and (7) serve as a surrogate end-point for therapeutic response.

Serologic and cellular immune markers have long been studied to predict the onset of acute and chronic GVHD and also to predict the severity of established disease [6]. Unfortunately, none of these markers meet all of the above criteria, or have been validated in a prospective manner. In this chapter, we will review the current literature summarizing immune cell and inflammatory mediators that have been studied as biomarkers for chronic GVHD.

Cellular Biomarkers

Table 2.1 lists immune cell populations associated with subsequent risk of cGVHD and Table 2.2 lists inflammatory biomarkers co-related with development of cGVHD.

Table 2.1 Immune cell populations associated with subsequent risk of cGVHD

Cell subset	Risk of cGVHD	References
Effector memory $CD4_{EM}$ T cells ($CCR7^{neg}$ $CD62L^{low}$)	Increase in this T-cell subset co-related with increased risk of cGVHD	Yamashita et al. [7]
CD8+ Central Memory T cells	Increase in this T-cell subset co-related with increased risk of cGVHD	Yamashita et al. [8]
CD4+CD27 – T cells	Increase in this T-cell subset co-related with increased risk of cGVHD	Fukunaga et al. [9]
Tregs CD4+CD25+	Increase in this T-cell subset co-related with decreased risk of cGVHD	Zorn et al. [10]
Host APCs	If activated with co-stimulatory molecules CD86/CD80 – co-related with increased risk of cGVHD	Schlomchik et al. [11]
CD3-CD16+/56+ NK-cell	Lower numbers in patients with cGVHD	Abrahamsen et al. [12]

APCs antigen-presenting cells, *CD* cluster of differentiation, *NK* natural killer

Table 2.2 Inflammatory biomarkers co-related with development of cGVHD

Inflammatory marker	Risk of cGVHD	References
TNFα	Levels increased in acute and cGVHD	Dander et al. [13]
IL-6 and IL-8	Levels increased in acute and cGVHD	Dander et al. [13]
IFNγ, IL-12	Increased levels co-relate with cGVHD	Rozmus et al. [12]
Day 7 IL-15 level	Low day 7 IL-15 levels correspond to subsequent cGVHD	Pratt et al. [14]
CXCL9 levels	Levels increased at onset of cGVHD	Kitko et al. [15]
ST2, CXCL9, MMP3, Osteopentin	Elevated serum levels at day 100 co-relate with cGVHD	Yu et al. [16]
BAFF (B-cell activating factor)	Levels elevated in cGVHD	Sarantopoulous et al. [17]

CXCL9 chemokine (C-X-C motif) ligand 9, *IFNγ* interferon gamma, *IL* interleukin, *MMP3* matrix metalloproteinase, *ST2* suppression of tumorigenicity 2, *TNFα* tumor necrosis factor alpha

T Cells

T-Cell Differentiation Status

Immune cell subsets have been studied extensively in patients to determine their predictive value in chronic GVHD. Most studies have focused on CD4+ (post-thymic) T cell subsets. Human peripheral blood CD4+ T cells are classified into three broad populations: (1) naive CD45RA+CCR7+ and two memory subsets; (2) CD45RA-CCR7+ (central memory); and (3) CD45RA-CCR7- (effector memory). Chemokine receptor CCR7 is required for migration of T cells into secondary lymphoid organs such as lymph nodes and the spleen. CD62L expression guides lymphocytes into lymphoid tissue and is tightly linked to CCR7 expression on memory CD4+ T cells. Yamashita et al. [7] studied relative proportions of effector memory $CD4_{EM}$ T cells (CCR7-$CD62L^{low}$ in patients with established cGVHD and compared these to $CD4_{EM}$ T cells in healthy controls and patients with no clinical signs of cGVHD. Chronic GVHD patients had a significantly higher percentage of CCR7-$CD62L^{low}$ cells compared with healthy controls (35.5 % vs 13.8 % respectively; $P < .0001$) or stem cell transplantation patients without cGVHD (35.5 % vs 21.7 % respectively; $P < .01$) in the total CD4+ population.

Changes in relative ratios of CD4 and CD8 T cell subsets and decrease in CD4+ central memory T cells has been noted in patients with chronic GVHD. Yamashita et al. [8] reported changes in T cell subsets in 37 patients who developed cGVHD after allogeneic HSCT. Specifically, an increase in central memory CD8+ cells with concomitant decline in CD4+ cells was noted. This immune cell pattern was not seen in patients who did not develop cGVHD post-HSCT or in patients who responded to immunotherapy with photopheresis. This finding indicates that the ratio of central and effector memory T cell subsets is altered in cGVHD and successful treatment leads to normalization of this ratio.

Fukunaga et al. [9] reported a unique subset of T cells, CD4+CD27−, which are seen in peripheral blood in increased frequency in patients with cGVHD (39.5 % compared to < 10 % in healthy adults). These T cells have shortened telomere length, increased susceptibility to activation-induced cell death and decreased clonal diversity. This depletion of central memory CD4+ T cell pool increases patients' susceptibility to recurrent infections, thereby increasing infectious morbidity. Patients who have decreasing numbers of CD4+CD27+ cells post-allogeneic HCT should be monitored closely for infectious complications and should remain on appropriate antimicrobial prophylaxis until immune recovery occurs post-HSCT.

CD4 T-Cell Cytokine Subsets (Th1, Th2, Th 17)

The CD4 T helper cells can be classified in to Th1 and Th2 based on cytokine secretion profiling, with Th1 cells secreting IFN-γ, IL-2 and TNFα. Th2 cells produce IL-4,IL-5,IL-6,IL-10 and IL-13. Th1 cells are responsible for delayed type hypersensitivity and are important in defense from infectious microorganisms. When exposed to foreign antigens, the APCs (macrophages and dendritic cells [DCs]) migrate to lymphoid organs and present antigens to naïve T cells and produce pro-inflammatory cytokines, such as IL-12, which leads to Th1 type response. Human and animal studies have shown that acute GVHD is a clinical syndrome caused by an imbalance between Th1 (pro-inflammatory cytokines) and Th2 response (anti-inflammatory cytokines) [18–20]. Chronic GVHD is a T cell mediated allo-reactive process and Th2 response dominates in cGVHD [21, 22]. Another subset of CD4 T cells which produce IL-17 (Th17) have been also implicated in development of cGVHD. Dander et al. [13] studied the role of IL-17 producing CD4+ T cells (Th17) in cGVHD in serum of 51 patients post-allo HSCT with clinical manifestations of cGVHD and compared this to 15 healthy donors (HD). Patients with cGVHD showed an increase of Th17 population compared with HD (mean SFU = 178/25,000 cells, n = 18, ANOVA $P < 0.001$). Importantly, by analyzing the proportion of Th17 cells according to the activation status of cGVHD (active vs. inactive phases), the authors were able to demonstrate that patients with active cGVHD show an increase of Th17 population (mean SFU = 237/25,000 cells, n = 13, ANOVA $P < 0.001$). Inflammatory cytokines produced by Th17 cells such as IL-6, TNF- α and IL-8 were also significantly elevated in patients with active cGVHD.

Therapeutic approaches: Based on the critical role played by CD4+ T cells in propagating cGVHD, attempts have been made to reduce these alloreactive T cells by inhibition of the Janus Kinase/Signal Transducer and Activator of Transcription (JAK/STAT) pathway. Common gamma chain signaling via JAK pathway leads to up-regulation of IL-2, IL-4, IL-7, IL-9, IL-15, and IL-21—this cytokine storm causes T cell activation, lineage commitment, and survival signaling. Patients with steroid refractory cGVHD who were treated with the commercially available JAK1/2 inhibitor ruxolitinib exhibited excellent clinical responses with an overall response rate of 85.4 %. These responses were independent of organ involvement [23]. Additional clinical trials are in progress to further study the role of this important class of medications in prevention of cGVHD (NCT02806375, NCT01790295).

Regulatory T Cells (Tregs)

Regulatory T cells, or Tregs, constitute 5–10 % of circulating CD4+ T cells, and suppress auto- and allo-reactive T cell clones. Tregs have also been associated with clinical symptoms of cGVHD. Immunophenotypically, Tregs are CD4+ and CD25+ and express forkhead transcription factor *FOXP3*. Zorn et al. [10] evaluated CD4+CD25+ Tregs in 30 patients with cGVHD after allogeneic HSCT, 27 patients without active cGVHD, and 26 healthy controls. They also evaluated T cell receptor excision circles (TREC) by peripheral blood polymerase chain reaction (PCR) as a marker of thymic activity in post-HCT patients. Patients with active cGVHD had significantly lower expression of FOXP3 when compared with patients without cGVHD (P = .009) or healthy donors (P = .01). Moreover, patients with active cGVHD had significantly lower expression of FOXP3 when compared with patients without cGVHD (P = .009) or healthy donors (P = .01). Patients with or without cGVHD showed a significant decrease in TRECs compared with healthy donors (P < .001), supporting that thymic function is substantially impaired following allogeneic HSCT.

Therapeutic approaches: Based on studies showing the role of IL-2 as a growth factor for Tregs, clinical trials have been reported with use of low-dose IL-2 in cGVHD setting with promising response rates [24, 25]. Additional combinations of IL-2 with Tregs (NCT01937468) and photopheresis (NCT02340676) are ongoing to see if therapeutic response can be augmented above that seen with IL-2 monotherapy.

Antigen-Presenting Cells

In addition to T cells, antigen-presenting cells (APCs), such as macrophages, dendritic cells, and B cells, play a critical role in initiating and propagating immune responses associated with cGVHD. Schlomchik et al. [11] demonstrated that host APCs are radio- and chemo-resistant post-conditioning regimens, and are critical for antigen presentation to incoming donor T cells, thereby proving the antigenic and co-stimulatory signals for T-cell activation and expansion leading to aGVHD. T-cell activation in the context of APC requires (1) antigen presentation with MHC class II molecules (MHC restriction) and (2) signal transduction via co-stimulatory molecules such as CD 80 and CD86. APCs are able to recognize the presence of microorganisms through the detection of conserved pathogen-associated molecular patterns (PAMP) and rapidly initiate tailored responses to these danger signals. Blockage of PAMP inducible co-stimulatory molecules such as CD40 or B7.1/B7.2 is effective in decreasing incidence of GVHD. She et al. [26] described the role of B cells primed for TLR9 (toll-like receptor 9), the response of which may play a role in pathophysiology of cGVHD. TLR9 expression has a significant correlation with expression of CD86 and CD80—furthermore, expression of these surface proteins was used as surrogate for TLR9 expression in this trial. A significantly greater percentage of B cells from and early cGVHD group (3–8 months post-HSCT; n = 19, 56.3 %) were capable of up-regulating CD86, compared to 6-month non-cGVHD controls (n = 9, 15.8 %; P = .0004) in response to PS-modified CpG. To confirm the B cell responses were mediated by TLR pathway, mRNA expression levels were checked in purified B cells by RT-PCR. There was a significant correlation (n = 12, r^2 = 0 .65, P = .002) between PS-modified CpG 2006 response and B cell TLR9 mRNA levels. Anderson et al. [27] further clarified the role of donor and host APCs in cGVHD. Both donor and host APCs can elicit cGVHD phenotype in setting of CD80/86 co-stimulation—in the absence of this co-stimulatory signal, no cGVHD developed. This process is CD4+ T cell mediated. Their findings show that donor APCs can cause late cGVHD in a CD4 cell dependent mechanism in setting of appropriate co-stimulatory signals. This finding provides additional therapeutic targets for prevention of cGVHD.

B Cells and Humoral Immunity

B Cell and B-Cell Activating Factor (BAFF)

The role of donor B cells in mediating chronic GVHD by antibody-mediated targeting of recipient tissues was first reported by Sarantopoulous et al. [17]. B-cell activating factor (BAFF) is known to be a key regulator of normal B-cell homeostasis in humans [28] and high BAFF levels have been found in patients with a variety of autoimmune diseases. A total of 104 patients who had undergone allogeneic HSCT between 1994 and 2005 for hematologic malignancies were studied. Enzyme-linked immunosorbent assay (ELISA) was used to measure plasma BAFF levels, and flow cytometry was used to assess BAFF receptor expression on B cells in patients with or without chronic GVHD. These plasma samples were collected prospectively at predetermined time points and BAFF levels were correlated with clinical outcomes. BAFF levels were significantly higher in patients with active chronic GVHD compared with those without disease (P = 0.02 and 0.0004, respectively). Patients treated with glucocorticoids showed reduction in BAFF levels, suggesting this correlation with disease severity. Furthermore, it was noted that BAFF levels were high post-HSCT and declined in patients who never developed chronic GVHD. In contrast, BAFF levels remained elevated in patients who developed clinical manifestations of cGVHD. Six-month BAFF levels ≥ 10 ng/mL were strongly associated with subsequent development of chronic GVHD (P < 0.0001). Following transplant, plasma BAFF levels correlated inversely with BAFF receptor expression on B cells (P = 0.01), suggesting that soluble BAFF affected B-cells through this receptor [29].

Fujii et al. [30] demonstrated variation in biomarker levels based on early (3–8 months post-HSCT) versus late ≥ 9 months post-HCT). Soluble B cell activation factor (sBAFF), anti-dsDNA antibody, soluble interleukin-2 receptor alpha (sIL-2Rα), and soluble CD13 (sCD13) were elevated in patients with early-onset cGVHD compared with

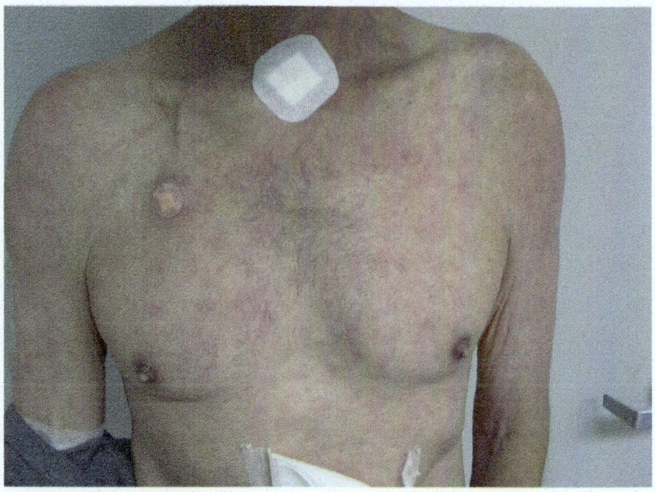

Fig. 3.6 Patchy erythema of the trunk and arms

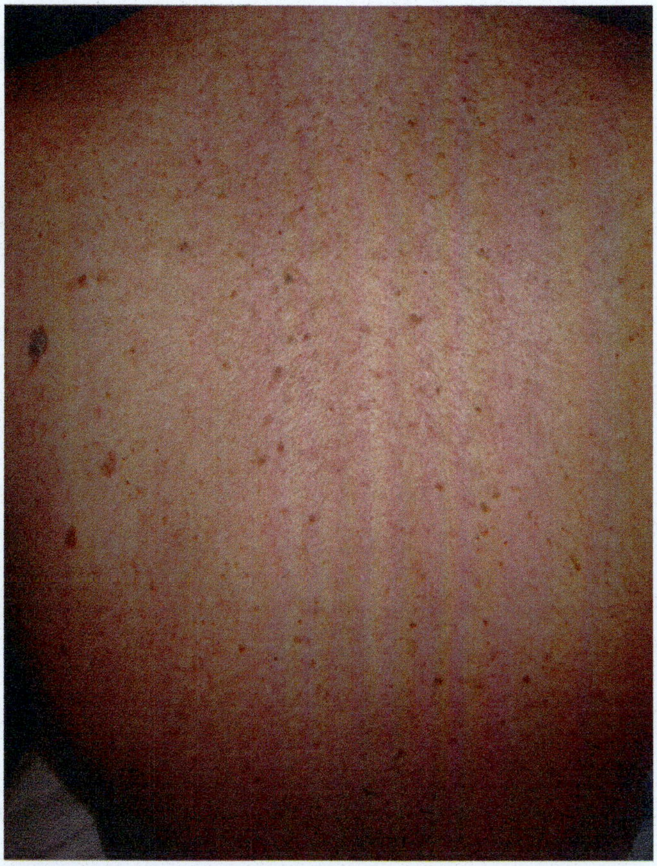

Fig. 3.7 Confluent erythema of the back

Follicular Accentuation

Prominence of hair follicles (whether overlying erythema is present or not) is typical of aGVHD [5]. Such prominence is often misdiagnosed as folliculitis, but it typically heralds the involvement of aGVHD within the follicular epithelium (Figs. 3.8 and 3.9).

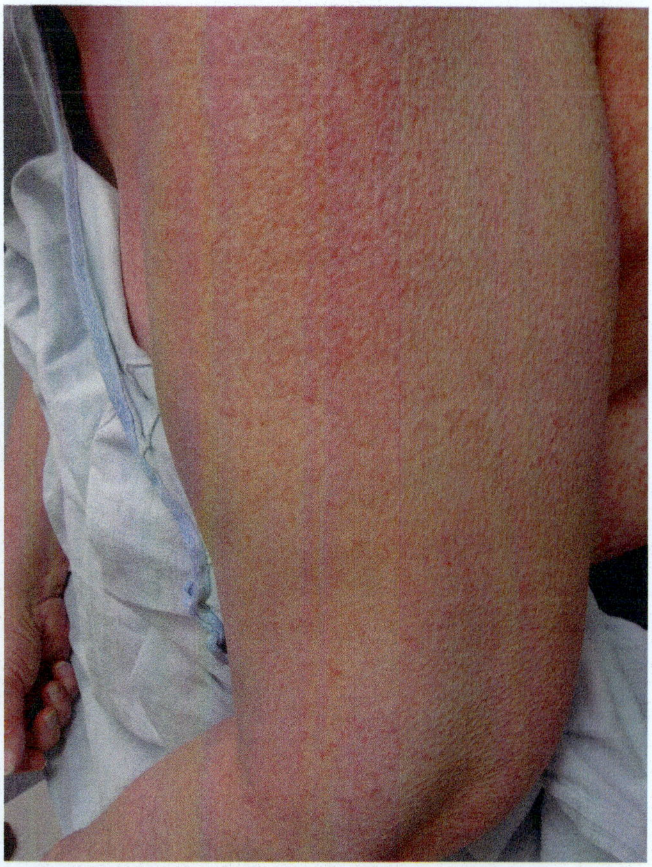

Fig. 3.8 Erythema of the arm with follicular accentuation

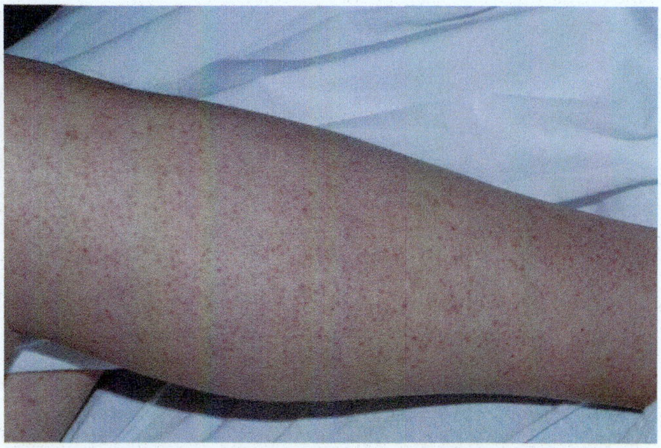

Fig. 3.9 Erythema with follicular accentuation of the leg

Morbilliform Lesions

Morbilliform aGVHD is among the most common presentations [6]. Eruptions are erythematous macules and papules that may coalesce into larger papules and plaques, which are symmetric and are often pruritic. This presentation may clinically mimic viral exanthema or drug eruptions (Figs. 3.10, 3.11, 3.12, and 3.13).

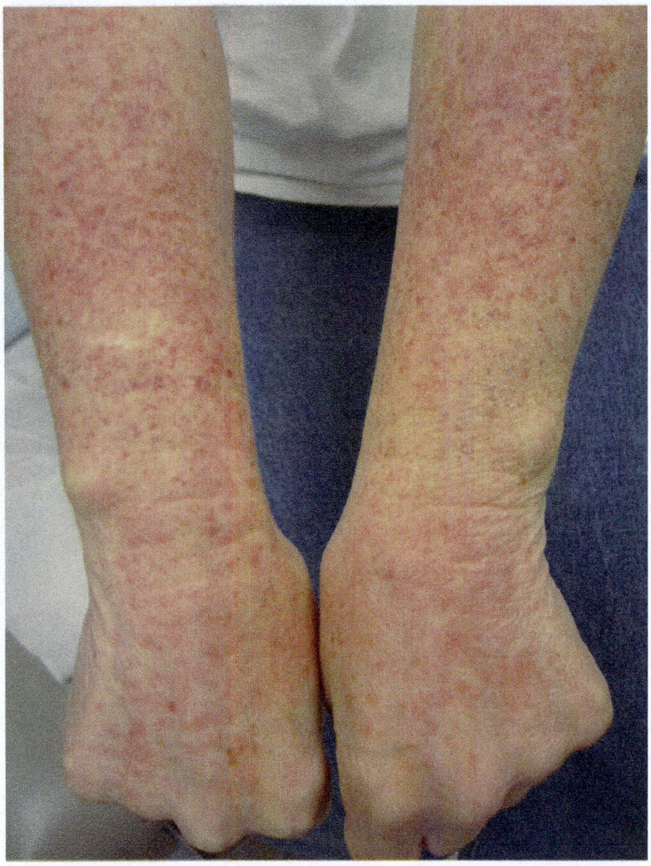

Fig. 3.10 Morbilliform lesions on the dorsal forearms/hands

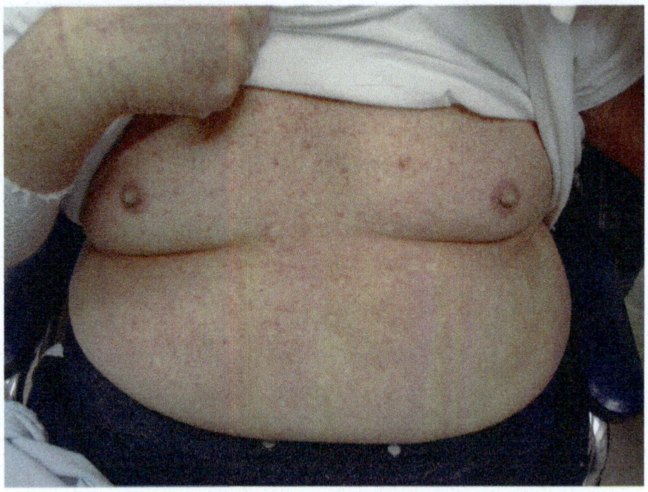

Fig. 3.11 Morbilliform lesions on the chest and abdomen

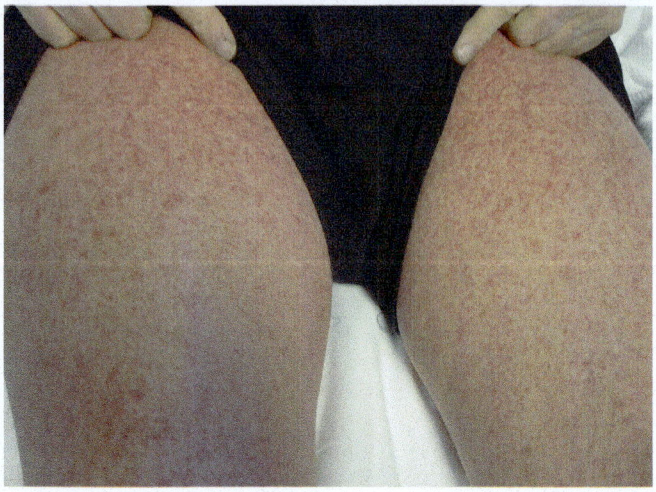

Fig. 3.12 Morbilliform lesions on the thighs

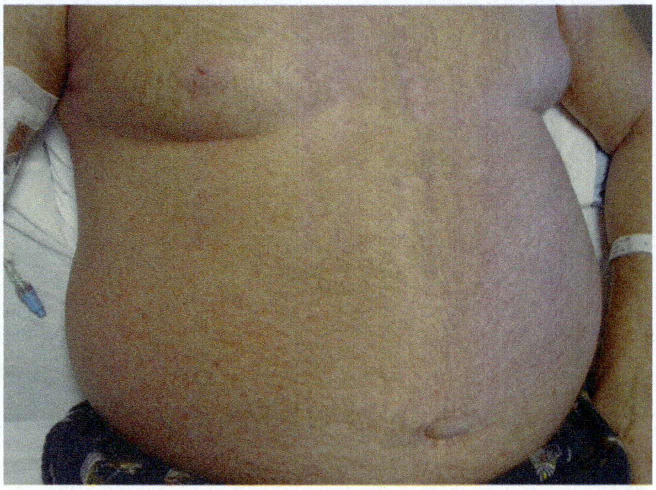

Fig. 3.13 Morbilliform lesions diffusely located on the trunk

Erythroderma

Erythrodermic aGVHD presents with confluent erythematous patches that mimic severe viral exanthema, drug reactions, psoriasis, eczematous dermatitis, cutaneous T-cell lymphoma, or staphylococcal scalded skin syndrome (SSSS) (Fig. 3.14). When mucous membrane lesions are present, there are no clinical or histologic differences between skin stage 4 aGVHD and toxic epidermal necrolysis (TEN) [7–9]. If extracutaneous features of aGVHD are present, diagnosis may be possible via tissue confirmation at involved sites. If extracutaneous features of aGVHD are absent, review of clinical symptoms and their development in relation to initiation of medications is mandatory. Viral serologies and/or quantification of viremia via polymerase chain reaction (PCR) testing of the blood may aid in the diagnosis of an erythrodermic viral exanthem, such as those caused by HHV-6. Concurrent empiric treatment of aGVHD, viral infection, and TEN may be necessary if a clear diagnosis cannot be rendered.

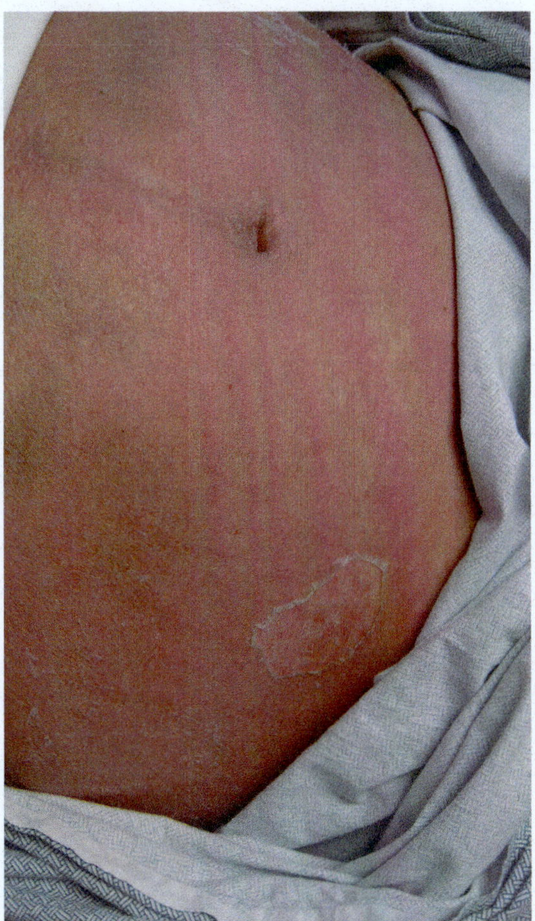

Fig. 3.14 Confluent erythema with scale mimicking staphylococcal scalded skin syndrome (SSSS)

Reticulated Patterns

Acute GVHD may present in a reticulated, netlike pattern (Fig. 3.15).

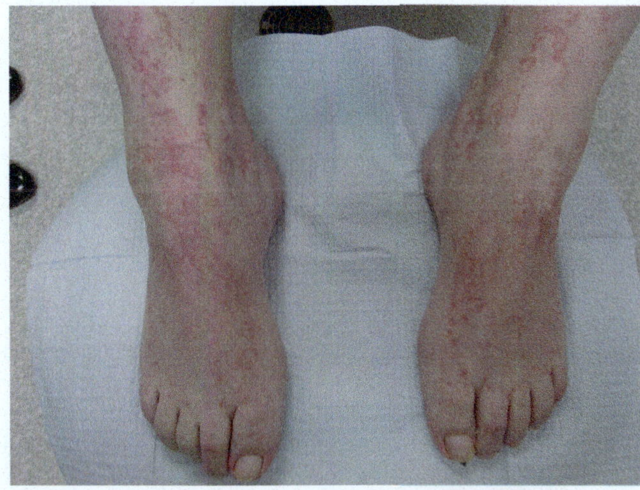

Fig. 3.15 Erythematous, reticulated patches on the distal legs and feet

Desquamation

Superficial desquamation is typical of a variety of inflammatory dermatoses, whether or not patients are hematopoietic stem cell transplantation (HSCT) recipients. In aGVHD, desquamation may develop as skin lesions resolve, or it may appear at presentation. Desquamation may be superficial, deep, focal, or more generalized, in which case it may mimic SJS, TEN, or SSSS (Figs. 3.16, 3.17, 3.18, and 3.19).

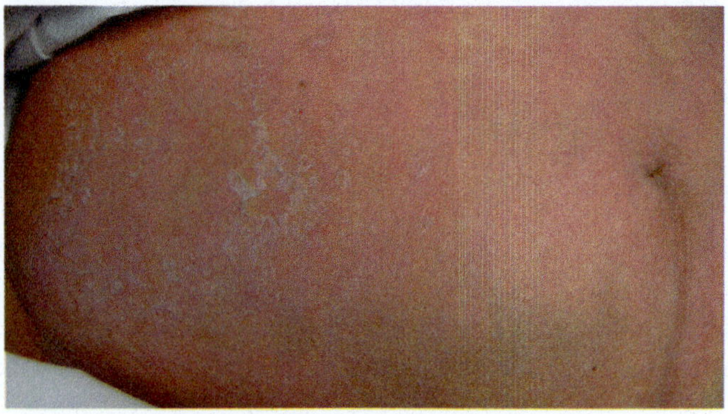

Fig. 3.16 Erythema and diffuse superficial desquamation

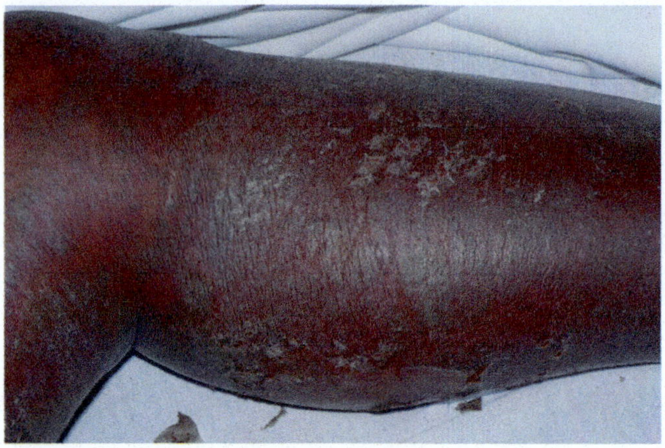

Fig. 3.17 Erythema with deeper desquamation

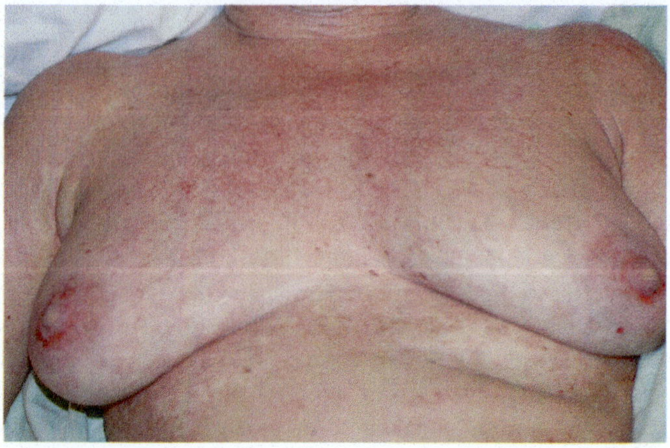

Fig. 3.18 Erythema with desquamation of the areolar regions

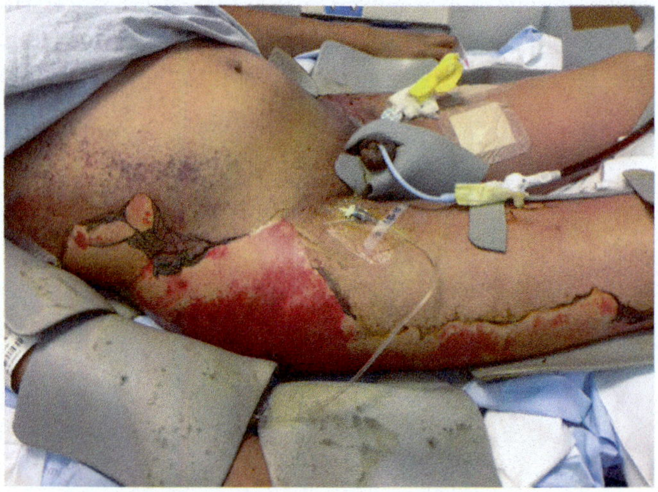

Fig. 3.19 Erythema with sheet-like desquamation mimicking toxic epidermal necrolysis (TEN)

Bullae

Rarely, bullous aGVHD may develop (Fig. 3.20).

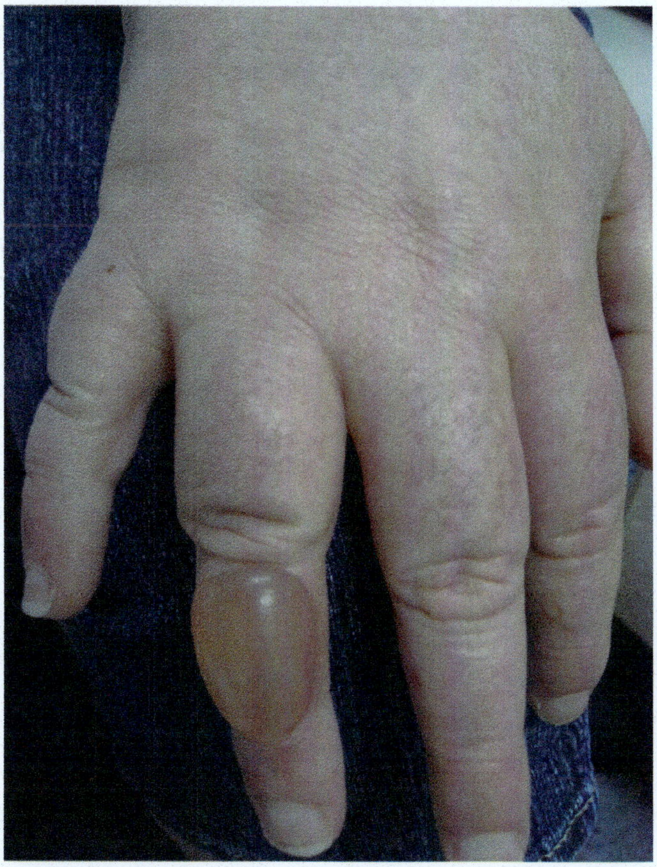

Fig. 3.20 Erythema of the right dorsal hand and fingers with a tense bulla on the fourth finger

Papules

Papular aGVHD may mimic papular eczema or papular urticaria (Figs. 3.21 and 3.22).

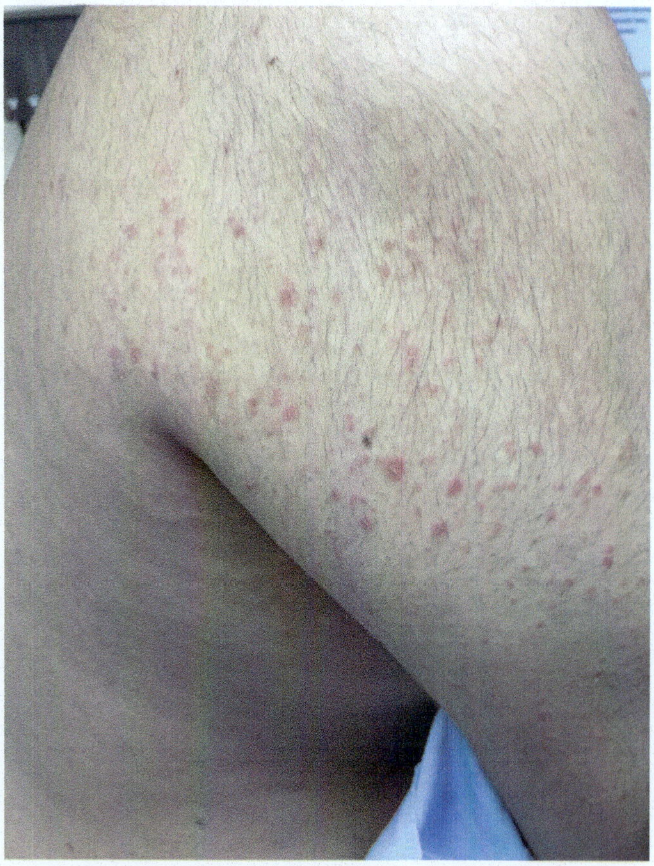

Fig. 3.21 Erythematous, scaly papules on the right arm and shoulder

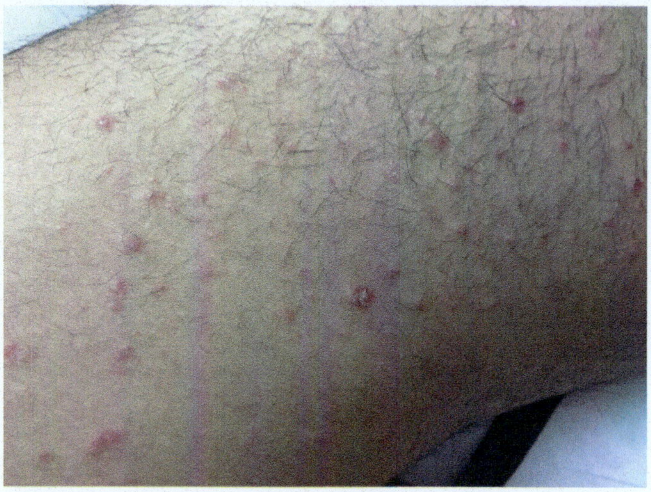

Fig. 3.22 Close-up image of erythematous, scaly papules on the thigh

Conclusion

Familiarity with the many presentations of aGVHD and its clinical spectrum is imperative in the care of patients after HSCT. Recognition of this variability can ensure that accurate and immediate treatment of aGVHD is initiated to improve outcomes for affected patients.

References

1. Ziemer M, Haeusermann P, Janin A, Massi D, Ziepert M, Wolff D, et al. Histopathological diagnosis of graft-versus-host disease of the skin: an interobserver comparison. J Eur Acad Dermatol Venereol. 2014;28:915–24.
2. Byun HJ, Yang JI, Kim BK, Cho KH. Clinical differentiation of acute cutaneous graft-versus-host disease from drug hypersensitivity reactions. J Am Acad Dermatol. 2011;65:726–32.
3. Mays SR, Kunishige JH, Truong E, Kontoyiannis DP, Hymes SR. Approach to the morbilliform eruption in the hematopoietic transplant patient. Semin Cutan Med Surg. 2007;26:155–62.
4. Hymes SR, Alousi AM, Cowen EW. Graft-versus-host disease: part I. Pathogenesis and clinical manifestations of graft-versus-host disease. J Am Acad Dermatol 2012;66:515.e1–18; quiz 533–4.
5. Friedman KJ, LeBoit PE, Farmer ER. Acute follicular graft-vs-host reaction. A distinct clinicopathologic presentation. Arch Dermatol. 1988;124:688–91.
6. Cornejo CM, Kim EJ, Rosenbach M, Micheletti RG. Atypical manifestations of graft-versus-host disease. J Am Acad Dermatol. 2015;72:690–5.
7. Macedo FI, Faris J, Lum LG, Gabali A, Uberti JP, Ratanatharathorn V, White MT. Extensive toxic epidermal necrolysis versus acute graft versus host disease after allogenic hematopoietic stem-cell transplantation: challenges in diagnosis and management. J Burn Care Res. 2014;35:e431–5.
8. Arvidson J, Kildal M, Linde T, Gedeborg R. Toxic epidermal necrolysis and hemolytic uremic syndrome after allogeneic stem-cell transplantation. Pediatr Transplant. 2007;11:689–93.
9. Correia O, Delgado L, Barbosa IL, Domingues JC, Azevedo R, Vaz CP, Pimentel P. CD8+ lymphocytes in the blister fluid of severe acute cutaneous graft-versus-host disease: further similarities with toxic epidermal necrolysis. Dermatology. 2001;203:212–6.

Clinical Presentation of Mucosal Acute and Chronic Graft-Versus-Host Disease

4

Lauren Curtis, Rachel I. Kornik, Jacqueline W. Mays, and Haley B. Naik

Graft-versus-host disease (GVHD) may affect any mucosal site and is a significant source of patient morbidity. Acute and chronic GVHD at various mucosal sites share similarities in symptoms, clinical signs, and histopathologic features. Early and accurate diagnosis of GVHD, in conjunction with timely intervention, is key to minimizing discomfort and unnecessary medication exposure, and to preventing irreversible organ damage and functional deficits. In stem cell transplant patients, GVHD must be distinguished from other causes of mucosal inflammation and discomfort, including medication effect, infection, and malignancy. Careful surveillance of mucosal sites is key to prevention, detection, and management of GVHD and other complications of stem cell transplantation. Significant advances in our understanding of the presentation and pathogenesis of GVHD continue to drive further clarification of classification, staging, and management of GVHD at mucosal sites (Figs. 4.1, 4.2, 4.3, 4.4, 4.5, and 4.6; Tables 4.1, 4.2, 4.3, 4.4, 4.5, and 4.6).

L. Curtis
Experimental Transplantation and Immunology Branch, National Cancer Institute, National Institutes of Health, Bethesda, MD, USA
e-mail: lauren.curtis@nih.gov

R.I. Kornik • H.B. Naik (✉)
Department of Dermatology, University of California, San Francisco, San Francisco, CA, USA
e-mail: rachel.kornik@ucsf.edu; haley.naik@ucsf.edu

J.W. Mays
Oral and Pharyngeal Cancer Branch, National Institute of Dental and Craniofacial Research, National Institutes of Health, Bethesda, MD, USA
e-mail: jacqueline.mays@nih.gov

J.A. Cotliar (ed.), *Atlas of Graft-versus-Host Disease*, DOI 10.1007/978-3-319-46952-2_4

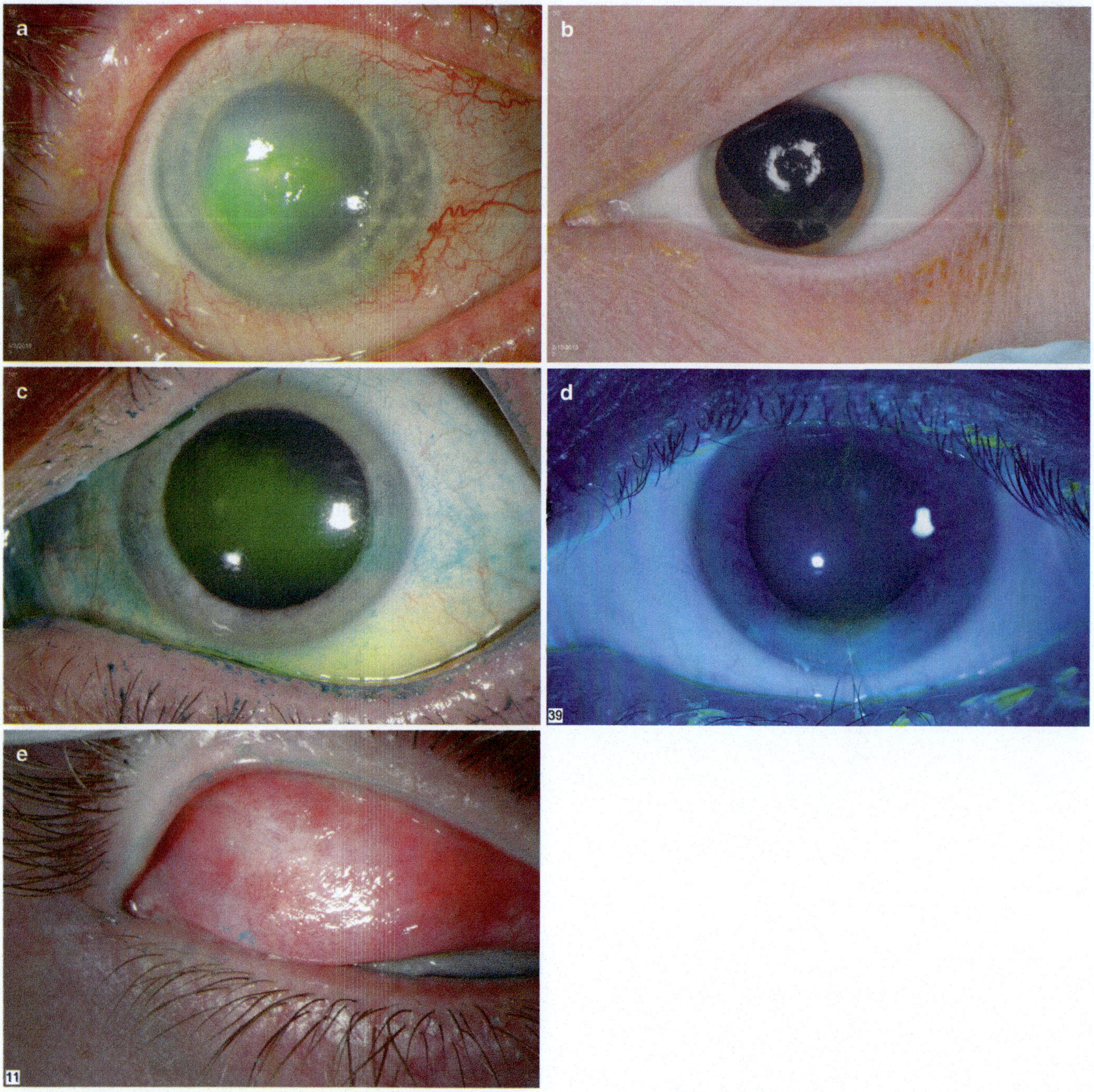

Fig. 4.1 Ocular graft-versus-host disease. Ocular GVHD can affect almost every structure of the eye. Distinctive characteristics of chronic ocular GVHD include keratoconjunctivitis sicca, confluent areas of punctate keratopathy, and cicatricial conjunctivitis. (**a**) Acute ocular GVHD can present with pseudomembranous conjunctivitis and sloughing of the cornea, which can be visualized using fluorescein dye staining or slit lamp examination. (**b**) Complete loss of eyelashes may also be seen in the setting of acute ocular GVHD. (**c**) In chronic ocular GVHD, punctate keratopathy involving the cornea and conjunctiva can be seen in the setting of keratoconjunctivitis sicca, or *dry eye syndrome*, and can be visualized with the aid of dyes including fluorescein, lissamine green (*as shown*), and rose Bengal. (**d**) Blepharitis, or inflammation of the eyelids, may also be observed and can lead to trichiasis—ingrowth or misdirection of eyelashes, which can result in corneal abrasion. (**e**) Chronic inflammation of the ocular mucosa can lead to conjunctival fibrosis, which can be visualized with eyelid eversion (*Photos courtesy of* Manuel B. Datiles III, MD)

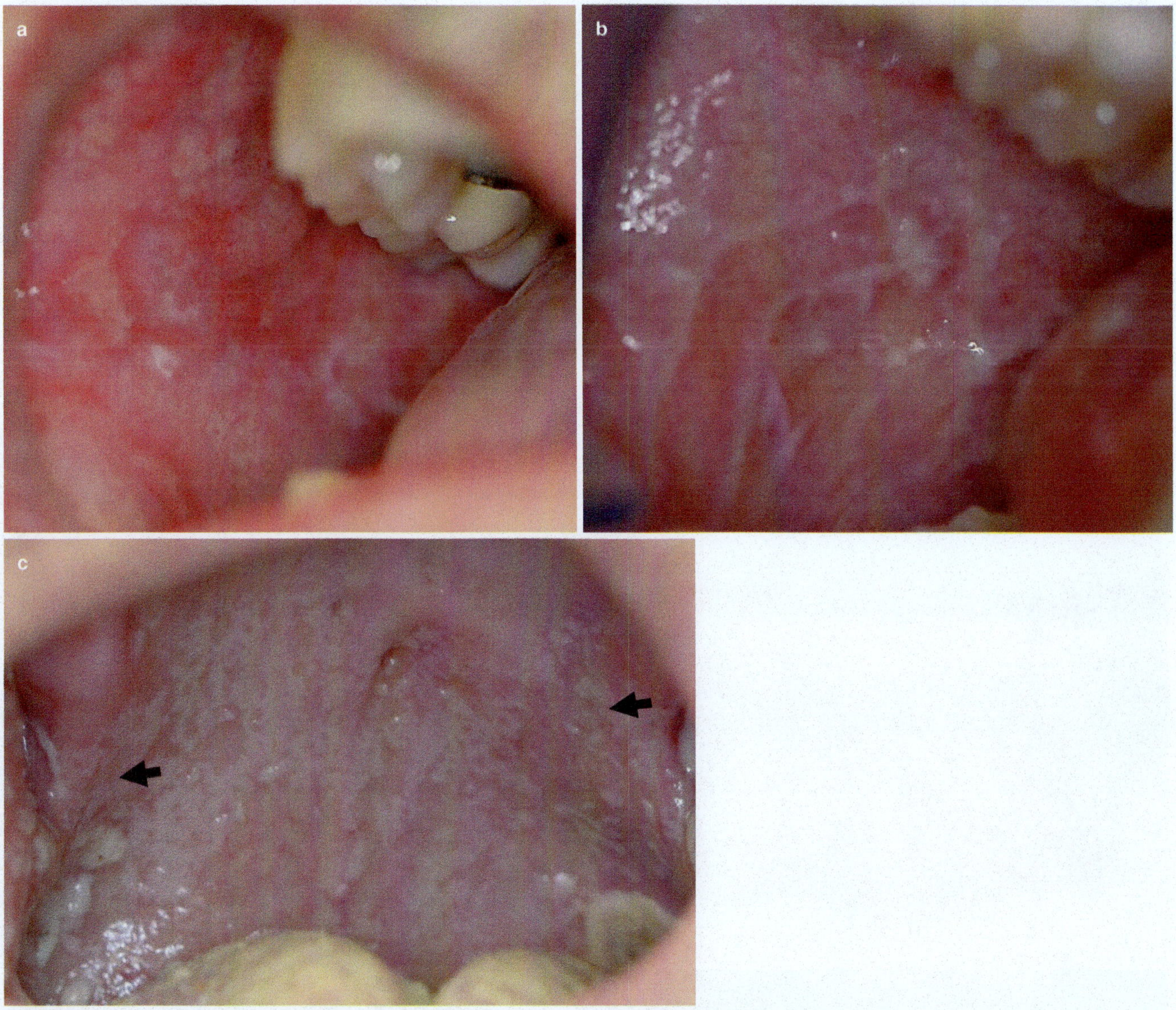

Fig. 4.2 Diagnostic and distinctive features of oral GVHD. Chronic GVHD may be clinically diagnosed by the presence of lichen planus–like hyperkeratosis on the oral mucosa in a patient who has undergone stem cell transplantation. (**a**) Chronic GVHD may present as white reticulate, hyperkeratotic plaques on the buccal mucosa. (**b**) Erythema, hyperkeratotic plaques, and pseudomembranous ulceration may be observed in chronic GVHD. Acute GVHD may have a similar ulcerated presentation with mild erythema and without hyperkeratotic plaques. (**c**) Mucocutaneous candidiasis, presenting here as white plaques on the posterior soft palate and anterior pillar of fauces (*arrows*) and yellow-coated tongue, can mimic acute or chronic GVHD but is generally accompanied by a burning sensation relieved with topical and systemic antifungal therapy

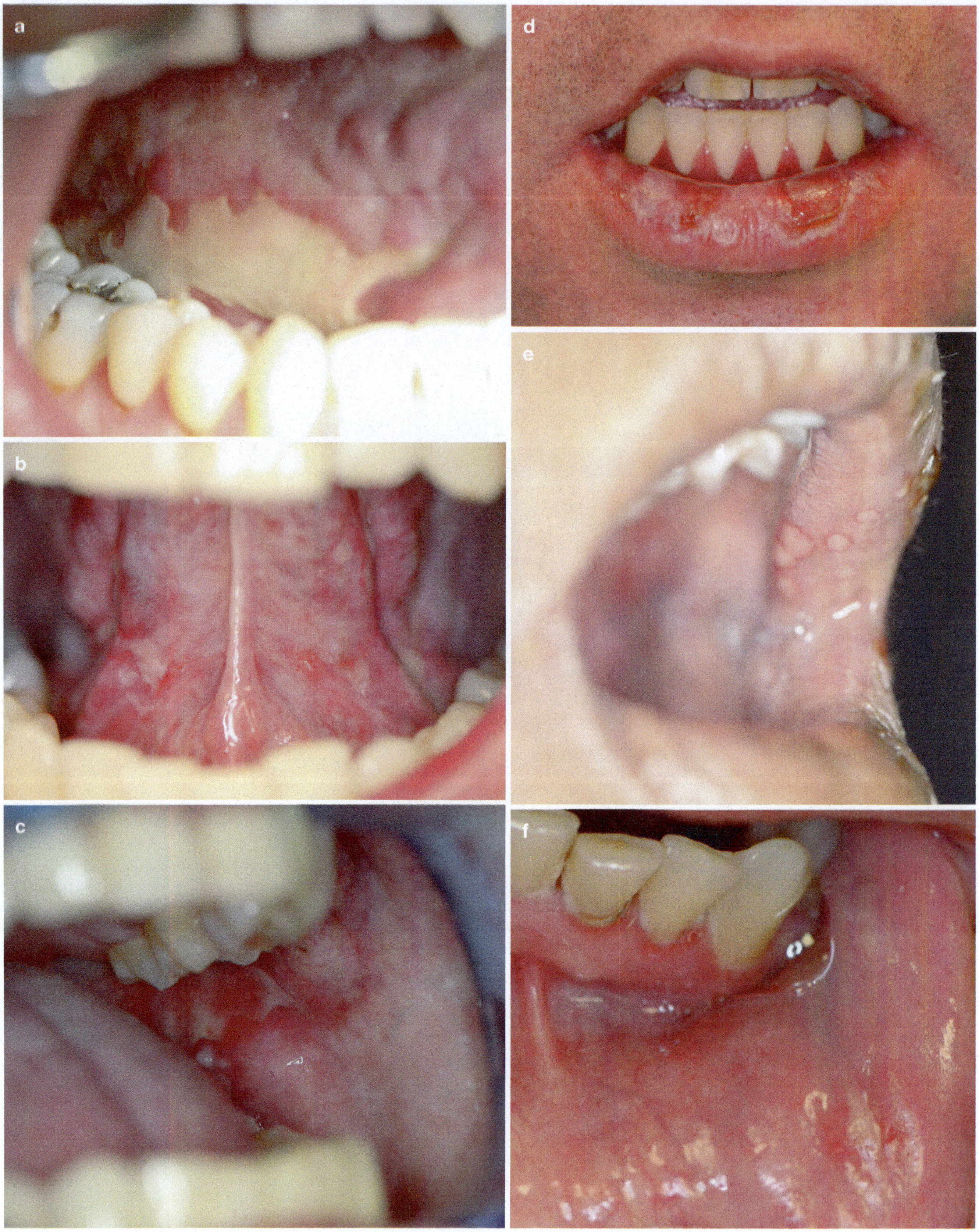
a
b
c
d
e
f

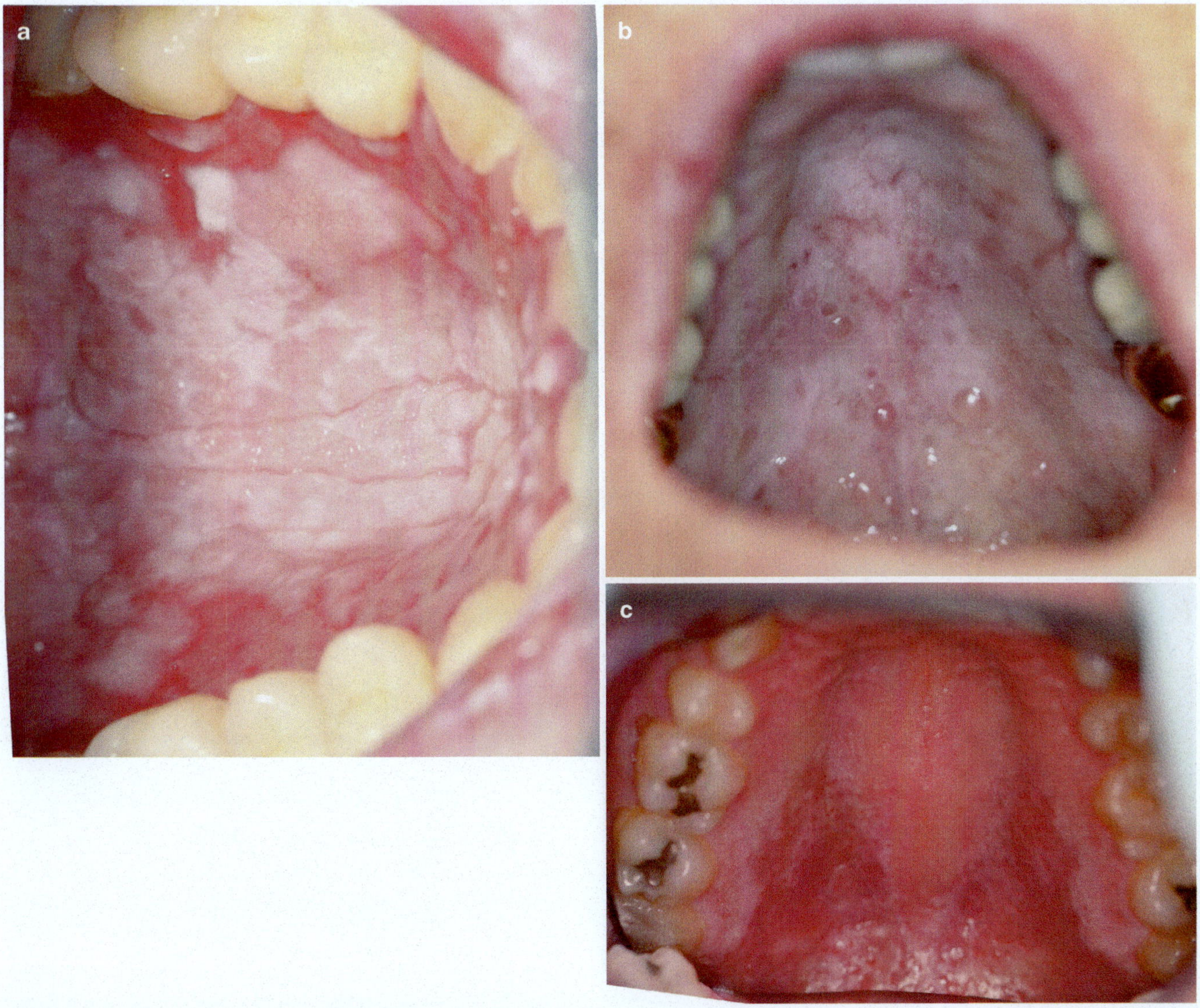

Fig. 4.4 Palatal changes in oral chronic GVHD. Alterations in the palatal mucosa may be seen in chronic GVHD. (**a**) Palatal hyperkeratosis, erythema, and ulceration may be present on the hard palate and soft palate in chronic GVHD. (**b**) The presence of mucoceles is a distinctive, but not diagnostic, sign of oral chronic GVHD. Mucoceles occur when the ductal openings of the minor salivary glands are blocked, either with foreign material or because of lymphocytic infiltrate in the underlying skin or salivary glands. These are most commonly seen on the lower labial mucosa and at the junction between the hard and soft palate. Though typically painless, mucoceles may be bothersome and slow to resolve. (**c**) Milder changes involving the palate, such as a mottled *red* and *white* discoloration, may also be seen in chronic GVHD

Fig. 4.3 Oral ulcerations in post-transplant patients. Ulcerations may occur at any site on the oral mucosa, including the roof of the mouth, buccal mucosa, tongue, gingiva, vestibules, and lips. Establishing a clear diagnosis is critical for successful treatment. Ulcers may result from GVHD, viral infection, systemic medications or other causes. (**a**) Acute GVHD may present as mucositis involving any site on the oral mucosa (*Photo courtesy of* Robert Range, DDS). (**b, c**) Pseudomembranous ulcerations in chronic GVHD occur in many forms, and may eventually lose their pseudomembranous covering. Common sites include the base of the ventral tongue and the buccal mucosa. (**d**) Chronic GVHD may present on the cutaneous lip as wide, irregularly shaped ulcers in the setting of white lacy lesions, chapping, or generalized superficial hyperkeratosis of the cutaneous lip. (**e**) Ulcerations on the cutaneous lip may also be caused by viruses, including herpes simplex virus (HSV). HSV presents as clustered vesicles that, when unroofed, leave punched-out ulcerations. (**f**) Sirolimus, and less frequently other mTOR inhibitors, may induce isolated painful oral ulcerations, mucositis, or stomatitis. These findings typically occur in the setting of supratherapeutic serum drug levels and resolve with adjustment of drug dose. Palliative care may be required to help reduce oral pain until resolution of the ulcers

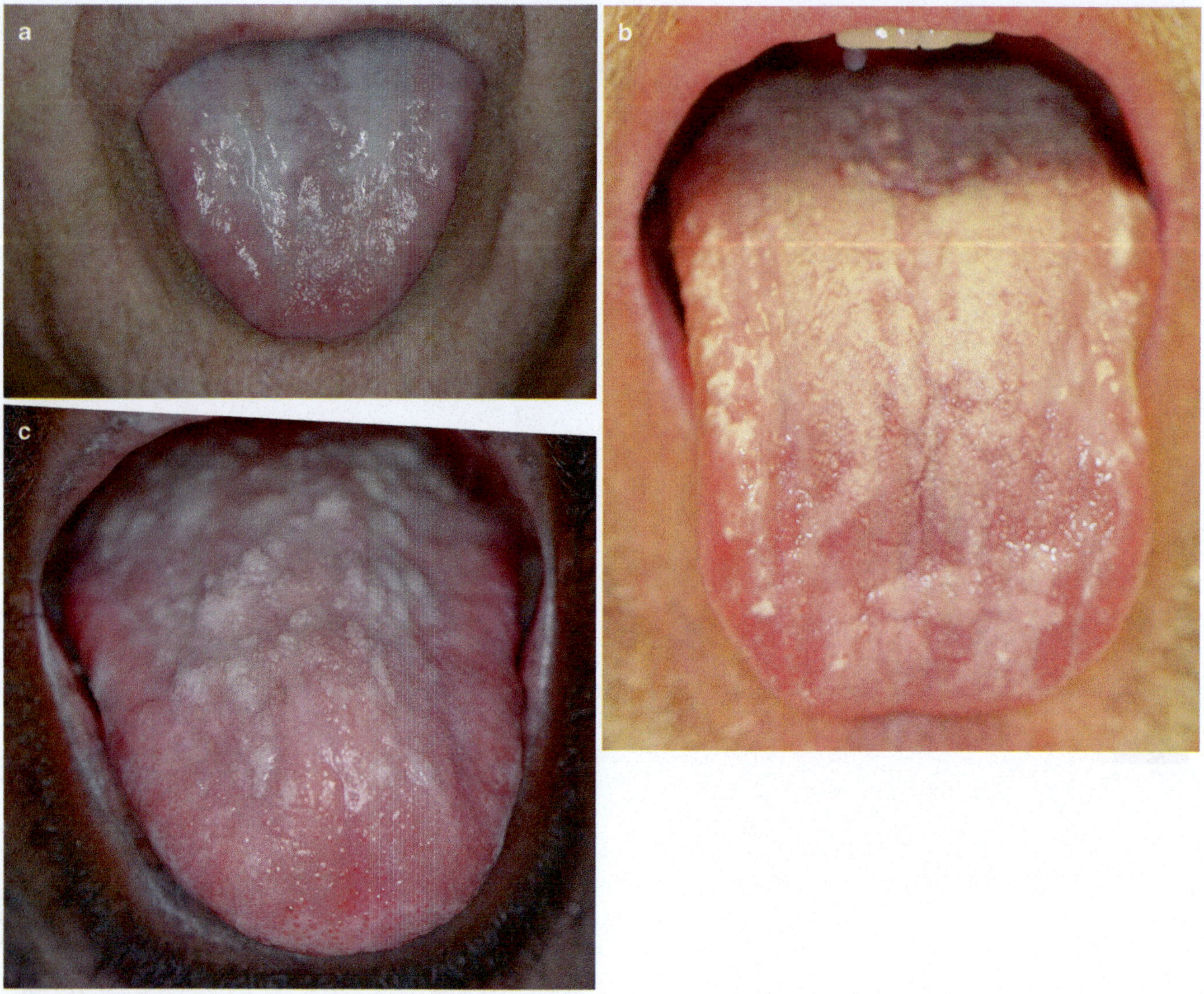

Fig. 4.5 Tongue changes in post-transplant patients. The tongue is a sensitive indicator of changes in the post-transplant period. In the setting of long-standing xerostomia or prolonged oral chronic GVHD, the tongue may lose its filiform and fungiform papillae, resulting in smooth appearance of the dorsal tongue. (**a**) When xerostomia is induced by chronic GVHD, associated white hyperkeratotic plaques may also be seen on the dorsal surface. (**b**) Hyperkeratotic plaques on the dorsal tongue may also be patchy and intermixed with patches of atrophy and erythema. (**c**) Chronic GVHD may induce isolated or multiple tufted, hyperkeratotic papules and plaques on the dorsal tongue, which require careful monitoring and evaluation with diagnostic biopsy to assess for human papillomavirus (HPV) or secondary malignancy

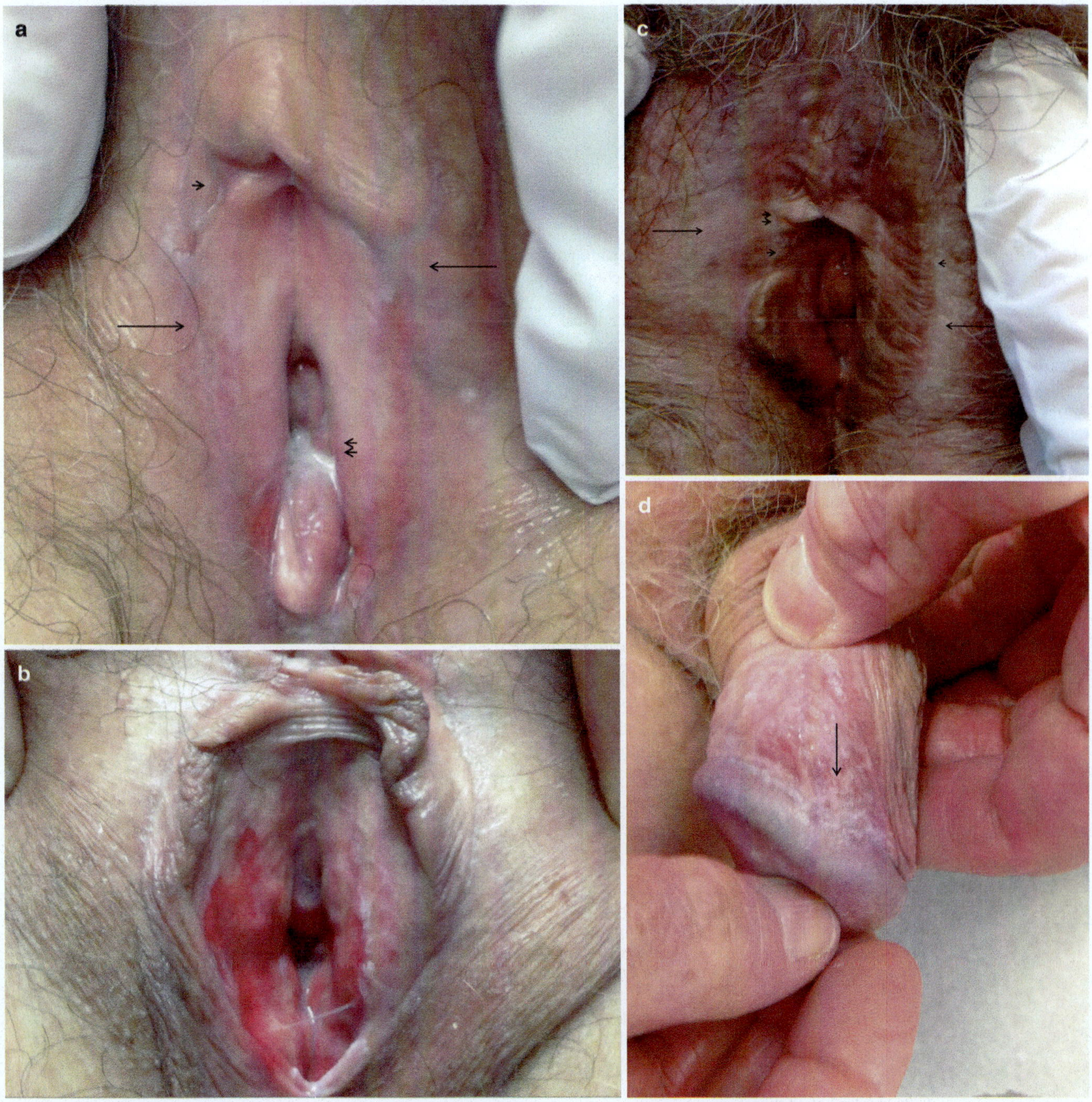

Fig. 4.6 Genital GVHD. Chronic GVHD of the genitals may manifest as erythema, white plaques, erosions, fissures, ulcerations, or significant scarring resulting in loss of normal genital anatomy if not diagnosed at an early stage. Symptoms include vaginal dryness, pruritus, dyspareunia, and pain to touch around the introitus, particularly concentrated at the Skene's and Bartholin's duct openings. Genital GVHD may occur alone, but typically is associated with involvement of other mucosal sites [1]. (**a**) Chronic lichen planus-like GVHD of the genital mucosa is characterized by reticulate leukokeratosis (Wickham striae) overlying erythematous patches or erosions and can lead to complete resorption of the labia minora (*arrow*), clitoral hood agglutination (*arrowhead*), and narrowing of the vaginal orifice (*double arrowhead*). The vagina should always be examined for involvement in all forms of GVHD. (**b**) Erosive GVHD is characterized by painful erosions and ulcerations favoring the modified mucous membranes of the labia minora, perineum, clitoral prepuce, vestibule, and vaginal mucosa. The resulting vaginal stenosis, synechiae, and labial adhesions often require surgical correction to maintain sexual and urinary function and to prevent hematocolpos [2]. (**c**) Lichen sclerosus–like GVHD is characterized by waxy, hypopigmented plaques (*arrow*) and loss of genital structures secondary to scarring. Agglutination of the labia minora (*arrowhead*) and clitoral hood scarring (*double arrowhead*) may be seen. (**d**) Male genital GVHD is not well characterized. Reported presentations include appearances resembling lichen planus (*arrow*) or lichen sclerosus, phimosis, meatal scarring [3], and Peyronie's disease [4]. Coronal fusion (*arrowhead*) may also be seen

Table 4.1 Differential diagnosis of ocular graft-versus-host disease by clinical features

	Xerophthalmia [5]	Ocular irritation or pain [5, 6]	Conjunctival injection ("Red Eye") [5]	Cicatricial conjunctivitis [7, 8]
DDx	Drug-induced[a] Injury secondary to total body irradiation Infection[b] Other medical conditions[c]	Infection[b] Trauma	Infection[b] Glaucoma Allergy Chemical irritant Corneal abrasion Subconjunctival hemorrhage	Autoimmune diseases (ocular cicatricial pemphigoid) Postinfectious conjunctivitis Ocular rosacea Atopic keratoconjunctivitis
Useful Tests	Schirmer tear test Tear film breakup time Meibomian gland exam Tear osmolarity measurement Corneal and/or conjunctival staining[d]	Slit lamp examination[e] Corneal and/or conjunctival staining[d] Conjunctival or corneal sampling for microbiological evaluation	Slit lamp examination[e] Measurement of intraocular pressure Corneal and/or conjunctival staining[d] Conjunctival or corneal sampling for microbiological evaluation	Slit lamp examination[e] Eversion of upper and lower lids Conjunctival or corneal sampling for microbiological evaluation Conjunctival biopsy ± direct immunofluorescence

DDx differential diagnosis

[a]Main culprits: antihistamines, beta-blockers, anticholinergics, thiazide diuretics, selective serotonin reuptake inhibitors [9]

[b]Bacterial (Streptococcus, Staphylococcus), viral (adenovirus, herpes simplex virus, cytomegalovirus), fungal (Fusarium, Aspergillus)

[c]Diabetes, thyroid disorder, vitamin A deficiency, environmental allergies

[d]With fluorescein (conjunctival and corneal staining), rose Bengal (conjunctival staining), and/or lissamine green (conjunctival staining), depending on availability and provider preference [10]

[e]To examine structures in the anterior eye

Table 4.2 Differential diagnosis of oral graft-versus-host disease by clinical features

	Xerostomia	Oral erosions and ulcerations	Mucosal erythema	White patches and plaques
DDx	Drug-induced hyposalivation[a] Dehydration Injury secondary to total body irradiation	Drug-induced[b] Viral infection[c]	Gingivitis Erythematous candidiasis Irritant or allergic contact mucositis	*Wipes away with gauze* Candidiasis/thrush Pseudomembrane *Fixed* HPV-reactive hyperkeratotic plaque Leukoplakia Secondary malignancy (SCC)
Useful tests	Increase patient liquid intake Review medication list for anticholinergic agents Palpate major salivary glands to observe saliva expression Minor labial salivary gland biopsy to assess for histopathologic features of GVHD Consider trial of cholinergic agonist drug	Assess plasma levels of offending drug[b] Viral direct fluorescent antibody, PCR and/or culture Incisional mucosal biopsy of affected, intact tissue adjacent to defect	Assess for local irritating factors (heavy dental calculus, poor oral hygiene) KOH preparation and fungal culture for *Candida* Incisional mucosal biopsy	KOH preparation and fungal culture for *Candida* Incisional mucosal biopsy

DDx differential diagnosis, *GVHD* graft-versus-host disease, *HPV* human papillomavirus, *KOH* potassium hydroxide, *PCR* polymerase chain reaction, *SCC* squamous cell carcinoma

[a]Main culprits: antidepressants, antihistamines, anxiolytics, decongestants, diuretics, muscle relaxants, and agents for neuropathic pain

[b]mTOR inhibitor

[c]Herpes simplex, herpes zoster, coxsackie, cytomegalovirus, Epstein-Barr virus

Table 4.3 Differential diagnosis of genital graft-versus-host disease by clinical features

	Vulvovaginal dryness [11]	Vulvovaginal erosions and ulcerations [12, 13]	Mucosal erythema [13]	White patches and plaques [13]	Vulvar pain and/or dyspareunia [14]	Vaginal discharge [15–17]
DDx	Estrogen deficiency Drug- induced[a]	Viral infection[b] Secondary malignancy Candidiasis Bacterial infection Sexually transmitted infections (STI)[c] Drug reaction[d]	Estrogen deficiency Erythematous candidiasis Bacterial infection Irritant or allergic contact dermatitis Vulvar intraepithelial neoplasia (VIN) Plasma cell mucositis	Lichen planus[e] Lichen sclerosus[e] Lichen simplex chronicus Vitiligo Postinflammatory pigment alteration Candidiasis Condyloma VIN/squamous cell carcinoma	Estrogen deficiency Vulvodynia[e]	Candidiasis Bacterial infection[f] Trichomoniasis Atrophic vaginitis Vaginal intraepithelial neoplasia Vaginal condyloma Cervicitis[g] Foreign body Irritant or allergic contact dermatitis
Useful tests	Consider trial of topical/ intravaginal estrogen if no contraindications Consider skin biopsy to assess for features of GVHD	Viral direct fluorescent antibody, PCR and/ or culture KOH preparation and fungal culture Bacterial culture STD testing as appropriate Diagnostic biopsy of affected, intact skin adjacent to defect	Assess for irritants[h] KOH preparation and fungal culture for *Candida* Bacterial culture Diagnostic skin biopsy	KOH preparation and fungal culture for *Candida* Diagnostic skin biopsy	Consider trial of topical/ intravaginal estrogen if no contraindications Consider skin biopsy to assess for features of GVHD	Saline wet mount KOH preparation and fungal culture for *Candida* Amine whiff test Vaginal pH Consider bacterial culture Consider vaginal biopsy

DDx differential diagnosis, *GVHD* graft-versus-host disease, *KOH*potassium hydroxide, *STD* sexually transmitted disease
[a]Main culprit medications with antiestrogen effect: tamoxifen, medroxyprogesterone, aromatase inhibitors
[b]Herpes simplex, herpes zoster, cytomegalovirus, Epstein-Barr virus, HIV
[c]Syphilis, HIV
[d]Fixed drug eruption, Stevens-Johnson syndrome, toxic epidermal necrolysis (TEN)
[e]Only if present prior to transplantation
[f]Bacterial vaginosis, *Staphylococcus aureus*, group A *Streptococcus*
[g]Gonorrhea, chlamydia, herpes simplex virus (HSV), trichomonas
[h]Personal care products, topical prescription preparations, urine, feces

Table 4.4 Clinical and histopathologic features of mucosal graft-versus-host disease

Organ/site	Features of acute GVHD[a]	Diagnostic features of cGVHD[b]	Distinctive features of cGVHD[c]	Other features of cGVHD[d]	Common findings in GVHD[e]	Histopathologic features [18, 19]
Eyes	*Conjunctivitis* Cicatrizing Hemorrhagic Pseudomembranous Serosanguinous Sloughing of corneal epithelium	No diagnostic features	New-onset dry, gritty, painful eyes Keratoconjunctivitis sicca Confluent areas of punctate keratopathy Cicatricial conjunctivitis	Photophobia Periorbital hyperpigmentation Blepharitis (erythema and edema of the eyelids)	Photophobia Erythema Pain	**Acute/Active** Lichenoid interface lymphocytes with infiltration of mucosa (exocytosis) Variable apoptosis **Chronic** *Conjunctiva:* Lymphocyte exocytosis Satellitosis Vacuolization of basal epithelium Epithelial cell necrosis *Lacrimal glands:* Periductal mononuclear cell infiltrate Loss of acinar lobules in the setting of fibrosis
Mouth	Mucositis Gingivitis Erythema Pain	Lichen planus–like changes	Xerostomia Mucoceles Mucosal atrophy Ulcers Pseudomembranes	Foamy or thick saliva [20, 21] Atrophic glossitis Difficulty chewing and swallowing food without water Oral mucosal sensitivity to foods that are spicy, salty, acidic, minty, or crunchy New-onset taste changes	Gingivitis Mucositis Erythema Pain	**Acute/Active** Lichenoid interface lymphocytes with infiltration of mucosa (exocytosis) Variable apoptosis **Chronic**[f] Periductal lymphocytic infiltrate with damaged intralobular ducts or acinar tissues Fibroplasia in periductal stroma Mixed lymphocytic and plasmacytic inflammation with destruction of acinar tissue
Genital Tract	Erosions/ulcerations Erythema Reticulate white plaques [22]	Lichen planus–like changes Lichen sclerosus–like changes *Female* Vaginal scarring Labial/clitoral hood agglutination *Male* Phimosis Urethral meatus scarring or stenosis	Erosions Fissures			**Acute and Chronic** Foci of chronic and acute inflammation within stroma and epithelium Lichenoid dermatitis Spongiotic dermatitis

Adapted from Jagasia et al. [23]
cGVHD chronic graft-versus-host disease
[a]Acute genital GVHD manifestations have not been described in the literaturea
[b]Diagnostic features are sufficient to establish the diagnosis of chronic GVHD
[c]Distinctive features are seen in chronic GVHD but are insufficient to establish diagnosis on their own
[d]Can be acknowledged as part of the chronic GVHD manifestations if diagnosis is confirmed
[e]*Common* refers to features shared by both acute and chronic GVHD
[f]These features are specific to chronic GVHD but apply only to the salivary gland. The oral mucosa shares histopathologic features between active acute and chronic GVHD.

Table 4.5 National Institutes of Health Guidelines for chronic graft-versus-host disease mucosal organ severity scoring

	Score 0	Score 1	Score 2	Score 3
Eyes	No symptoms	Mild dry eye symptoms not affecting ADL (requiring eyedrops <3 × per day)	Moderate dry eye symptoms partially affecting ADL (requiring drops >3 × per day or punctal plugs), *without* new vision impairment due to KCS	Severe dry eye symptoms significantly affecting ADL (special eyewear to relieve pain) *or* unable to work because of ocular symptoms *or* loss of vision caused by KCS
Mouth	No symptoms	Mild symptoms with disease signs but not limiting oral intake significantly	Moderate symptoms with disease signs with partial limitation of oral intake	Severe symptoms with disease signs on examination with major limitation of oral intake
Genital (male or female)	No signs	Mild signs, and females may have symptoms[a] with discomfort on exam[b] *Females (any of following):* Erythema on vulvar mucosal surfaces Vulvar lichen planus Vulvar lichen sclerosis *Males:* Lichen planus–like features	Moderate signs, and may have symptoms with discomfort on exam[b] *Females (any of following):* Erosive inflammatory changes of the vulvar mucosa Fissures in vulvar folds *Males (any of following):* Lichen sclerosus–like features Moderate erythema	Severe signs, with or without symptoms *Females (any of following):* Labial fusion Clitoral hood agglutination Fibrinous vaginal adhesions Circumferential fibrous vaginal banding Vaginal shortening Synechia Dense sclerotic changes Complete vaginal stenosis *Males (any of following):* Phimosis Urethral/meatal scarring

Adapted from Jagasia et al. [23]
ADL activities of daily living, *KCS* keratoconjunctivitis sicca.
[a]Symptoms are not specific and can represent premature gonadal failure or infection
[b]To be determined by specialist or trained medical provider; discomfort is defined as vulvar pain elicited by gentle touch with cotton swab to any of the following sites: vestibular glands, labia minora or majora

Table 4.6 Topical therapies[a] and recommended prevention and monitoring for mucosal graft-versus-host disease

	Ocular	Oral	Genital
Acute GVHD	**Conjunctivitis** [6, 24] Topical steroids Topical tacrolimus or cyclosporine	**Mucositis** Cryotherapy [25, 26] Supersaturated calcium phosphate rinses [27, 28] Pain control [27]	**Lichen planus like-changes or erosions involving the vulva or penis** [14] Topical steroids
Chronic GVHD	**Keratoconjunctivitis** [6] Topical steroids Cyclosporine ophthalmic emulsion (0.05, 0.1 %) Autologous serum eye drops **Xerophthalmia** [6] Lubricating eye drops Punctal plugs Selective muscarinic agonists (pilocarpine, cevimeline) Bandage contact lenses Scleral lenses **Conjunctival scarring** Topical steroids	**Lichen planus–like changes** [28] Steroid rinses Calcineurin-inhibitor rinses **Oral ulcers (isolated)** [28] Topical steroid gel[b] Tacrolimus gel Intralesional triamcinolone injection **Xerostomia** [28] Oral lubricants Salivary stimulants (sugar-free gum/lozenges) Cholinergic agonists (pilocarpine, cevimeline) **Reduced oral aperture (sclerosis)** [28, 29] Progressive stretching regimen Peri-oral steroid injections Surgical intervention	**Lichen sclerosus/lichen planus–like changes or erosions involving the vulva or penis** [14, 29, 30] Correction of estrogen deficiency with topical estrogen if no contraindications, *plus*: High-potency topical steroid ointment Addition of tacrolimus ointment 0.1 % **Female genital lichen planus–like changes or erosions also involving vaginal mucosa** [14, 29] Correction of estrogen deficiency with topical estrogen if no contraindicatiions, *plus:* Consider referral to a specialist Intravaginal estrogen if no contraindication Intravaginal high-potency steroid or suppository Tacrolimus cream/suppository 0.1 % (2 mg tacrolimus per 2 g suppository)[c] Dilator therapy **Female genital: Vaginal stenosis/synechiae (fibrosis)** [14, 29]**:** As above, *plus* Surgical intervention for lysis of adhesions or vaginal reconstruction as necessary Dilator therapy to prevent recurrence
Preventive/Supportive Measures [29]	Photoprotection Surveillance for infection, cataract formation, and increased intraocular pressure	Strict oral/dental hygiene Routine dental cleaning with endocarditis prophylaxis Surveillance for infection and malignancy	**Females:** Surveillance for estrogen deficiency Vulvar hygiene to minimize irritation Use of nonirritating personal lubricants Simple emollient to the vulva **Females & Males**: Surveillance for infection and secondary malignancy

Recommended Monitoring [29]	Ophthalmologic exams every 3–12 months during systemic immunosuppressive therapy for chronic GVHD *Flare:* rule out infectious conjunctivitis	Dental exam and prophylaxis every 6 months with annual oral cancer screen and interproximal radiographs [28] *Flare:* rule out infection and gastric reflux [28]	**Females** [30, 31]**:** Genital exam, including inspection of vulva, vaginal mucosa, and cervix at 3–6 months following transplantation or sooner based on symptoms, then at least annually Consider gynecologic exam every 3 months for patients with known genital GVHD Cervical cytology testing annually or more frequently based on results Consider HPV vaccination *Flare:* rule out infection and allergic or irritant contact dermatitis

GVHD graft-versus-host disease, *HPV* human papillomavirus

[a]Topical therapy is most effective for GVHD involving isolated mucosal sites or for GVHD of isolated sites that is recalcitrant to systemic therapy. Topical therapies may need to be used in combination with systemic agents for management of severe localized GVHD or multiorgan involvement of GVHD.

[b]Initiating with World Health Organization Class V moderate-potency agents and increasing in strength

[c]Intravaginal preparations must be specially compounded, and patients should be monitored for systemic absorption

References

1. Hirsch P, Leclerc M, Rybojad M, Petropoulou AD, Robin M, Ribaud P, et al. Female genital chronic graft-versus-host disease: importance of early diagnosis to avoid severe complications. Transplantation. 2012;93:1265–9.
2. Kim TH, Lee HH, Chung SH. Hematocolpos as a complication of chronic graft-versus-host disease. Taiwan J Obstet Gynecol. 2012; 51:292–3.
3. Mueller SM, Haeusermann P, Rovo A, Halter JP, Passweg J, Itin P, et al. Genital chronic GVHD in men after hematopoietic stem cell transplantation: a single-center cross-sectional analysis of 155 patients. Biol Blood Marrow Transplant. 2013;19: 1574–80.
4. Jain NA, Venkatesan K, Anandi P, Ito S, Kumar D, Lu K, et al. A rare consequence of chronic graft versus host disease – Peyronie's disease. Arch Cancer Res. 2015;3(2)
5. Shikari H, Antin JH, Dana R. Ocular graft-versus-host disease: a review. Surv Ophthalmol. 2013;58:233–51.
6. Kim SK, Smith JA, Dunn Jr JP. Chronic ocular graft versus host disease. In: Vogelsang GB, Pavletic SZ, editors. Chronic graft versus host disease: interdisciplinary management. New York: Cambridge University Press; 2009. p. 199–206.
7. Faraj HG, Hoang-Xuan T. Chronic cicatrizing conjunctivitis. Curr Opin Ophthalmol. 2001;12:250–7.
8. Marzano AV, Facchetti M, Berti E, Caputo R. Chronic graft-vs.-host disease with severe cicatrizing conjunctivitis mimicking cicatricial pemphigoid. Br J Dermatol. 2000;143:209–10.
9. Fraunfelder FT, Sciubba JJ, Mathers WD. The role of medications in causing dry eye. J Ophthalmol. 2012;2012:285851.
10. Methodologies to diagnose and monitor dry eye disease: report of the Diagnostic Methodology Subcommittee of the International Dry Eye WorkShop (2007). Ocul Surf. 2007;5(2):108–52.
11. Mac Bride MB, Rhodes DJ, Shuster LT. Vulvovaginal atrophy. Mayo Clin Proc. 2010;85:87–94.
12. Bohl TG. Vulvar ulcers and erosions–a dermatologist's viewpoint. Dermatol Ther. 2004;17:55–67.
13. Edwards L, Lynch PJ. Genital dermatology atlas. Philadelphia: Lippincott Williams and Wilkins; 2011.
14. Stratton P, Turner ML, Childs R, Barrett J, Bishop M, Wayne AS, et al. Vulvovaginal chronic graft-versus-host disease with allogeneic hematopoietic stem cell transplantation. Obstet Gynecol. 2007;110:1041–9.
15. Frega A, Sopracordevole F, Assorgi C, Lombardi D, De Sanctis V, Catalano A, et al. Vaginal intraepithelial neoplasia: a therapeutical dilemma. Anticancer Res. 2013;33:29–38.
16. Smith L, Angarone MP. Sexually transmitted infections. Urol Clin North Am. 2015;42:507–18.
17. Sobel JD. Vaginitis. N Engl J Med. 1997;337:1896–903.
18. Shulman HM, Cardona DM, Greenson JK, Hingorani S, Horn T, Huber E, et al. NIH consensus development project on criteria for clinical trials in chronic graft-versus-host disease: II. The 2014 Pathology Working Group Report. Biol Blood Marrow Transplant. 2015;21:589–603.
19. Shulman HM, Kleiner D, Lee SJ, Morton T, Pavletic SZ, Farmer E, et al. Histopathologic diagnosis of chronic graft-versus-host disease: National Institutes of Health consensus development project on criteria for clinical trials in chronic graft-versus-host disease: II. Pathology Working Group Report. Biol Blood Marrow Transplant. 2006;12:31–47.
20. Mays JW, Fassil H, Edwards DA, Pavletic SZ, Bassim CW. Oral chronic graft-versus-host disease: current pathogenesis, therapy, and research. Oral Dis. 2013;19:327–46.
21. Treister N, Duncan C, Cutler C, Lehmann L. How we treat oral chronic graft-versus-host disease. Blood. 2012;120:3407–18.
22. Stratton P. Personal communication (Kornik RI, editor, 2015).
23. Jagasia MH, Greinix HT, Arora M, Williams KM, Wolff D, Cowen EW, et al. National Institutes of Health consensus development project on criteria for clinical trials in chronic graft-versus-host disease: I. The 2014 Diagnosis and Staging Working Group report. Biol Blood Marrow Transplant. 2015;21:389–401.
24. Nassar A, Tabbara KF, Aljurf M. Ocular manifestations of graft-versus-host disease. Saudi J Ophthalmol. 2013;27:215–22.
25. Riley P, Glenny AM, Worthington HV, Littlewood A, Clarkson JE, McCabe MG. Interventions for preventing oral mucositis in patients with cancer receiving treatment: oral cryotherapy. Cochrane Database Syst Rev. 2015;(12):CD011552.
26. Worthington HV, Clarkson JE, Bryan G, Furness S, Glenny AM, Littlewood A, et al. Interventions for preventing oral mucositis for patients with cancer receiving treatment. Cochrane Database Syst Rev. 2011;(4):CD000978.
27. Clarkson JE, Worthington HV, Furness S, McCabe M, Khalid T, Meyer S. Interventions for treating oral mucositis for patients with cancer receiving treatment. Cochrane Database Syst Rev. 2010;(8):CD001973.
28. Markiewicz M, Dzierzak-Mietla M, Frankiewicz A, Zielinska P, Koclega A, Kruszelnicka M, et al. Treating oral mucositis with a supersaturated calcium phosphate rinse: comparison with control in patients undergoing allogeneic hematopoietic stem cell transplantation. Support Care Cancer. 2012;20:2223–9.
29. Carpenter PA, Kitko CL, Elad S, Flowers ME, Gea-Banacloche JC, Halter JP, et al. National Institutes of Health consensus development project on criteria for clinical trials in chronic graft-versus-host disease: V. The 2014 Ancillary Therapy and Supportive Care Working Group Report. Biol Blood Marrow Transplant. 2015;21:1167–87.
30. Shanis D, Merideth M, Pulanic TK, Savani BN, Battiwalla M, Stratton P. Female long-term survivors after allogeneic hematopoietic stem cell transplantation: evaluation and management. Semin Hematol. 2012;49:83–93.
31. Markowitz LE, Dunne EF, Saraiya M, Chesson HW, Curtis CR, Gee J, et al.; Centers for Disease Control and Prevention (CDC). Human papillomavirus vaccination: recommendations of the Advisory Committee on Immunization Practices (ACIP). MMWR Recomm Rep. 2014;63:1–30. Erratum in: MMWR Recomm Rep. 2014;63:1182.

Histopathology of Cutaneous Graft-Versus-Host Disease

5

Cuong V. Nguyen, Christiane Querfeld, and Daniel D. Miller

Precise diagnosis of graft-versus-host disease (GVHD) remains elusive. The skin is one of the major organ systems affected by GVHD, but diagnosis of this entity in a timely manner is often hindered by clinical and histopathologic mimickers, such as drug hypersensitivity reactions, viral exanthema, and toxic erythema of chemotherapy. Microscopic findings in acute and chronic cutaneous GVHD are reviewed here, as are features of other entities in the clinical and histopathologic differential diagnosis.

Acute Graft-Versus-Host Disease

The fundamental inflammatory process in acute graft-versus-host disease (GVHD) is that of a vacuolar interface dermatitis—that is, a cytotoxic T-cell attack directed at epidermal keratinocytes and other cutaneous epithelial structures. According to the NIH Pathology Working Group [1], histologic confirmation of acute GVHD, regardless of staging, requires the presence of necrotic keratinocytes. Apoptosis can be present at the Malpighian layer (basal epidermis), the follicular outer root sheath, or the acrosyringium. In acute GVHD (aGVHD), features of chronic GVHD (cGVHD) should be absent (see below for details of histologic diagnosis of cGVHD). However, in patients diagnosed clinically with late-onset aGVHD (>100 days), histologic features of cGVHD have been concurrently identified in up to 40 % of patients [2]. These patients are at greater risk of complete progression to cGVHD.

Consensus on the utility of cutaneous biopsy to evaluate for aGVHD remains inconsistent. Of clinicians from 25 centers in Germany, Austria, and Switzerland, only 62 % felt that skin biopsy was necessary for diagnosis of aGVHD [3]. Disagreement was based on (1) lack of discriminating features to distinguish aGVHD from other diagnoses, (2) opinion that biopsy is necessary only when atypical clinical features are present, and (3) center policy to perform a biopsy only if the clinical course warrants it. The decision to treat aGVHD is often more dependent on the clinical picture than on biopsy findings, which correlate poorly with clinical severity [4]. This discrepancy is likely to be partially the result of high interobserver variability in the histopathologic diagnosis of aGVHD.

In a 2013 study, four expert pathologists reviewed 15 biopsies of aGVHD and its histologic mimickers [5]. When the pathologists were blinded to the clinical data, diagnostic concordance was only 53 %, with the correct diagnosis rendered in 33 % of cases. When detailed clinical information was provided, concordance and correct diagnosis were achieved in 80 %. Other studies have suggested that skin biopsy is most useful in guiding treatment in patient populations with an aGVHD incidence less than 30 %. In populations where the incidence is greater than 30 %, patient outcomes were better for those treated empirically without skin biopsy [6]. However, the Consensus Conference held in 2012 by the Cutaneous Pathology Group continues to recommend skin biopsy in aiding the diagnosis of aGVHD [3].

If skin biopsy is performed, at minimum a 4-mm punch biopsy should be obtained [3]. Specimens should be acquired prior to the initiation of systemic or topical therapies that may alter histopathologic features. There is no consensus as to the optimal timing of the biopsy. It has been suggested that that biopsies should be delayed until 21 days post-transplantation, as donor lymphocytes are not typically seen

C.V. Nguyen
Department of Dermatology, University of Minnesota, 516 Delaware Street SE, Minneapolis, MN, USA
e-mail: nguy2291@umn.edu

C. Querfeld
Division of Dermatology, City of Hope Comprehensive Cancer Center, 1500 East Duarte Road, Duarte, CA, USA
e-mail: cquerfeld@coh.org

D.D. Miller (✉)
Department of Dermatology, University of Minnesota Medical Center, 4-240 Phillips Wangensteen Building, 516 Delaware Street SE, Minneapolis, MN, USA
e-mail: mill0581@umn.edu

J.A. Cotliar (ed.), *Atlas of Graft-versus-Host Disease*, DOI 10.1007/978-3-319-46952-2_5

in the epidermis within the first 14 days [7, 8], though this timeline is clearly patient-dependent.

Concept of Interface Dermatitis

An inflammatory dermatosis is defined as an *interface dermatitis* when dermal-epidermal junction degenerative change is present. The terms "liquefactive degeneration," "hydropic degeneration," and "vacuolar alteration" have all been used synonymously in reference to this degenerative change. "Vacuolar alteration" was popularized by Ackerman et al. [9] and is now the preferred term. Some authors further separate interface dermatitis into lichenoid versus vacuolar types [10]. In both, lymphocytes are the predominant cell type. A robust band-like inflammatory infiltrate is present in the lichenoid type. In contrast, a sparser inflammatory infiltrate is seen in the vacuolar type, with spaces separating the basal layer from the papillary dermis. These terms are not mutually exclusive, however, as vacuolar spaces in the basal layer can often be found concurrently with a lichenoid infiltrate.

Histologic Grading and Microscopic Findings

In 1974, Lerner first developed a histopathologic grading system for aGVHD [11]. This system was modified 20 years later by Horn and Haskell [7] (Table 5.1). However, the NIH Pathology Working Group does not recommend the use of any preexisting grading scheme, as schemata do not correlate with any clinical end points and are often affected by immunosuppressive status [1]. Instead, they recommend four categories of histologic sign-out:

1. No evidence of GVHD
2. Possible GVHD
3. Consistent with or highly suggestive of GVHD
4. GVHD without equivocation

The histologic diagnosis of GVHD can be limited by findings suggestive of concurrent infection or drug eruption, by recent chemotherapy or radiotherapy, or by minimal foci to suggest unequivocal GVHD.

Acute GVHD is characterized histologically by basal cell vacuolar alteration, and may be accompanied by varying degrees of a lymphocytic lichenoid infiltrate [12]. In contrast, numbers of Langerhans cells (epidermal antigen-presenting cells) are reduced [13]. In early aGVHD, the vacuolar change may be very subtle, and the dermis often features only a sparse perivascular lymphocytic infiltrate (Fig. 5.1) [14]. During this stage, orthokeratosis, parakeratosis (apoptotic, cornified cells with retained nuclei), or both can be seen overlying a hypergranular layer. As the clinical severity of aGVHD progresses, necrotic or dyskeratotic keratinocytes (Fig. 5.2) are more frequently found and may be present in any epidermal layer, including the follicular epithelium (Fig. 5.3) [1, 15, 16]. Cytoid bodies, or "eosinophilic bodies" (*i.e.*, necrotic keratinocyte debris), are often present either within the affected epidermis or in the immediately subjacent papillary dermis [7]. Lymphocytic exocytosis and satellite cell necrosis (lymphocytes in close apposition to apoptotic keratinocytes) are inconsistent features [16, 17]. There may frequently be a background of cytotoxic effects including loss of epidermal polarity with dysmaturation and atypical mitoses, often resembling low-grade squamous dysplasia; these cutaneous toxic effects of chemotherapy often partially limit interpretation, as cytotoxic agents may also produce necrotic keratinocytes [14]. Spongiosis is variable, and microvesiculation can occur [14, 18]. Vascular proliferation has been described in association with perivascular edema, a lymphocytic infiltrate, and prominent mast cells [19, 20]. On direct immunofluorescence, deposition of C3 and IgM at the dermal-epidermal junction is present in up to 39 % of aGVHD [21].

Table 5.1. Histologic grading scheme for acute graft-versus-host disease

	Lerner grading system [11]	Horn grading system [7]
Grade 0		Normal skin or unrelated cutaneous disease
Grade 1	Vacuolar alteration	Vacuolar alteration
Grade 2	Spongiosis and dyskeratosis (eosinophilic bodies)	Epidermal or follicular dyskeratotic cells, dermal lymphocytic infiltration
Grade 3	Epidermolysis and formation of bulla	Formation of subepidermal clefts and microvesicles
Grade 4	Total epidermal denudation	Epidermal separation from dermis

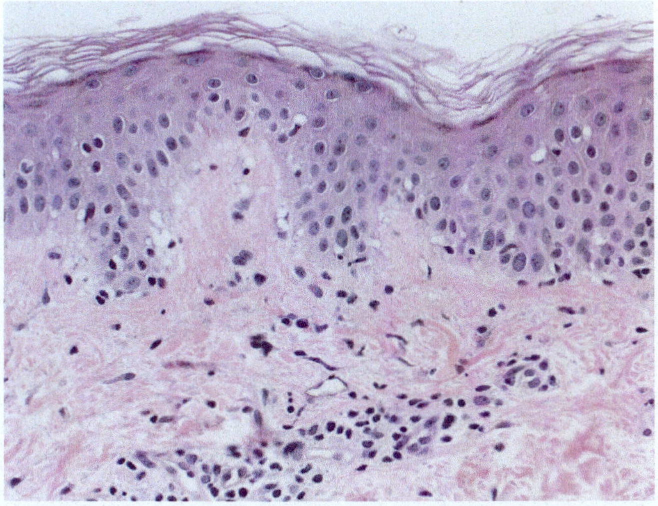

Fig. 5.1 Acute vacuolar interface dermatitis. Basal keratinocyte vacuolization is present, with cytotoxic lymphocytes aligned along the basal layer. Overtly necrotic keratinocytes are absent. These findings correspond to acute graft-versus-host disease (aGVHD) histologic grade I, changes considered insufficiently specific to make a definitive GVHD diagnosis (H&E-stained section, 200× magnification)

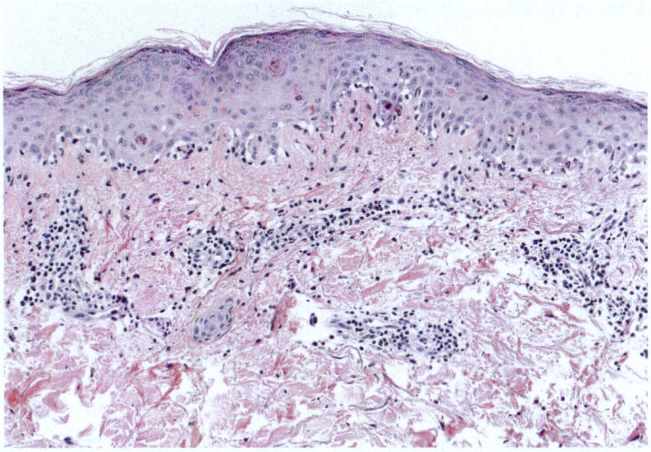

Fig. 5.2 Interface dermatitis with necrotic keratinocytes at and above the epidermal basal layer, corresponding to aGVHD histologic grade II (H&E, 100× magnification)

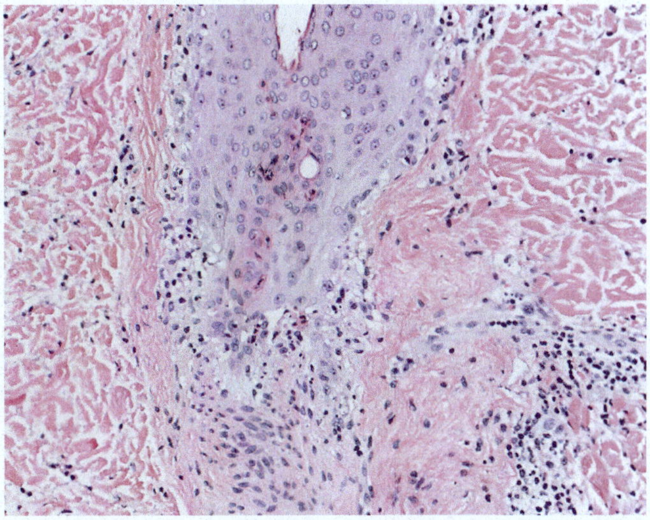

Fig. 5.3 Vacuolar interface change with necrotic keratinocytes within follicular epithelium in aGVHD (H&E, 200× magnification)

Clues to Histologic Diagnosis

Definitive diagnosis of aGVHD is more readily made when histologic Grade 3 or 4 changes are identified (Fig. 5.4). In less severe cases, given the lack of pathognomonic findings, histologic diagnosis of aGVHD can be difficult. However, there are several features that when taken into constellation may help in the diagnosis of aGVHD.

Though interface dermatitis may be encountered in GVHD, drug hypersensitivity, and viral exanthema (all clinical considerations in the acute post-transplant period), vacuolar alteration of adnexal structures is uncommon in cutaneous pathology and is not typically seen in most drug eruptions [22]. GVHD represents a prime example in which vacuolar alteration of adnexae, principally of follicular units, may be encountered (Fig. 5.3) [23]. However, adnexal vacuolar change also may be found in systemic lupus erythematosus (SLE) and toxic erythema of chemotherapy (TEC). Theoretically, it may also be found in dermatomyositis, but this has not been consistently reported in the literature. Because of the uneven distribution of cutaneous adnexal structures, level sections should be obtained to search for follicular units and sweat gland epithelium when there is a high clinical index of suspicion for aGVHD.

In addition to involvement of the follicular epithelium, diagnosis of aGVHD is more suggestive in the absence of eosinophils. However, the presence of eosinophils does not completely exclude a diagnosis of aGVHD until more than 16 eosinophils per 10 high power fields (HPF) are found (Fig. 5.5) [24]. The presence of >16 eosinophils per 10 HPF is 100 % specific for a cutaneous drug eruption, whereas >3.5 eosinophils per 10 HPF has 93 % specificity. In the context of aGVHD, a specificity of 93 % is likely inadequate, as a false negative diagnosis can result in significant morbidity and mortality. However, finding at least 4 eosinophils per 10 HPF should prompt consideration of "possible GVHD" rather than "consistent with or highly suggestive of GVHD" as the final diagnosis.

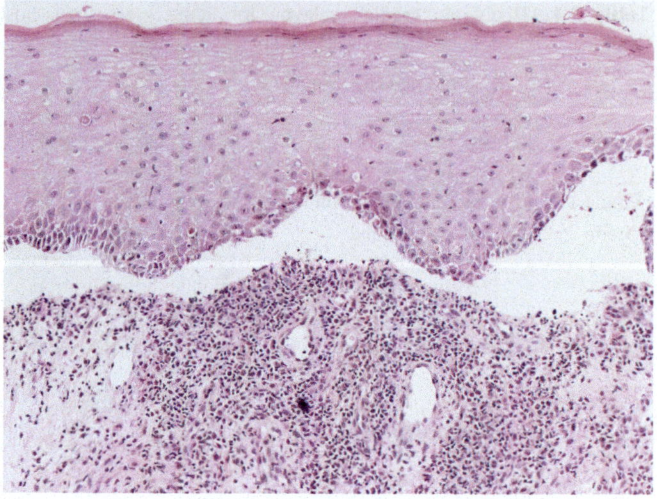

Fig. 5.4 Interface dermatitis (lichenoid type) with subepidermal clefting, corresponding to aGVHD histologic grade III (H&E, 100× magnification)

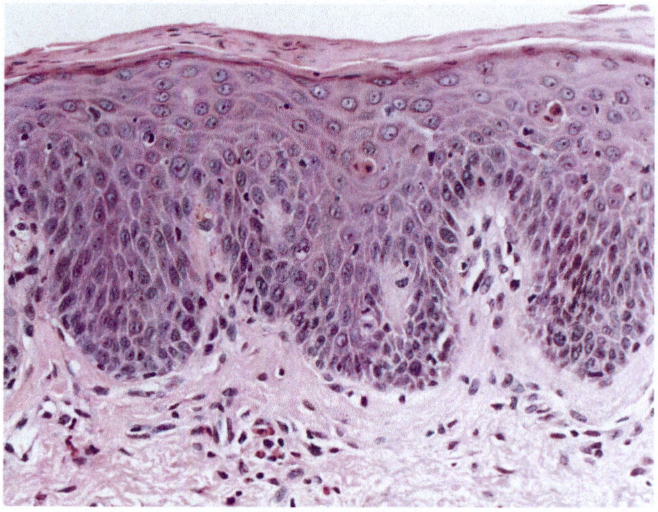

Fig. 5.5 Interface dermatitis with perivascular eosinophils. These findings may be seen in aGVHD, but the presence of more than 4 eosinophils per 10 HPF around the superficial perivascular plexus makes a drug hypersensitivity reaction more likely. A diagnosis of "possible GVHD" with a comment regarding tissue eosinophilia is likely the most appropriate approach in this setting (H&E, 200× magnification)

Differential Diagnosis of Acute GVHD

The histologic features of aGVHD are mimicked by several entities (Table 5.2). The microscopic features of aGVHD are largely identical to engraftment syndrome (and likely pre-engraftment syndrome), which requires clinicopathologic correlation. Unlike aGVHD, however, engraftment syndrome typically occurs 10–14 days after transplantation, specifically 48 hours before or after the first appearance of neutrophils in peripheral blood (absolute neutrophil count >500) [25]. This event usually precedes the appearance of peripheral lymphocytes.

Similar to aGVHD, toxic erythema of chemotherapy (TEC) can also present in the post-transplantation period with necrotic keratinocytes involving the epidermis and adnexal structures (Fig. 5.6), especially eccrine epithelium (likely owing to the fact that chemotherapy may concentrate in eccrine sweat). Significant keratinocyte dysmaturation and/or cytologic atypia leans toward the diagnosis of TEC [22]. In addition, TEC also may show dermal edema, eccrine squamous syringometaplasia, and peri-eccrine neutrophils [26]. Theoretically, TEC is a direct toxicity effect, a nonimmunologic process that should be minimally inflammatory, but in practice, biopsies often demonstrate mild perivascular lymphocytic inflammation that does not differ significantly from that seen in many aGVHD cases.

As discussed under clues to diagnosis, drug hypersensitivity reactions such as morbilliform drug eruption are favored in the presence of eosinophils, with >16 eosinophils per 10 HPF ruling out aGVHD [24]. Erythema multiforme and Stevens-Johnson syndrome/toxic epidermal necrolysis spectrum disorders may be indistinguishable from aGVHD, but involvement of adnexal structures and involvement of follicular epithelium is more likely in aGVHD, as noted above. In addition, squamatization of the basal layer and parakeratosis or compact hyperkeratosis are more likely to be seen in aGVHD than in erythema multiforme [27]. The presence of bile pigment has been suggested as a marker to differentiate aGVHD from erythema multiforme, though its sensitivity is only 6 % [28].

Viral exanthems may also commonly mimic aGVHD microscopically, with basal layer vacuolization seen in up to 40 % of cases [29]. Some histopathologic clues may provide a specific viral diagnosis in limited cases. Multinucleate keratinocytes are suggestive of herpes simplex or varicella infection. Human herpes virus-6 may show distinctive viral inclusions within lymphocytes: a halo surrounds the irregularly shaped nuclei, which contain a central basophilic inclusion [30]. Cytomegalic endothelial cell nuclei, or "owl's eyes," may be found in dermal blood vessels in cytomegalovirus infections [31]. Serum polymerase chain reaction (PCR) studies can be performed for confirmation when skin biopsies suggest viral infection.

Other interface dermatoses must also be excluded from the differential. Acute systemic lupus erythematosus (SLE) may be the most difficult to distinguish from aGVHD, with each revealing a sparse lymphocytic interface dermatitis, though SLE is not a common clinical consideration in the period immediately after transplantation. Findings of increased mucin in the superficial dermis may help to distinguish the two [32]. In discoid lupus or other lesions of chronic cutaneous lupus, more prominent superficial and deep lymphocytic infiltrates, follicular plugging, and increased dermal mucin deposition can be seen. Dermatomyositis may be distinguishable from GVHD only by the presence of increased dermal mucin and/or C5b-9 deposition at the dermo-epidermal junction on direct immunofluorescence [33]. Both pityriasis lichenoides et varioliformis acuta (PLEVA) and pityriasis lichenoides chronica (PLC) reveal a sparse vacuolar interface in early lesions. As PLEVA continues to develop, vacuolar change becomes more extensive, and parakeratosis, a dense wedge-shaped lymphocytic infiltrate, and prominent erythrocyte extravasation may be found [34]. Within the parakeratosis, there may be an inflammatory infiltrate composed of neutrophils or sometimes lymphocytes. Unlike PLEVA, PLC is more likely to have broad parakeratosis without neutrophils and with fewer necrotic keratinocytes.

Table 5.2. Histologic differential diagnosis of acute graft-versus-host disease

			aGVHD	ES	TEC	SJS/TEN
Epidermis	Keratinocytes	Necrotic	+[a]	+	+	+
		Atypical			+	
	Lymphocytic exocytosis		+			+
	Basal vacuolization		+	+	+	+
Dermis	Perivascular lymphocytes		+	+		±
	Eosinophils		±			+
	Neutrophils				±	
	Edema				+	+
Adnexae	Vacuolar alteration		+		+	+
	Necrotic keratinocytes		+			+
	Peri-eccrine neutrophils				+	
	Squamous syringometaplasia				+	

aGVHD acute graft-versus-host disease, *ES* engraftment syndrome, *TEC* toxic erythema of chemotherapy, *SJS/TEN* Stevens-Johnson syndrome/toxic epidermal necrolysis

[a]Necrotic keratinocytes present at all epidermal layers

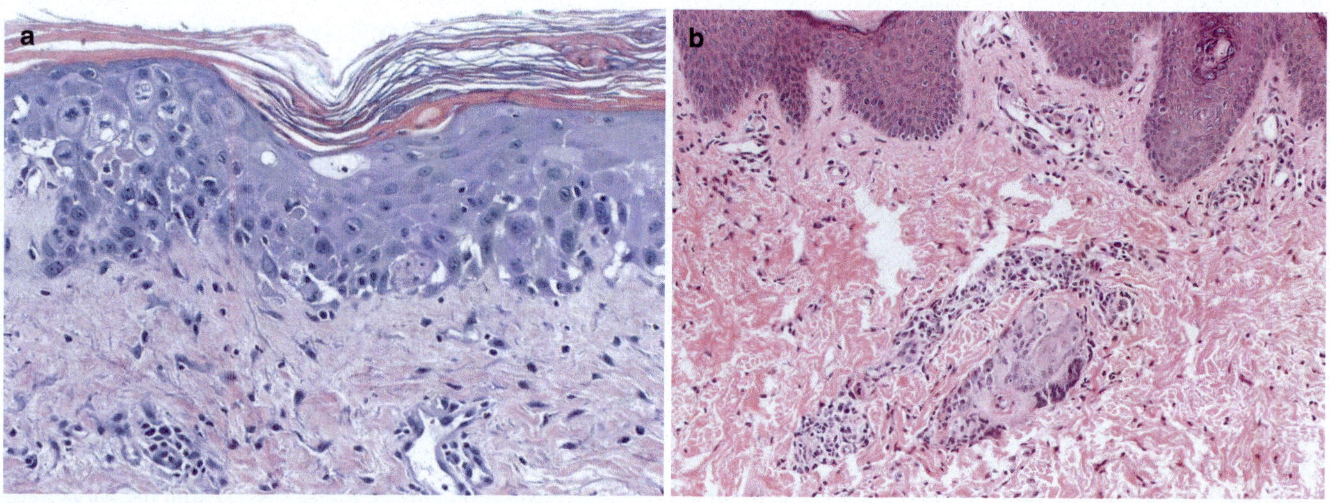

Fig. 5.6 Toxic erythema of chemotherapy. (**a**) Atypia of epidermal keratinocytes and multiple mitotic figures, resulting from accumulation of cytotoxic agents within the skin. Note basal layer vacuolization and necrotic keratinocytes mimicking aGVHD (H&E, 200× magnification). (**b**) Interface dermatitis with focal necrosis isolated to eccrine sweat duct epithelium only. The absence of overlying epidermal changes is a clue to the diagnosis in this specimen (H&E, 100× magnification)

Potential Adjunctive Tests

Given the significant adverse outcomes that can occur in untreated aGVHD, several tools have surfaced as aids in the diagnosis of GVHD. HLA immunostaining is utilized in some centers, with HLA-DR staining of keratinocytes found to be up to 100 % specific [13]. Significant recent research has focused on identifying biomarkers of prognostic and diagnostic significance in GVHD. Biomarker assays commonly utilize serum, but they can also be performed on tissue via immunostains or cytogenetic tests.

The biomarker thymic stromal lymphoprotein (TSLP) may be helpful in predicting which patients are likely to develop aGVHD. TLSP is a keratinocyte-derived cytokine that skews the immune response toward a Th_2 phenotype. In cutaneous specimens taken 20 to 30 days after transplantation, elevated TSLP has been found in patients who later develop aGVHD [35]. TLSP levels were not elevated in patients who did not develop cutaneous aGVHD. A TSLP immunostain is available as an investigational assay and labels epidermal keratinocytes.

Of the biomarkers studied, elafin, an elastase inhibitor expressed by the inflamed epidermis, has emerged as a reliable marker of aGVHD activity [36, 37]. Evaluation of elafin can be performed on both serum and histologic skin specimens. It is unclear whether elafin levels can help differentiate aGVHD from other diagnoses, but once a diagnosis of aGVHD has been unequivocally made, measurement of elafin levels via serum ELISA can help prognosticate disease; increased elafin levels portend a poorer prognosis [37].

Given the utility of elafin, it has recently been included in a six-marker panel in the evaluation of aGVHD [38]. Also included in this panel were previously validated diagnostic biomarkers IL-2 receptor-α, tumor necrosis factor receptor-1, hepatocyte growth factor, IL-8, and regenerating islet–derived 3-α (reg3α). The six-biomarker panel was able to predict two clinical outcomes: which patients would be nonresponsive at day 28 post-therapy, and mortality risk at day 180 from aGVHD onset. The use of this biomarker panel may aid in determining patients at high risk for treatment nonresponse and mortality, supporting the potential for earlier intervention and change in therapeutics.

Special Situations

In patients with hematologic malignancies, the use of T-cell–depleted (TCD) bone marrow transplants is an effective method of reducing the risk of GVHD [39]. Similarly to T-cell–replete transplant recipients (TCR) who develop aGVHD, TCD patients who develop aGVHD share conserved histologic features [40]. In these patients, a diagnosis of aGVHD was made on the findings of diffuse basal layer vacuolar alteration, more than three necrotic keratinocytes per HPF, and necrosis involving all layers of the epidermis. In contrast to TCR patients, however, TCD patients with aGVHD were more likely to have follicular involvement (77 % *vs* 16 %), dermal eosinophils (31 % *vs* 3 %), dermal neutrophils (31 % *vs* 0 %), satellitosis (77 % *vs* 24 %), lymophocyte exocytosis (92 % *vs* 37 %), and extravasated erythrocytes (69 % *vs* 13 %). The significance of these variations has not been determined, and further studies are needed to assess whether clinical outcomes are correlated with these histologic differences.

Recently, children with dystrophic and junctional epidermolysis bullosa have been treated with stem cell transplants. From October 2007 to August 2009, seven children with recessive dystrophic epidermolysis bullosa were treated with a co-infusion of mesenchymal stromal cells and hematopoietic stem cells [41]. None of the seven patients developed acute or chronic GVHD in up to 2 years of follow-up. It is unclear why these patients have a decreased GVHD incidence. It has been suggested that the decreased incidence of GVHD may be from the presence of mesenchymal stromal cells or from an inherent defect in the skin of patients with recessive dystrophic epidermolysis bullosa [42]. Further histopathologic evaluation and studies may be helpful in the development of tools or conditioning regimens to prevent GVHD onset.

Chronic Graft-Versus-Host-Disease

Broad diagnostic criteria make it difficult to estimate the exact incidence and prevalence of cGVHD. The NIH Pathology Working Group is striving to create more uniform criteria to help establish the diagnosis. At this time, it is estimated that the prevalence of cGVHD is approximately 50 % [1, 43]. The skin is the most frequent organ site to be involved in cGVHD, with cutaneous disease occurring in up to 75 % of patients at the time of diagnosis [44]. The presence of at least one *diagnostic* clinical feature of cutaneous cGVHD negates the need for biopsy (Table 5.3) [1]. Biopsy is recommended to help confirm the diagnosis of cGVHD in the presence of only *distinctive* clinical features—those that are seen in cGVHD but are insufficient as isolated findings to definitively diagnose cGVHD. In the skin, the most common distinctive feature is depigmentation, but other features that may be present include hypopigmentation, hyperpigmentation, ichthyosis, keratosis pilaris, or sweat impairment (hypohidrosis) [1]. Other distinctive features involving the nails, hair, oral mucosa, and genitalia are discussed in further detail in the clinical chapters of this book.

Biopsy can be an invaluable tool in confirming suspicion for cGVHD. The size of the biopsy specimen is dependent on the clinical picture. For patients with non-sclerotic cGVHD, the specimen should be at least 4 mm in size, preferably from a palpable lesion without overlying secondary change [3]. In sclerotic lesions, an excisional biopsy is preferred. However, a punch biopsy of 6–8 mm is also an acceptable alternative [3]. Biopsy of a bullous or vesicular lesion should be done at the edge of the blister and should include surrounding erythema. Although biopsy can be a significant diagnostic aide, its use in long-term follow-up to assess treatment response has not been validated.

Table 5.3. Diagnostic clinical criteria seen in chronic graft-versus-host disease [1]

	Cutaneous	Oral mucosa	Genitalia
Poikiloderma	+		
Lichen planus–like features	+	+	+
Sclerotic features	+	+[a]	+
Morphea-like features	+		
Lichen sclerosus–like features	+		
Hyperkeratotic plaques		+	

[a]Mouth opening is restricted by sclerosis

Main Histologic Patterns in cGVHD: Lichenoid and Sclerodermoid

Classically, chronic cutaneous GVHD has been clinically and histologically classified into two subtypes: an early lichenoid stage and a later sclerotic stage. In early cGVHD, patients clinically present with lichen planus-like papules with histopathologic findings nearly identical to aGVHD (Fig. 5.7) [45]. The epidermis shows irregular acanthosis, parakeratosis, hypergranulosis, vacuolar alteration, and variable keratinocyte necrosis (again, a key feature of GVHD). A bandlike lymphocytic infiltrate may obscure the dermal-epidermal junction with evidence of basal vacuolar degeneration, though many biopsies of lichenoid GVHD demonstrate a dermal lymphocytic infiltrate that is significantly sparser than lichen planus and other lichenoid dermatitis. Squamous eccrine metaplasia can be seen in the transition from acute to chronic GVHD [46].

In sclerotic cGVHD, patients can present with cutaneous sclerodermatous changes resembling systemic sclerosis, but they typically lack visceral organ involvement. Two recent studies estimate a 3- to 5-year incidence of sclerotic cGVHD between 20–22.6 %, occurring after a median 18 months [47, 48]. Historically, it has been presumed that lichenoid cGVHD precedes sclerotic cGVHD, but cases have been described of the processes occurring independently [49, 50]. In the initial descriptions of sclerotic cGVHD that followed lichenoid cGVHD, fibrosis progressed from the papillary dermis downward into the reticular dermis [51]. The histologic variants of sclerotic cGVHD are unified by the presence of sclerosis and homogenization of dermal collagen (Fig. 5.8). The level by which sclerosis appears in the skin determines its clinical morphology. Epidermal atrophy, a mild lichenoid infiltrate, and loss of elastic fibers is more typical of lichen sclerosus–like cGVHD than morphea-like cGVHD [52]. Patients with a morphea-like clinical morphology display more prominent reticular sclerosis microscopically, with little involvement of the papillary dermis or the epidermis. In the fasciitis-like variant, the sclerosis may be confined to the fascia but may also involve the subcutaneous septae [52, 53].

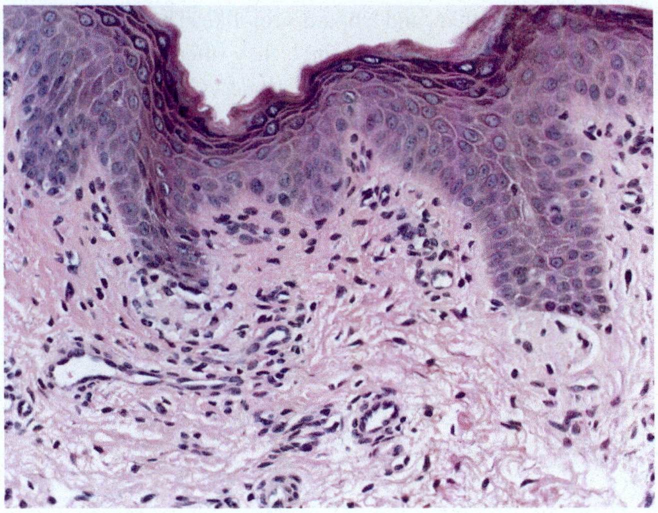

Fig. 5.7 Early lichenoid-type chronic graft-versus-host disease (cGVHD). These findings do not differ significantly from many specimens of aGVHD, although the presence of clusters of necrotic keratinocytes at the bases of rete ridges, epidermal acanthosis, and hypergranulosis all suggest a more chronic inflammatory process (H&E, 200× magnification)

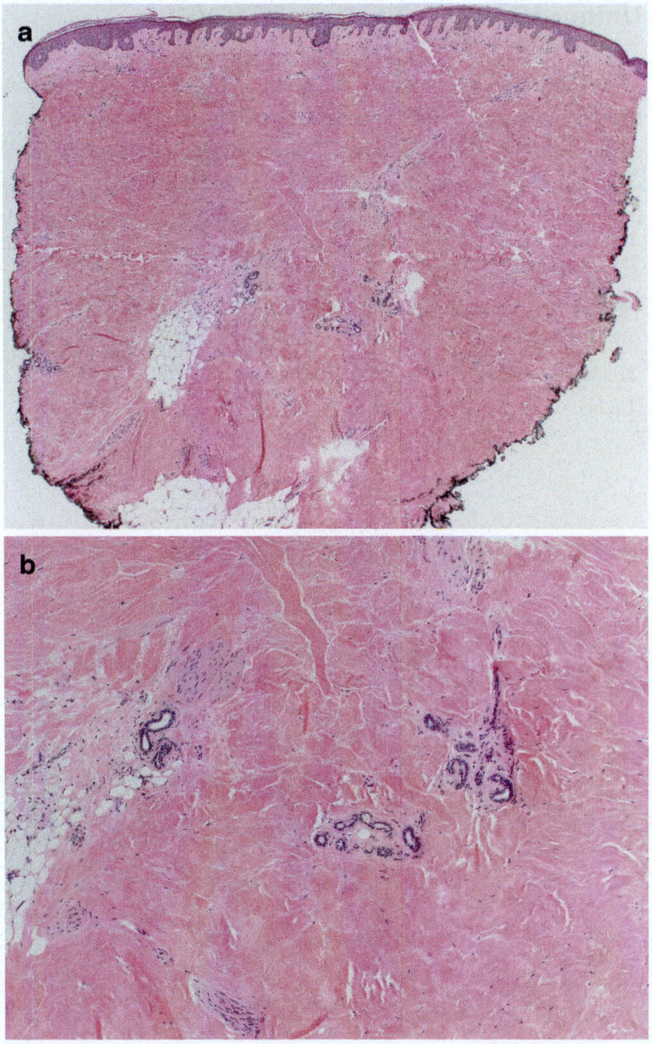

Fig. 5.8 Sclerotic cGVHD. (**a**) The biopsy specimen exhibits a markedly expanded, highly sclerotic dermis with densely packed, hypocellular, hyalinized collagen accentuated within the deeper aspects of the specimen (H&E, 40× magnification). (**b**) Higher power demonstrates hyalinized, hypocellular collagen with "trapping" of eccrine sweat glands and loss of peri-eccrine fat, findings indistinguishable from idiopathic morphea or scleroderma (H&E, 100× magnification)

Unique Histologic Features of cGVHD

With the increased number of patients requiring bone marrow transplantation, more and more morphologic variants of cGVHD have been described. These clinical patterns include eczematous, atopic dermatitis–like, psoriasiform, pityriasis rosea–like, lupus-like, comedonal, follicular keratosis or keratosis pilaris–like, and leopard skin–like. Though these entities may appear clinically distinct, they often share histologic features of either lichenoid or sclerotic cGVHD (Table 5.4). However, unlike more classic lichenoid or sclerotic cGVHD, these morphologic variants may display certain histologic features that could distinguish them as unique clinical and histopathologic variants of cGVHD.

Table 5.4 Common clinical variants of lichenoid/vacuolar and sclerotic chronic GVHD

Histologic subtype	Clinical variant	Comments on clinical features	Comments on histopathologic features
Lichenoid or vacuolar	Lichen planus–like	Violaceous papules	Lichenoid
	Psoriasiform	Annular, guttate, or confluent	Vacuolar change with psoriasiform epidermal hyperplasia
	Eczematous	Can appear erythrodermic	Vacuolar change with spongiosis
	Atopic dermatitis–like	Pruritic, dry skin, perifollicular accentuation	Vacuolar change with spongiosis
	Lupus-like	Malar erythema, lichenoid papules in photodistribution	Lichenoid
	Pityriasis rosea–like	Can appear in inverse location	Vacuolar change with pigment incontinence
	Comedone-like	Acneiform papules and comedones	Follicular vacuolar change, dilated pore, and sclerosis
	Keratosis pilaris–like	Follicular erythema or keratosis	Both lichenoid and sclerotic
Sclerotic	Sclerodermatous	Tightened skin often with poikiloderma	Superficial dermal collagen homogenization
	Lichen sclerosus	Atrophic, pearly-white to violaceous plaques	Superficial dermal sclerosis and epidermal atrophy
	Morphea-like	Indurated, brown to violaceous plaques	Pandermal or deep dermal sclerosis
	Panniculitis/fasciitis	Clinically appears rippled	Deep dermal sclerosis, fasciitis, panniculitis
	Leopard skin	Well-defined, hyperpigmented macules with scale, precedes clinical sclerosis	Dermal reticular sclerosis with sparse vacuolar change
	Comedone-like	Acneiform papules and comedones	Follicular vacuolar change, dilated pore, and sclerosis
	Keratosis pilaris–like	Follicular erythema or keratosis	Both lichenoid and sclerotic

Psoriasiform Pattern

Like psoriasis, psoriasiform cGVHD reveals epidermal acanthosis with regular elongation of rete ridges, parakeratosis, and loss of the granular layer [54–56]. Neutrophilic abscesses can also be found in the stratum corneum. Unlike psoriasis, the presence of focal satellite cell necrosis, dyskeratosis, lymphocytic exocytosis, and basal layer vacuolar change helps to confirm the diagnosis of cGVHD.

Eczematous Pattern

Vacuolar degeneration can be seen admixed with spongiosis (*i.e.*, intercellular edema within the epidermis) in this uncommon cGVHD variant. Dermal eosinophils may also be increased. In a study of 10 patients with eczematoid cGVHD, 4 were found to have eosinophils interspersed within a sparse perivascular lymphocytic infiltrate [57]. Interestingly, all 10 patients clinically progressed to erythroderma, and this variant may be predictive of erythrodermic cGVHD. As discussed in the histopathologic findings of aGVHD, the presence of eosinophils does not exclude a diagnosis of GVHD. Spongiosis may also be present as a minor feature in many cases of aGVHD. As such, the eczematous pattern of cGVHD is not universally agreed upon as a unique variant.

Lupus-like Pattern

Prior reports have described violaceous papules in a malar distribution in patients following bone marrow transplantation [58]. Biopsies of these lichenoid papules revealed necrotic keratinocytes and surrounding lymphocytes in the epidermis and follicular epithelium. Vacuolar change was also identified at the basal layer. These findings were consistent with lichenoid cGVHD. Though a nonspecific finding, follicular plugging, as seen in lupus, could be occasionally identified. There has also been one case report of a patient who clinically and histopathologically resembled hypertrophic lupus [59]. Pseudoepitheliomatous hyperplasia, follicular plugging, thickened basement membrane, and dermal mucin deposition were accompanied by more typical findings of cGVHD, including a paucicellular, lymphocytic, patchy lichenoid infiltrate at the dermal-epidermal junction and along follicular epithelium. None of the patients described subsequently developed other symptoms to support a diagnosis of lupus. However, at least three of the five patients in the original case series described did progress to sclerotic cGVHD [58].

Pityriasis Rosea–like Pattern

In pityriasis rosea–like cGVHD, microscopic features of pityriasis rosea can be seen, including focal spongiosis with overlying mounded parakeratosis [60]. In addition, Civatte bodies and superficial dermal melanophages may be present. Concurrent satellite cell necrosis and an interface dermatitis help to confirm the diagnosis of cGVHD. Clinically, the papules appear along skin tension lines and may occur in an inverse distribution [61].

Comedone-like Pattern

Both sclerotic and lichenoid features can be found in comedone-like cGVHD [62]. Sclerosis can be found expanding and filling nearly the entirety of the epidermis. Comedone-like dilated follicles demonstrate keratotic plugging, hypergranulosis, and hydropic degeneration of the follicular basal layer. Scattered lymphocytes and melanophages may be seen in the superficial dermis.

Follicular Keratosis or Keratosis Pilaris–like Pattern

Follicular keratosis–like cGVHD presents clinically with hyperkeratotic follicular papules or pink cutaneous spicules [61, 62]. Histologically, it is nearly identical to comedone-like cGVHD, but lacks the dilated, comedone-like follicle. It also has both follicular lichenoid and sclerotic features.

cGVHD-associated Angiomatosis

A case series of 11 patients documented the development of cutaneous vascular proliferations exclusively within areas of sclerotic cGVHD, mostly on the lower extremities or trunk, at a median of 44 months after transplantation (Fig. 5.9) [63]. Six biopsies from four patients were initially diagnosed as traumatized pyogenic granulomas, cavernous hemangioma, angiokeratoma, and lymphangiomas. HHV-8 staining was completed for one patient and was negative. Vascular endothelial cells did not appear atypical in any case. As these vascular proliferations occurred in a background of preexisting sclerotic cGVHD, it was hypothesized that they represented a reactive process.

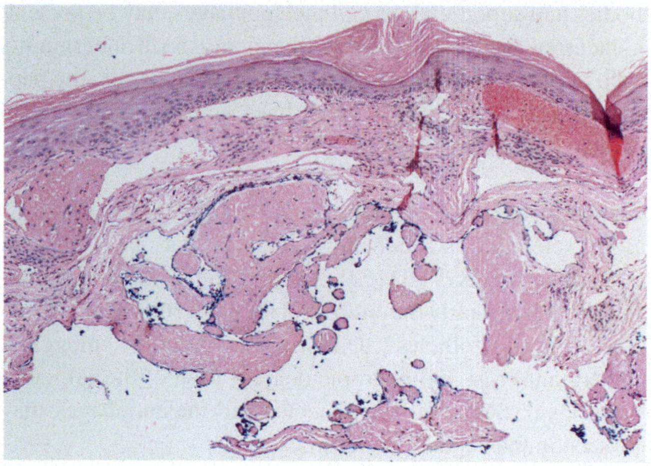

Fig. 5.9 GVHD-associated angiomatosis. The specimen exhibits a benign vascular proliferation with luminal thrombosis arising in a background of sclerodermoid GVHD (H&E, 100× magnification)

Differential Diagnosis of cGVHD

As discussed, the histopathology of early lichenoid cGVHD can resemble aGVHD. The differential diagnosis is mainly that of lichen planus, but unlike lichen planus, the lymphocytic infiltrate at the dermal-epidermal junction is typically less robust and may reveal scattered eosinophils. In addition, the presence of satellite cell necrosis may be a helpful marker of GVHD, especially when features seen in the pattern variants of cGVHD discussed above are seen. Unfortunately, sclerotic cGVHD can be nearly indistinguishable from morphea or scleroderma. As there is no pathognomonic histologic finding in GVHD, clinical correlation is extremely important. A negative biopsy cannot exclude the diagnosis of GVHD. A pathologist can help guide clinical decision making by utilizing the four-tier grading system: no evidence of GVHD, possible GVHD, consistent with or highly suggestive of GVHD, or GVHD without equivocation. Given the significant morbidity and mortality that can be associated with untreated GVHD, high clinical suspicion should result in consideration of empiric treatment, continued investigation, and close clinical monitoring.

References

1. Shulman HM, Kleiner D, Lee SJ, Morton T, Pavletic SZ, Farmer E, et al. Histopathologic diagnosis of chronic graft-versus-host disease: National Institutes of Health Consensus Development Project on Criteria for Clinical Trials in Chronic Graft-versus-Host Disease: II. Pathology Working Group Report. Biol Blood Marrow Transplant. 2006;12:31–47.
2. Bridge AT, Nelson RP, Schwartz JE, Mirowski GW, Billings SD. Histological evaluation of acute mucocutaneous graft-versus-host disease in nonmyeloablative hematologic stem cell transplants with

an observation predicting an increased risk of progression to chronic graft-versus-host disease. Am J Dermatopathol. 2007;29:1–6.
3. Hillen U, Häusermann P, Massi D, Janin A, Wolff D, Lawitschka A, et al. Consensus on performing skin biopsies, laboratory workup, evaluation of tissue samples and reporting of the results in patients with suspected cutaneous graft-versus-host disease. J Eur Acad Dermatol Venereol. 2015;29:948–54.
4. Zhou Y, Barnett MJ, Rivers JK. Clinical significance of skin biopsies in the diagnosis and management of graft-vs-host disease in early postallogeneic bone marrow transplantation. Arch Dermatol. 2000;136:717–21.
5. Ziemer M, Haeusermann P, Janin A, Massi D, Ziepert M, Wolff D, et al. Histopathological diagnosis of graft-versus-host disease of the skin – an interobserver comparison. J Eur Acad Dermatol Venereol. 2014;28:915–24.
6. Firoz BF, Lee SJ, Nghiem P, Qureshi AA. Role of skin biopsy to confirm suspected acute graft-vs-host disease: results of decision analysis. Arch Dermatol. 2006;142:175–82.
7. Horn TD, Haskell J. The lymphocytic infiltrate in acute cutaneous allogeneic graft-versus-host reactions lacks evidence for phenotypic restriction in donor-derived cells. J Cutan Pathol. 1998;25:210–4.
8. Kuykendall TD, Smoller BR. Lack of specificity in skin biopsy specimens to assess for acute graft-versus-host disease in initial 3 weeks after bone-marrow transplantation. J Am Acad Dermatol. 2003;49:1081–5.
9. Ackerman AB, Penneys NS, Clark WH. Erythema multiforme exudativum: distinctive pathological process. Br J Dermatol. 1971;84:554–66.
10. Alsaad KO, Ghazarian D. My approach to superficial inflammatory dermatoses. J Clin Pathol. 2005;58:1233–41.
11. Lerner KG, Kao GF, Storb R, Buckner CD, Clift RA, Thomas ED. Histopathology of graft-vs.-host reaction (GvHR) in human recipients of marrow from HL-A-matched sibling donors. Transplant Proc. 1974;6:367–71.
12. Dickinson AM, Sviland L, Dunn J, Carey P, Proctor SJ. Demonstration of direct involvement of cytokines in graft-versus-host reactions using an in vitro human skin explant model. Bone Marrow Transplant. 1991;7:209–16.
13. Dreno B, Milpied N, Harousseau JL, Stalder JF, Bureau B, Milpied B, Barriere H. Cutaneous immunological studies in diagnosis of acute graft-versus-host disease. Br J Dermatol. 1986;114:7–15.
14. Canninga-van Dijk MR, Sanders CJ, Verdonck LF, Fijnheer R, van den Tweel JG. Differential diagnosis of skin lesions after allogeneic haematopoietic stem cell transplantation. Histopathology. 2003;42:313–30.
15. Ruffin N, Ahmed SS, Osorio LM, Wang XN, Jackson GH, Collin MP, et al. The involvement of epithelial Fas in a human model of graft versus host disease. Transplantation. 2011;91:946–51.
16. Langley RG, Walsh N, Nevill T, Thomas L, Rowden G. Apoptosis is the mode of keratinocyte death in cutaneous graft-versus-host disease. J Am Acad Dermatol. 1996;35:187–90.
17. Goiriz R, Peñas P, Pérez-Gala S, Delgado-Jiménez Y, Aragüés M, García-Diez A, et al. Stage IV cutaneous acute graft-versus-host disease. Clinical and histological study of 15 cases. J Eur Acad Dermatol Venereol. 2009;23:1398–404.
18. Sviland L, Pearson AD, Eastham EJ, Hamilton PJ, Proctor SJ, Malcolm AJ. Histological features of skin and rectal biopsy specimens after autologous and allogeneic bone marrow transplantation. J Clin Pathol. 1988;41:148–54.
19. Sale GE, Lerner KG, Barker EA, Shulman HM, Thomas ED. The skin biopsy in the diagnosis of acute graft-versus-host disease in man. Am J Pathol. 1977;89:621–36.
20. Dumler JS, Beschorner WE, Farmer ER, Di Gennaro KA, Saral R, Santos GW. Endothelial-cell injury in cutaneous acute graft-versus-host disease. Am J Pathol. 1989;135:1097–103.
21. Tsoi MS, Storb R, Jones E, Weiden PL, Shulman H, Witherspoon R, et al. Deposition of IgM and complement at the dermoepidermal junction in acute and chronic cutaneous graft-vs-host disease in man. J Immunol. 1978;120:1485–92.
22. McCalmont TH. TEC. J Cutan Pathol. 2013;40:785–787.
23. Goddard DS, Horn BN, McCalmont TH, Cordoro KM. Clinical update on graft-versus-host disease in children. Semin Cutan Med Surg. 2010;29:92–105.
24. Weaver J, Bergfeld WF. Quantitative analysis of eosinophils in acute graft-versus-host disease compared with drug hypersensitivity reactions. Am J Dermatopathol. 2010;32:31–4.
25. Spitzer TR. Engraftment syndrome following hematopoietic stem cell transplantation. Bone Marrow Transplant. 2001;27:893–8.
26. Parker TL, Cooper DL, Seropian SE, Bolognia JL. Toxic erythema of chemotherapy following i.v. BU plus fludarabine for allogeneic PBSC transplant. Bone Marrow Transplant. 2012;48:646–50.
27. LeBoit PE. Interface dermatitis. How specific are its histopathologic features? Arch Dermatol. 1993;129:1324–8.
28. Dilday BR, Smoller BR. Intraepidermal bile pigment in skin biopsy specimens for graft-versus-host disease versus erythema multiforme. Mod Pathol. 1998;11:1005–9.
29. Wang ECE, Lee JSS, Tan AWH, Tang MBY. Fas-ligand staining in non-drug- and drug-induced maculopapular rashes. J Cutan Pathol. 2011;38:196–201.
30. Roux J, Battistella M, Fornecker L, Legoff J, Deau B, Houhou N, et al. Human Herpesvirus-6 cytopathic inclusions: an exceptional and recognizable finding on skin biopsy during HHV6 reactivation after autologous stem-cell transplantation. Am J Dermatopathol. 2012;34:e73–6.
31. Choi YL, Kim JA, Jang KT, Kim DS, Kim WS, Lee JH, et al. Characteristics of cutaneous cytomegalovirus infection in non-acquired immune deficiency syndrome, immunocompromised patients. Br J Dermatol. 2006;155:977–82.
32. Clark WH, Reed RJ, Mihm MC. Lupus erythematosus. Histopathology of cutaneous lesions. Hum Pathol. 1973;4:157–63.
33. Crowson AN, Magro CM. The role of microvascular injury in the pathogenesis of cutaneous lesions of dermatomyositis. Hum Pathol. 1996;27:15–9.
34. Longley J, Demar L, Feinstein RP, Miller RL, Silvers DN. Clinical and histologic features of pityriasis lichenoides et varioliformis acuta in children. Arch Dermatol. 1987;123:1335–9.
35. Brüggen MC, Klein I, Greinix H, Bauer W, Kuzmina Z, Rabitsch W, et al. Diverse T-cell responses characterize the different manifestations of cutaneous graft-versus-host disease. Blood. 2014;123:290–9.
36. Paczesny S, Braun TM, Levine JE, Hogan J, Crawford J, Coffing B, et al. Elafin is a biomarker of graft-versus-host disease of the skin. Sci Transl Med. 2010;2:13ra2.
37. Brüggen MC, Petzelbauer P, Greinix H, Contassot E, Jankovic D, French L, et al. Epidermal elafin expression is an indicator of poor prognosis in cutaneous graft-versus-host disease. J Invest Dermatol. 2015;135:999–1006.
38. Levine JE, Logan BR, Wu J, Alousi AM, Bolaños-Meade J, Ferrara JL, et al. Acute graft-versus-host disease biomarkers measured during therapy can predict treatment outcomes: a Blood and Marrow Transplant Clinical Trials Network study. Blood. 2012;119:3854–60.
39. Goldberg JD, Linker A, Kuk D, Ratan R, Jurcic J, Barker JN, et al. T cell-depleted stem cell transplantation for adults with high-risk acute lymphoblastic leukemia: long-term survival for patients in first complete remission with a decreased risk of graft-versus-host disease. Biol Blood Marrow Transplant. 2013;19:208–13.
40. Fischer A, Jakubowski AA, Lacouture ME, Hollmann TJ, Drucker AM, Maloy M, et al. Histopathologic features of cutaneous acute graft-versus-host disease in T-cell-depleted peripheral blood stem cell transplant recipients. Am J Dermatopathol. 2015;37:523–9.

41. Wagner JE, Ishida-Yamamoto A, McGrath JA, Hordinsky M, Keene DR, Woodley DT, et al. Bone marrow transplantation for recessive dystrophic epidermolysis bullosa. N Engl J Med. 2010;363:629–39.
42. Tolar J, Wagner JE. Allogeneic blood and bone marrow cells for the treatment of severe epidermolysis bullosa: repair of the extracellular matrix. Lancet. 2013;382:1214–23.
43. Linhares YPL, Pavletic S, Gale RP, Chronic GVHD. Where are we? Where do we want to be? Will immunomodulatory drugs help? Bone Marrow Transplant. 2013;48:203–9.
44. Hymes SR, Alousi AM, Cowen EW. Graft-versus-host disease. J Am Acad Dermatol. 2012;66:515.e1–18.
45. Aractingi S, Chosidow O. Cutaneous graft-versus-host disease. Arch Dermatol. 1998;134:602–12.
46. Shulman HM, Sale GE, Lerner KG, Barker EA, Weiden PL, Sullivan K, et al. Chronic cutaneous graft-versus-host disease in man. Am J Pathol. 1978;91:545–70.
47. Inamoto Y, Storer BE, Petersdorf EW, Nelson JL, Lee SJ, Carpenter PA, et al. Incidence, risk factors, and outcomes of sclerosis in patients with chronic graft-versus-host disease. Blood. 2013;121:5098–103.
48. Uhm J, Hamad N, Shin EM, Michelis FV, Shanavas M, Gupta V, et al. Incidence, risk factors, and long-term outcomes of sclerotic graft-versus-host disease after allogeneic hematopoietic cell transplantation. Biol Blood Marrow Transplant. 2014;20:1751–7.
49. Peñas PF, Jones-Caballero M, Aragüés M, Fernández-Herrera J, Fraga J, García-Díez A. Sclerodermatous graft-vs-host disease: clinical and pathological study of 17 patients. Arch Dermatol. 2002;138:924–34.
50. Chosidow O, Bagot M, Vernant JP, Roujeau JC, Cordonnier C, Kuentz M, et al. Sclerodermatous chronic graft-versus-host disease. Analysis of seven cases. J Am Acad Dermatol. 1992;26:49–55.
51. Shulman HM, Sullivan KM, Weiden PL, McDonald GB, Striker GE, Sale GE, et al. Chronic graft-versus-host syndrome in man. A long-term clinicopathologic study of 20 Seattle patients. Am J Med. 1980;69:204–17.
52. Schaffer JV, McNiff JM, Seropian S, Cooper DL, Bolognia JL. Lichen sclerosus and eosinophilic fasciitis as manifestations of chronic graft-versus-host disease: expanding the sclerodermoid spectrum. J Am Acad Dermatol. 2005;53:591–601.
53. Janin A, Socie G, Devergie A, Aractingi S, Esperou H, Vérola O, Gluckman E. Fasciitis in chronic graft-versus-host disease. A clinicopathologic study of 14 cases. Ann Intern Med. 1994;120:993–8.
54. Jang S, Kim IS, Youn SW. Chronic graft-versus-host disease mimicking psoriasis in a patient with hemophagocytic lymphohistiocytosis. Ann Dermatol. 2016;28:90–3.
55. Matsushita T, Hasegawa M, Shirasaki F, Fujimoto M, Yamazaki H, Sato S, Takehara KA. A case of acute cutaneous graft-versus-host disease mimicking psoriasis vulgaris. Dermatology. 2008;216:64–7.
56. Taguchi S, Kawachi Y, Fujisawa Y, Nakamura Y, Furuta J, Otsuka F. Psoriasiform eruption associated with graft-versus-host disease. Cutis. 2013;92:151–3.
57. Creamer D, Martyn-Simmons CL, Osborne G, Kenyon M, Salisbury JR, Devereux S, et al. Eczematoid graft-vs-host disease: a novel form of chronic cutaneous graft-vs-host disease and its response to psoralen UV-A therapy. Arch Dermatol. 2007;143:1157–62.
58. Goiriz R, Peñas PF, Delgado-Jiménez Y, Fernández-Herrera J, Aragüés-Montañés M, Fraga J, García-Díez A. Cutaneous lichenoid graft-versus-host disease mimicking lupus erythematosus. Lupus. 2008;17:591–5.
59. SW H, Myskowski PL, Papadopoulos EB, Busam KJ. Chronic cutaneous graft-versus-host disease simulating hypertrophic lupus erythematosus–a case report of a new morphologic variant of graft-versus-host disease. Am J Dermatopathol. 2012;34:e81–3.
60. Spelman LJ, Robertson IM, Strutton GM, Weedon D. Pityriasis rosea-like eruption after bone marrow transplantation. J Am Acad Dermatol. 1994;31:348–51.
61. Cornejo CM, Kim EJ, Rosenbach M, Micheletti RG. Atypical manifestations of graft-versus-host disease. J Am Acad Dermatol. 2015;72:690–5.
62. Llamas-Velasco M, Solano-López Morel GE, Gruber-Wackernagel A, Concha-Garzón MJ, Requena L, Cerroni L. Comedonal graft-vs-host disease: a distinct clinical expression of a lichenoid follicular GVHD. J Cutan Pathol. 2014;41:853–8.
63. Kaffenberger BH, Zuo RC, Gru A, Plotner AN, Sweeney SA, Devine SM, et al. Graft-versus-host disease-associated angiomatosis: a clinicopathologically distinct entity. J Am Acad Dermatol. 2014;71:745–53.

Grading and Treatment of Acute Graft-Versus-Host Disease

6

Anar Mikailov, Molly Plovanich, and Arturo P. Saavedra

Acute graft-versus-host disease (aGVHD) remains a major complication and is the leading cause of nonrelapse mortality after allogeneic hematopoietic stem cell transplantation (HSCT). The most commonly involved organ is the skin, providing an opportunity for clinicians to recognize and intervene in this potentially fatal process. Appropriate grading of severity is critical to determine treatment. Therapy for advanced aGVHD is challenging. This chapter reviews the evidence for commonly studied and novel approaches that hold promise.

Diagnosis and Grading of aGVHD

Physiology Overview

aGVHD is an immunologic process that is the most common undesirable effect encountered after HSCT [1]. Immune competent donor T-cells are the primary mediators that initiate an inflammatory cascade after recognizing host tissue protein as foreign antigens [1, 2]. This response is a double-edged sword. Fundamentally, it is appropriate for a functioning immune repertoire (that from the donor) to seek and destroy host antigens not previously encountered by the donor, although this leads to the unwanted phenomenon of GVHD. On the other hand, the same immunologic process also attacks remaining malignant cells; a desirable phenomenon termed graft-versus-leukemia/malignancy (GVL) [1, 2]. Human leukocyte antigens (HLA) are the most important proteins that determine donor T-cell acceptance or rejection of the host, and in effect, HLA disparity between donor and host is the most important independent factor that predicts acute and chronic GVHD. Skin is the most commonly affected organ in GVHD, and it is incumbent on dermatologists to play a critical role in diagnosis and management [3, 4]. In the past 30 years, the development of improved HLA-matching techniques, along with introduction of selective immunosuppressive therapies, has attenuated the unwanted GVHD phenomenon and, as a result, has increased the popularity of HSCT.

A. Mikailov (✉) • M. Plovanich
Department of Dermatology, Brigham and Women's Hospital and Harvard Medical School,
75 Francis Street, Boston, MA 02115, USA
e-mail: amikailov@partners.org; mplovanich@partners.org

A.P. Saavedra
Department of Dermatology, Massachusetts General Hospital and Harvard Medical School, 55 Fruit Street, Boston, MA 02114, USA
e-mail: asoavedra@partners.org

Diagnosis

aGVHD was originally distinguished from chronic GVHD by classic signs and symptoms that presented within 100 days of HSCT, although recent guidelines from the National Institutes of Health deemphasize time-based criteria and instead place much more importance on clinical findings [3, 5–8].

Classic aGVHD manifests within the first 3 or 4 months after HSCT and includes a combination of the following symptoms: erythematous maculopapular eruption, gastrointestinal disease (e.g. diarrhea), and cholestatic liver disease (i.e. elevated conjugated bilirubin and alkaline phosphatase) [7, 8]. The temporal onset of aGVHD is heavily influenced by factors that alter the immunologic interplay between the donor and host, including the conditioning regimen before transplantation, the degree of HLA compatibility, immunosuppression, and immunomodulation with interventions such as donor lymphocyte infusions [9]. As a result, the onset of aGVHD can be delayed or accelerated and does not always occur within the first 100 days after HSCT [6]. With an understanding of this complexity, the current aGVHD subtypes include: classic, persistent, recurrent, and late-onset (Table 6.1) [6]. Additionally, overlap GVHD is a newly observed subtype defined by features of aGVHD in a patient previously diagnosed with chronic GVHD [3, 6]. It is worthwhile to note that both late-onset and overlap aGVHD are more frequently observed after reduced-intensity conditioning [6].

J.A. Cotliar (ed.), *Atlas of Graft-versus-Host Disease*, DOI 10.1007/978-3-319-46952-2_6

In aGVHD, skin is the most commonly affected organ, followed by the gastrointestinal tract and lastly the liver [10]. Early harbingers of cutaneous disease include pruritus and erythema of the ears, face, palms, and soles [8, 9]. Often, subsequent cutaneous finings include folliculocentric blanching macular erythema, which ultimately progresses to a diffuse and symmetric morbilliform eruption (Fig. 6.1). Skin tenderness is not uncommon and often an ominous sign of severe cutaneous disease. In severe cutaneous aGVHD, the eruption progresses to erythroderma followed by bullae formation with epidermal detachment, mimicking toxic epidermal necrolysis (TEN) (Fig. 6.2). In addition to the skin, the mucous membranes, particularly the conjunctivae and oral mucosa, can become markedly inflamed (Fig. 6.3). It should be noted that, in contrast to the protean presentations of cutaneous chronic GVHD (see Chap. 10), cutaneous aGVHD invariably presents as aforementioned.

Table 6.1 Subtypes of acute GVHD: classic, persistent, recurrent, and late-onset

Category	Symptoms after DLI or HSCT	Acute features	Chronic features
Classic acute	< 100 days	Yes	No
Persistent, recurrent and late-onset	> 100 days	Yes	No
Overlap	> 100 days	Yes	Yes

Note: certain individuals demonstrate "overlap" GVHD, which is defined by features of aGVHD in a patient previously diagnosed with chronic GVHD [3, 6]
DLI donor lymphocyte infusion, *HSCT* hematopoietic stem cell transplant

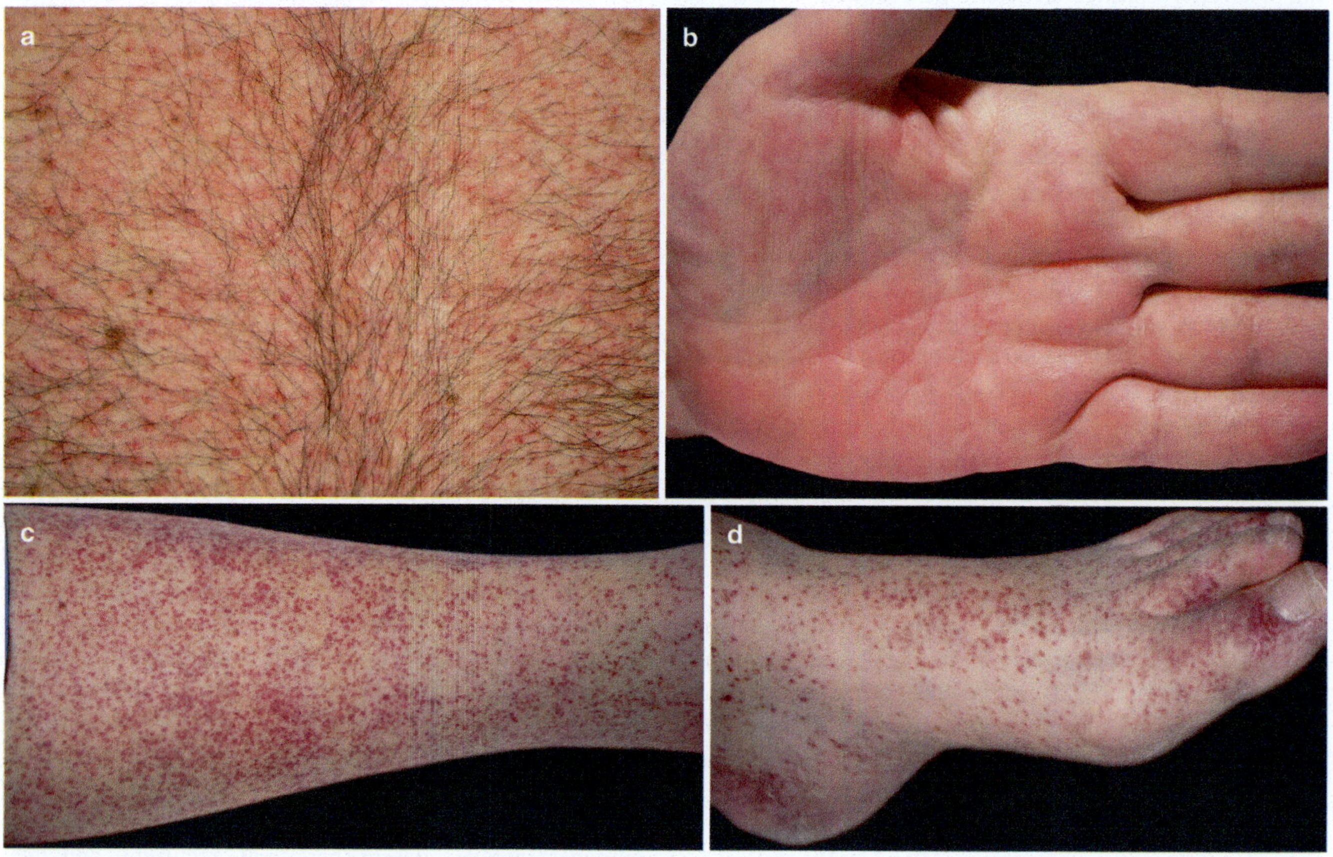

Fig. 6.1 Manifestations of stage II acute cutaneous GVHD. A morbilliform and folliculocentric eruption on the trunk (**a**), palmar involvement (**b**), folliculocentric involvement of the lower leg (**c**) and foot (**d**) (*Courtesy of* Dr. Ryan Trowbridge)

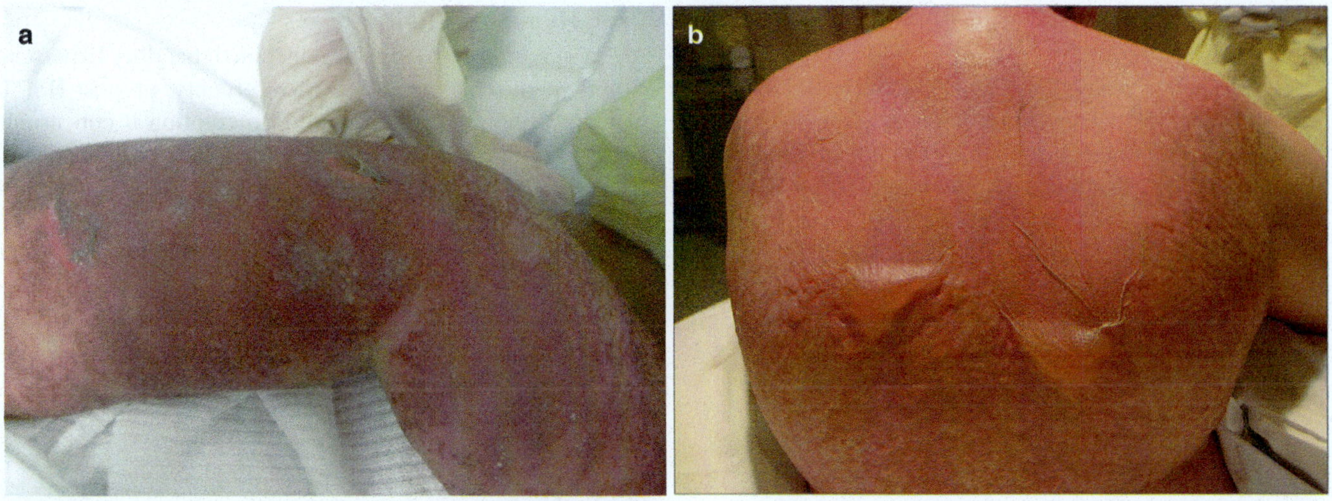

Fig. 6.2 Manifestations of stage IV acute cutaneous GVHD. Large bullae (**a**) and diffuse (**b**) purple-dusky hue, tenderness and sloughing (*Courtesy of* Dr. Jennifer Tan)

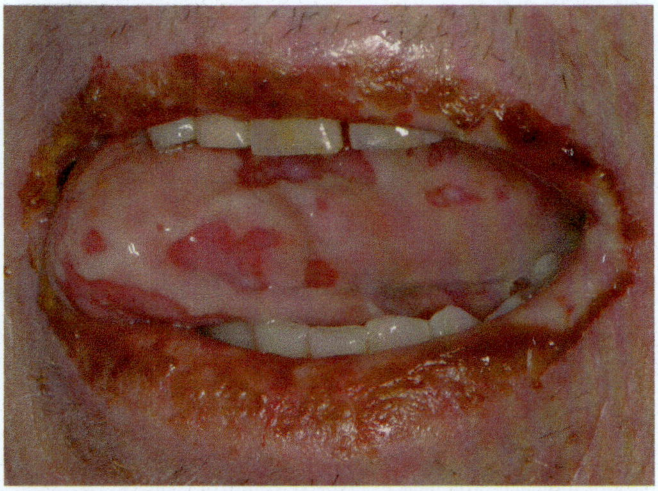

Fig. 6.3 Oral acute GVHD presenting with diffuse ulceration of the ventrolateral tongue, as well as ulceration and crusting of the lips (*Reprinted from* Ion et al. [11]; *with permission*)

Differential Diagnosis

During complete evaluation of aGHVD, the alternative diagnoses to consider include: engraftment syndrome, toxic erythema of chemotherapy, viral exanthem, and drug hypersensitivity, the most common alternative diagnosis (Table 6.2) [8, 9, 12]. A diagnosis of aGVHD is supported by an eruption that involves acral sites and is folliculotropic, with concomitant cholestatic liver damage and gastrointestinal manifestations. However, this triad is not specific to the diagnosis of aGVHD.

Table 6.2 Alternative diagnoses to consider in the evaluation of aGVHD [8, 9]

Diagnosis	Clinical presentation	Onset	Treatment
Drug hypersensitivity (Fig. 6.4)	Morbilliform, lack of peri-follicular accentuation	Anytime	Withdrawal of medication
Viral exanthem	Morbilliform	Anytime	Supportive
Toxic erythema of chemotherapy (Fig. 6.5)	Variable, often acral	2–3 weeks after chemotherapy	Supportive
Engraftment syndrome (Fig. 6.6)	Morbilliform, may begin in acral sites. Concurrent cytokine storm with capillary leak syndrome leading to anasarca and respiratory distress	~14 days after transplantation	Systemic corticosteroids leads to complete resolution

Drug Hypersensitivity

A recent retrospective review concluded that drug hypersensitivity could be excluded with certainty in post-HSCT patients who develop a morbilliform eruption if concurrent hyperbilirubinemia and diarrhea are present [12]. The distribution and onset of the cutaneous eruption in drug hypersensitivity often spares acral sites, particularly the palms and soles, and lacks the folliculocentric erythema of aGVHD eruptions (Fig. 6.4) [12].

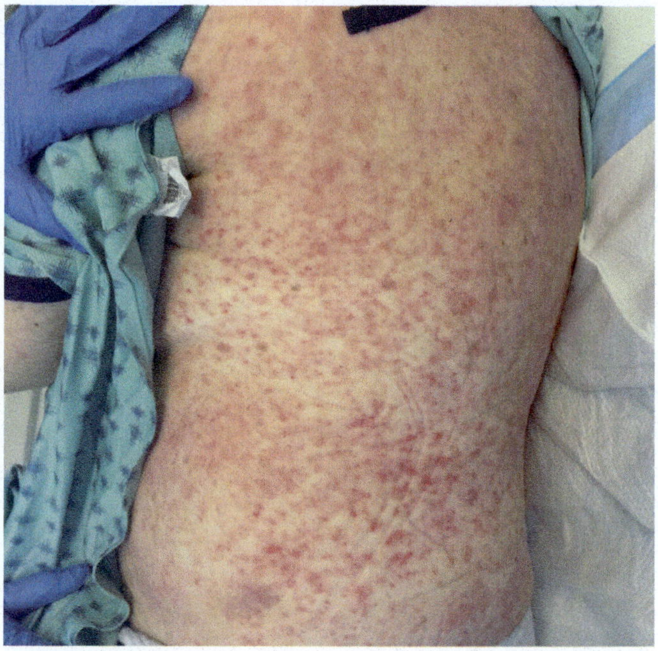

Fig. 6.4 Drug hypersensitivity reaction to vancomycin presenting as a diffuse morbilliform eruption on the trunk early after HSCT. Note the lack of follicular prominence, a typical feature of acute GVHD

Toxic Erythema of Chemotherapy

This diagnosis is suggested by blanching erythema that is painful and limited to palms and soles (most common) or flexural sites (Fig. 6.5). The pathophysiology is hypothesized to be a result of toxic metabolite accumulation in eccrine-rich sites [13].

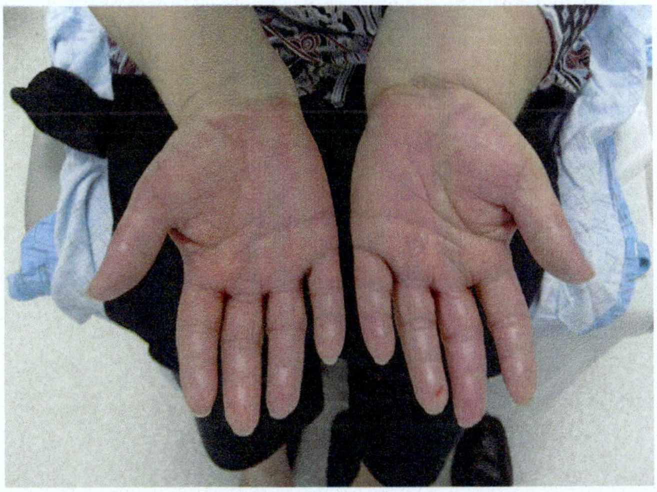

Fig. 6.5 Toxic erythema of chemotherapy due to cytarabine presenting as confluent erythema and edema of the palms

Engraftment Syndrome

Engraftment syndrome (ES) may be favored in patients who received an autologous transplant and develop symptoms reminiscent of capillary leak syndrome with cytokine storm [14, 15]. ES has also been described in allogeneic HSCT [16]. Clinical findings include non-infectious fever (persistently negative culture data and no response to empiric antibiotics), hypoxemia, diarrhea, weight gain, anasarca, and a morbilliform cutaneous eruption (Fig. 6.6). Timing of onset is, by definition, in the peri-engrafment period. ES is remarkably responsive to systemic corticosteroids, and in a recent retrospective review, 41 of 42 patients with ES showed rapid symptoms resolution leading to hospital discharge in a median of 10 days [15]. The same review found excellent correlation between markedly elevated C-reactive protein (CRP) and ES diagnosis (Table 6.2) [15].

Many studies have investigated the utility of a diagnostic skin biopsy for aGVHD. The histological findings are often non-specific and do not reliably improve diagnostic distinction between aGVHD and drug hypersensitivity, particularly in early GVHD [17–19]. The results of a decision analysis showed that a skin biopsy should be performed only in cases in which the pretest probability for aGVHD is exceptionally low [20, 21].

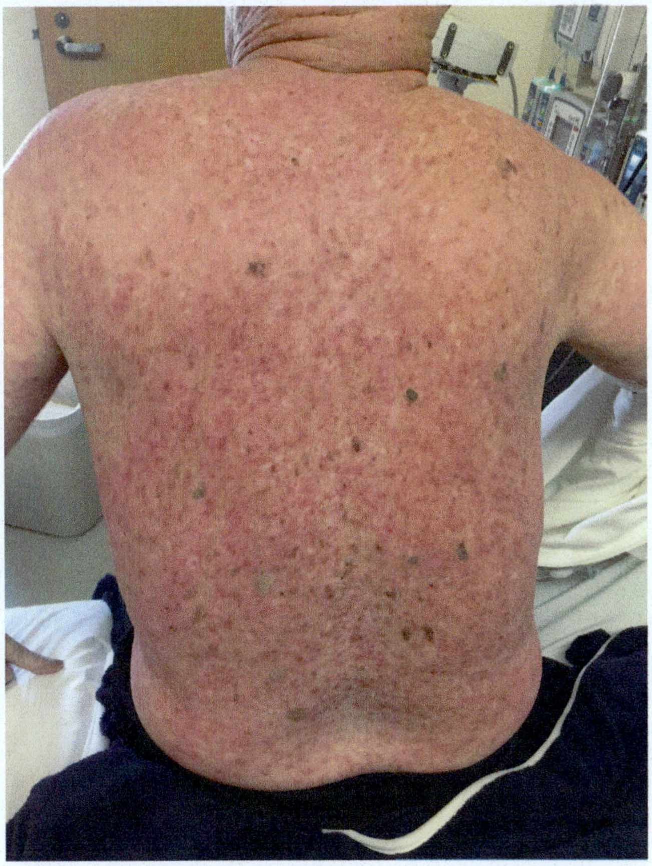

Fig. 6.6 Engraftment syndrome. Diffuse morbilliform eruption mimicking acute GVHD early after allogeneic HSCT

Grading and Prognostication

The most commonly utilized aGVHD grading system is the modified Seattle Glucksberg system (Tables 6.3 and 6.4), which is an evolution from the original 1974 Glucksberg study [5, 7]. The key variables that determine staging of aGVHD include: amount of body surface area of skin involvement, extent of elevation in serum bilirubin for hepatic involvement, and stool output volume for gastrointestinal involvement (Table 6.3). The integration of stages determines the grade, which is closely correlated with mortality (Table 6.4) [22].

A recently developed and validated Ann Arbor aGHVD severity score utilizes biomarkers alone and showed excellent concordance with response to therapy at 28 days as well as non-relapse mortality at 6 months [23]. The three biomarker (TNFR1, ST2, and REG3a) plasma concentrations are combined to create a single score (Table 6.5), which subsequently stratifies the patient as Ann Arbor score 1 (likelihood of complete or partial response to treatment, 81 % at day 28) to score 3 (likelihood of complete or partial response to treatment, 46 % at day 28) [23].

Interestingly, the Ann Arbor severity score more accurately predicted non-relapse mortality when compared with the Seattle Glucksberg grading system [23]. Although the Ann Arbor score is not a practical tool at the bedside, it will be essential for patient stratification and surrogate endpoint outcome analysis in future interventional studies.

Table 6.3 Modified Glucksberg criteria stages of aGVHD and transplant-related mortality [7, 8, 22]

Stage	Skin (% BSA)	Liver (bilirubin)	Gastrointestinal	Non-relapse mortality at 100 days [21]
1	Maculopapular rash < 25 %	2.0–2.9 mg/dL	Diarrhea 0.5–1 L/day or nausea/emesis with positive gut biopsy	27 %
2	Maculopapular rash 25–50 %	3.0–5.9 mg/dL	Diarrhea 1–1.5 L/day	43 %
3	Maculopapular rash >50 %	6.0–14.9 mg/dL	Diarrhea > 1.5 L/day	68 %
4	Generalized erythema (i.e. erythroderma) with desquamation or bullae	>14.9 mg/dL	Severe abdominal pain with or without ileus	92 %

BSA body surface area

Table 6.4 Glucksberg grading of aGVHD [7]

Grade	Skin stage	Liver stage	Gastrointestinal stage
I	1–2	0	0
II	3 or	1 or	1
III	0–3 and	2–3 or	2–4
IV	4 or	4 or	0–4 with Grade 4 skin or liver

Table 6.5 Ann Arbor Risk Score for aGVHD based on plasma concentrations of three biomarkers: TNFR1, REG3α, and ST2

Ann Arbor Score	CR/PR at 28 days	Non-relapse mortality at 12 months, % (95 % CI)
1	81 %	8 % (3–16)
2	68 %	27 % (20–24)
3	46 %	46 % (33–58)

The difference in CR/PR as well as the non-relapse mortality between each Ann Arbor score is statistically significant [23]
Algorithm: $Log[-log(1\text{-}p)] = -9.169 + 0.598(log2TNFR1) - 0.028(log2REG3\alpha) + 0.189(log2ST2)$
CI confidence interval, *CR* complete remission, *PR* partial remission

Treatment of aGVHD

The incidence of aGVHD after allogeneic HSCT is between 10 and 80 %, and ongoing research in HLA matching, conditioning and prophylactic regimens holds promise to decrease that rate [4, 8, 9, 24]. In newly diagnosed aGVHD, early recognition, intervention, and close monitoring are the cornerstones of effective management. The most recent 2012 guidelines from Haemato-oncology Task Force of the British Committee for Standards in Haematology (BCSH) and the British Society for Blood and Marrow Transplantation (BSBMT) and the American Society of Blood and Marrow Transplantation (ASBMT) emphasize that therapeutic choice should be in accordance with proper staging and grading, in conjunction with the rate of disease progression [8, 24]. Treatment strategies discussed here are primarily based on cutaneous aGVHD staging, although it is imperative to utilize the grade of aGVHD as defined earlier.

Brief Note on the Prevention of aGVHD

A noteworthy area of research revolves around the use of mammalian target of rapamycin (mTOR) inhibitors instead of calcineurin inhibitors after allogeneic HSCT for GVHD prophylaxis. In 2002, Hoffmann et al. [25] showed that transfer of donor CD4+ CD25+ regulatory T Cells (Tregs) after allogeneic HSCT can prevent severe aGVHD while maintaining graft-versus-leukemia effect in mice. More recent work by Satake et al. [26] showed (in mice) that the mTOR inhibitor sirolimus in combination with low dose IL-2 showed Treg expansion and decreased risk of aGVHD. Peccatori et al. [27] showed that use of sirolimus prophylaxis led to a much lower than expected incidence of GVHD in patients receiving high GVHD risk transplants (peripheral blood stem cell grafts from partially HLA-matched family donors). Prophylactic use of mTOR inhibitors in combination of Tregs modulation is a very active area of research with multiple ongoing trials (NCT02528877, NCT01795573, NCT02118311, NCT00105001, NCT01251575, NCT01903473, NCT00406393, NCT00993343, NCT00602693).

Treatment of Grade I aGVHD

General consensus guidelines from the BCSH, BSBMT, and ASBMT recommend management of grade I aGVHD (<50 % body surface area involvement) with topical therapies in addition to optimization of prophylactic immunosuppression [8, 9, 28]. The most common approach to grade I aGVHD includes topical corticosteroids and/or topical calcineurin inhibitors (CNIs). However, for cases in which 25–50 % of body surface area is involved, progression must be monitored closely and early initiation of first-line systemic therapy should be considered. Additionally, patients who have a clinical grade of I, although an Ann Arbor risk score of 3, are at a significantly increased risk for aGVHD to involve more organs and should be considered for systemic therapy [22]. It is foreseeable that the Ann Arbor score will play a larger role in early grade aGVHD management, particularly for cases with clinical and biomarker discordance.

High-potency topical corticosteroids (class 1 or 2), the cornerstone for therapy on the extremities and trunk, can be considered for short periods of time on the face, major body folds, and genital region with close monitoring. Topical CNIs, such as tacrolimus or pimecrolimus, provide benefits equivalent to class 4 or class 5 topical corticosteroids and they should be employed in tandem, especially to the face and genital region (Table 6.6) [29].

In addition to topical corticosteroids and CNIs, clinicians should stress skin hygiene and sun-safe practices. Excellent skin hygiene (i.e. use of emollients at least once per day) will optimize skin barrier function and minimize transepidermal water loss; recommendations include: minimize the duration of showers, minimize the use of soaps or other skin cleansers, favor skin care products that are unscented, and use thick emollients immediately after showers plus at least one other time per day. Regular use of sun protection factor creams and appropriate clothing, in addition to avoidance of high-intensity sun exposure will minimize the potential for additional keratinocyte damage.

If aGVHD involves the liver or gastrointestinal system, regardless of cutaneous involvement, or if cutaneous involvement is more than 50 % body surface area (BSA), management should be more aggressive with systemic therapies, as discussed in the next section.

Table 6.6 Therapeutic options in aGVHD and key studies or reviews

Therapeutic options	Key studies, reviews, and notable results
aGVHD grade I	
Daily preventative skin care (frequent emollient use, minimize ultraviolet exposure)	[4, 46, 47]
Topical corticosteroids (Class 1 or 2 to the trunk and extremities, less potent to the face/folds/genitalia)	[4, 8, 9, 46]
Topical calcineurin inhibitors (tacrolimus, pimecrolimus)	[4, 8, 9]
aGVHD grade II or greater	
Systemic corticosteroids	ORR 41–44 % [46, 48, 49]; 5 year survival 51 % vs 32 % steroid responders to non-responder [48]; Dose of 2 mg/kg equivalent to 10 mg/kg (prednisolone equivalent) [30]; Dose of 1 mg/kg equivalent to 2 mg/kg (prednisolone equivalent) [50]
Extracorporeal photopheresis (ECP)	CR 52–82 % in steroid-refractory aGVHD [33, 36]; ORR 75–86 % in steroid-refractory cutaneous aGVHD [34, 35]
Sirolimus	ORR 57–76 % in steroid-refractory aGVHD [51, 52]; CR 50–72 % in steroid-refractory aGVHD [53, 54]
Anti-thymocyte globulin (ATG)	ORR 54 % at 28 days with equine-ATG in steroid-refractory aGVHD [55]; Two trials showed surprisingly high mortality (90–95 %) with equine-ATG in steroid-refractory aGVHD [44, 56], while another trial showed equivalent survival at 2 years between equine-ATG plus prednisone vs. prednisone alone [57]; Low dose rabbit-ATG showed 90 % response for skin and gut aGVHD and an overall 1 year survival of 55 % [45]
Mycophenolate mofetil	ORR 47–65 % in prospective trials of steroid-refractory aGVHD [58, 59]; ORR 60 % in a retrospective study of steroid-refractory aGVHD [60]; CR 26–60 % CR in steroid-refractory aGVHD [61, 62]; MMF plus methylprednisolone as initial aGVHD therapy was not superior to methylprednisolone plus placebo [63]
Methotrexate	ORR 58–95 % in steroid-refractory aGVHD using 5 or 10 mg/m^2 IV every 3–10 days [64–66]; ORR 70 % in a pediatrics trial of steroid-dependent or steroid-refractory aGVHD [67]; CR 42 % in steroid-refractory aGVHD using weekly 5 mg/m^2 infusion [64]
TNFαi	Etanercept: CR 26–79 % in combination with methylprednisolone as initial aGVHD therapy [62, 77] Infliximab plus methylprednisolone was not superior to methylprednisolone alone in a phase III prospective trial [68]
Alemtuzumab	ORR 83–95 % for steroid-refractory aGVHD [69, 70], though only 33 % alive at 2 years [70]; another retrospective study showed ORR 70 % in steroid-refractory gastrointestinal aGVHD with 50 % survival at 1 year [71]
IL-2 inhibition (Denileukin diftitox, Basiliximab)	Denileukin diftitox: ORR 68–71 % in phase 1 [72] and phase 2 trials [73] of steroid-refractory aGHVD; Basiliximab: ORR 71–87 % in steroid-refractory aGVHD [74–76]
CD26 Antibody	Small study from 1985 showed 50 % (4/8) CR, with all 4 patients alive without GVHD 25 years later [42]. Phase 3 trial is underway [NCT02411084]
Ex vivo expanded, Tregs infusion	Single report of therapeutic adaptive Tregs transfer in patient with grade IV aGVHD showed transient benefit [39]; trials in animal models show promise [38]

ATG antithymocyte globulin, *BSA* body surface area, *CR* complete response, *ECP* extracorporeal photopheresis, *ORR* overall response rate, *PR* partial response, *TNFαi* tumor necrosis factor-α inhibitor

Grade II or Greater aGVHD

For grade II or greater aGVHD consensus recommendations support initiation of systemic corticosteroid therapy in addition to optimization of prophylactic immunosuppression as the first-line standard of care [8, 23]. Initial therapy with a prednisone-equivalent dose of 2.5 mg/kg/day is an accepted strategy and multiple landmark studies are referenced in Table 6.6. Studies evaluating higher doses have not shown an outcome advantage. A recently completed phase III randomized trial of low-dose systemic corticosteroids has not published a final analysis [8, 23, 30]. The largest retrospective review of first-line corticosteroid monotherapy in aGVHD found that about one half of patients have a complete response, which is also in line with the ASBMT consensus statement [23, 31]. In addition to systemic corticosteroids, adjuvant use of topical medications, as described earlier, is symptomatically helpful but does not affect internal organ response. Systemic combination therapies, such as corticosteroids plus a second agent, have not definitively shown superiority over corticosteroid monotherapy for first-line aGVHD treatment, although trials are ongoing [8, 24].

Corticosteroid-Refractory aGVHD

Corticosteroid-refractory aGVHD portends a worse prognosis and in general is more challenging to treat. There is no consensus on specific treatment and direct comparison of therapeutic studies is difficult as outcome criteria and patient inclusion characteristics are highly variable. Nevertheless, a review of recent literature shows some notable approaches.

The primary physiologic target of the second-line agents is T-cell pathway suppression or modulation, and possible options include systemic CNIs, tumor necrosis factor alpha inhibitors (TNFαi), extracorporeal photopheresis (ECP), sirolimus (mTOR inhibitor), interleukin-2 (IL-2) receptor antibodies, alemtuzumab, methotrexate, Treg infusion, and antithymocyte globulin (ATG) [8, 24, 32]. This list is not all-encompassing and additional therapies are continuously evaluated [32]. Three treatment modalities are reviewed below based on remarkable clinical data (ECP) or potential for benefit in the near future (anti-CD26 antibody and rabbit ATG). Additional studies and reviews are referenced in Table 6.6.

Extracorporeal Photopheresis

The process of ECP involves the isolation of a patient's leukocytes, followed by ex-vivo exposure of these cells to UV-A light and 8-methoxypsoralen with transfusion of the altered leukocytes back into the patient [33–36]. This process has no known immunosuppressive effects and instead leads to immune tolerance via an increase in Treg cell counts [34–37].

ECP was originally studied and used in T-cell mediated processes with low Tregs counts such as cutaneous T-cell lymphoma, and for prevention of rejection in solid organ transplantation [33–35, 37]. More recently, ECP has become one of the most promising and commonly studied second-line treatment modalities for corticosteroid-refractory aGVHD [24, 34, 36]. In a 2014 systematic review by Knobler et al. [34], complete or partial responses of cutaneous aGVHD were between 50 % and 100 % (median 75 %). In a 2015 meta-analysis by Zhang et al. [35], which only included prospective studies of corticosteroid-refractory aGVHD, complete or partial responses of cutaneous aGVHD were between 79 % and 93 % (median 86 %). In both the Knobler et al. [34] review and the Zhang et al. [35] meta-analysis, ECP was most successful for cutaneous aGVHD followed by gastrointestinal and then liver aGVHD. Further review of ECP clinical trials shows that early initiation and a more frequent ECP schedule correspond to higher response rates [35]. Perhaps the largest advantage of ECP is the favorable side-effect profile; because ECP is not immunosuppressive, there are no reports of severe World Health Organization grade III–IV side effects [34]. Lastly, newer modified ECP methodologies have the potential for even greater efficacy in high-grade aGVHD [36].

As noted in Table 6.6, ex-vivo expansion of Tregs populations is yet another independent treatment under investigation. Based on the principles of Tregs expansion with ECP, current research is evaluating the potential to directly infuse Tregs cell lines without the need for intermediary steps (e.g. ECP) [38–40].

Anti-CD26 Antibody

CD26 is expressed on a subset of CD4+ memory T helper cell, and this CD4+ $CD26^{high}$ T-cell population has been shown to respond maximally to recall antigens leading to high IL-2 production [41]. Given the implications in autoimmune disease and GVHD, Bacigalupo et al. [42] studied the use of a monoclonal antibody (mAB) blocking CD26 (BT 5/9) for treatment of corticosteroid-refractory grade II or greater aGVHD. The results showed complete remission in 4 of 8 patients with a 25-year follow-up noting 100 % survival in the original 4 patients; all are without GVHD [42, 43]. A phase 3 study is now enrolling patients to study a newer version of the anti-CD26 mAB [NCT02411084].

Rabbit Antithymocyte Globulin

Based on the extensive review by Martin et al. [24], horse-derived antithymocyte globulin (ATG) was the most extensively studied second-line option for corticosteroid-refractory aGVHD. Many trials showed poor response and high rates of infection [24, 44]. Interestingly, using very low-dose rabbit-derived ATG in corticosteroid-refractory aGVHD, Nishimoto et al. [45] reported an excellent response in 11 patients.

Three patients with isolated cutaneous aGVHD (one of each, stage 2–4) had either partial or complete response, including survival of 992 days in the patient with stage 4 cutaneous aGVHD [45]. Future studies are ongoing.

Table 6.6 reviews therapeutic options and key literature.

References

1. Ferrara JL, Deeg HJ. Graft-versus-host disease. N Engl J Med. 1991;324(10):667–74.
2. Ferrara JL, Levine JE, Reddy P, Holler E. Graft-versus-host disease. Lancet. 2009;373(9674):1550–61.
3. Jagasia MH, Greinix HT, Arora M, Williams KM, Wolff D, Cowen EW, et al. National institutes of health consensus development project on criteria for clinical trials in chronic graft-versus-host disease: I. The 2014 diagnosis and staging working group report. Biol Blood Marrow Transplant. 2015;21(3):389–401. e1
4. Hymes SR, Alousi AM, Cowen EW. Graft-versus-host disease: part I. Pathogenesis and clinical manifestations of graft-versus-host disease. J Am Acad Dermatol 2012;66(4):515 e1–515 18; quiz 533–4.
5. Glucksberg H, Storb R, Fefer A, Buckner CD, Neiman PE, Clift RA, et al. Clinical manifestations of graft-versus-host disease in human recipients of marrow from HL-A-matched sibling donors. Transplantation. 1974;18(4):295–304.
6. Filipovich AH, Weisdorf D, Pavletic S, Socie G, Wingard JR, Lee SJ, et al. National institutes of health consensus development project on criteria for clinical trials in chronic graft-versus-host disease: I. Diagnosis and staging working group report. Biol Blood Marrow Transplant. 2005;11(12):945–56.
7. Przepiorka D, Weisdorf D, Martin P, HG K, Beatty P, Hows J, et al. 1994 consensus conference on acute GVHD grading. Bone Marrow Transplant. 1995;15(6):825–8.
8. Dignan FL, Clark A, Amrolia P, Cornish J, Jackson G, Mahendra P, et al. Diagnosis and management of acute graft-versus-host disease. Br J Haematol. 2012;158(1):30–45.
9. SW H, Cotliar J. Acute graft-versus-host disease following hematopoietic stem-cell transplantation. Dermatol Ther. 2011;24(4):411–23.
10. Harris AC, Young R, Devine S, Hogan WJ, Ayuk F, Bunworasate U, et al. International, multicenter standardization of acute graft-versus-host disease clinical data collection: a report from the Mount Sinai acute GVHD international consortium. Biol Blood Marrow Transplant. 2016;22(1):4–10.
11. Ion D, Stevenson K, Woo SB, Ho VT, Soiffer R, Antin JH, et al. Characterization of oral involvement in acute graft-versus-host disease. Biol Blood Marrow Transplant. 2014;20(11):1717–21.
12. Byun HJ, Yang JI, Kim BK, Cho KH. Clinical differentiation of acute cutaneous graft-versus-host disease from drug hypersensitivity reactions. J Am Acad Dermatol. 2011;65(4):726–32.
13. Bolognia JL, Cooper DL, Glusac EJ. Toxic erythema of chemotherapy: a useful clinical term. J Am Acad Dermatol. 2008;59(3):524–9.
14. Maiolino A, Biasoli I, Lima J, Portugal AC, Pulcheri W, Nucci M. Engraftment syndrome following autologous hematopoietic stem cell transplantation: definition of diagnostic criteria. Bone Marrow Transplant. 2003;31(5):393–7.
15. Carreras E, Fernández-Avilés F, Silva L, Guerrero M, Fernández de Larrea C, Martínez C, et al. Engraftment syndrome after auto-SCT: analysis of diagnostic criteria and risk factors in a large series from a single center. Bone Marrow Transplant. 2010;45(9):1417–22.
16. Gorak E, Geller N, Srinivasan R, Espinoza-Delgado I, Donohue T, Barrett AJ, et al. Engraftment syndrome after nonmyeloablative allogeneic hematopoietic stem cell transplantation: incidence and effects on survival. Biol Blood Marrow Transplant. 2005;11: 542–50.
17. Sale GE, Lerner KG, Barker EA, Shulman HM, Thomas ED, et al. The skin biopsy in the diagnosis of acute graft-versus-host disease in man. Am J Pathol. 1977;89(3):621–36.
18. Zhou Y, Barnett MJ, Rivers JK. Clinical significance of skin biopsies in the diagnosis and management of graft-vs-host disease in early postallogeneic bone marrow transplantation. Arch Dermatol. 2000;136(6):717–21.
19. Kuykendall TD, Smoller BR. Lack of specificity in skin biopsy specimens to assess for acute graft-versus-host disease in initial 3 weeks after bone-marrow transplantation. J Am Acad Dermatol. 2003;49(6):1081–5.
20. Firoz BF, Lee SJ, Nghiem P, Qureshi AA. Role of skin biopsy to confirm suspected acute graft-vs-host disease: results of decision analysis. Arch Dermatol. 2006;142(2):175–82.
21. Barksdale SK, Oberlender SA, Barnhill RL. "Rush" skin biopsy specimens in a tertiary medical center: diagnostic yield and clinical utility. J Am Acad Dermatol. 1998;38(4):548–54.
22. Gratwohl A, Hermans J, Apperley J, Arcese W, Bacigalupo A, Bandini G, et al. Acute graft-versus-host disease: grade and outcome in patients with chronic myelogenous leukemia. Working party chronic leukemia of the European group for blood and marrow Transplantation. Blood. 1995;86(2):813–8.
23. Levine JE, Braun TM, Harris AC, Holler E, Taylor A, Miller H, et al. A prognostic score for acute graft-versus-host disease based on biomarkers: a multicentre study. Lancet Haematol. 2015;2(1): e21–9.
24. Martin PJ, Rizzo JD, Wingard JR, Ballen K, Curtin PT, Cutler C, et al. First- and second-line systemic treatment of acute graft-versus-host disease: recommendations of the American Society of Blood and Marrow Transplantation. Biol Blood Marrow Transplant. 2012;18(8):1150–63.
25. Hoffmann P, Ermann J, Edinger M, Fathman CG, Strober S, et al. Donor-type CD4(+)CD25(+) regulatory T cells suppress lethal acute graft-versus-host disease after allogeneic bone marrow transplantation. J Exp Med. 2002;196(3):389–99.
26. Satake A, Schmidt AM, Nomura S, Kambayashi T, et al. Inhibition of calcineurin abrogates while inhibition of mTOR promotes regulatory T cell expansion and graft-versus-host disease protection by IL-2 in allogeneic bone marrow transplantation. PLoS One. 2014;9(3):e92888.
27. Peccatori J, Forcina A, Clerici D, Crocchiolo R, Vago L, Stanghellini MT, et al. Sirolimus-based graft-versus-host disease prophylaxis promotes the in vivo expansion of regulatory T cells and permits peripheral blood stem cell transplantation from haploidentical donors. Leukemia. 2015;29(2):396–405.
28. Penas PF, Fernandez-Herrera J, Garcia-Diez A. Dermatologic treatment of cutaneous graft versus host disease. Am J Clin Dermatol. 2004;5(6):403–16.
29. Frankel HC, Qureshi AA. Comparative effectiveness of topical calcineurin inhibitors in adult patients with atopic dermatitis. Am J Clin Dermatol. 2012;13(2):113–23.
30. Van Lint MT, Uderzo C, Locasciulli A, Majolino I, Scimé R, Locatelli F, et al. Early treatment of acute graft-versus-host disease with high- or low-dose 6-methylprednisolone: a multicenter randomized trial from the Italian group for bone marrow transplantation. Blood. 1998;92(7):2288–93.
31. MacMillan ML, DeFor TE, Weisdorf DJ. The best endpoint for acute GVHD treatment trials. Blood. 2010;115(26):5412–7.
32. Holtan SG, Pasquini M, Weisdorf DJ. Acute graft-versus-host disease: a bench-to-bedside update. Blood. 2014;124(3):363–73.
33. Greinix HT, Volc-Platzer B, Knobler RM. Extracorporeal photochemotherapy in the treatment of severe graft-versus-host disease. Leuk Lymphoma. 2000;36(5–6):425–34.
34. Knobler R, Berlin G, Calzavara-Pinton P, Greinix H, Jaksch P, Laroche L et al. Guidelines on the use of extracorporeal photopheresis. J Eur Acad Dermatol Venereol 2014;28 Suppl 1:1–37.

35. Zhang H, Chen R, Cheng J, Jin N, Chen B. Systematic review and meta-analysis of prospective studies for ECP treatment in patients with steroid-refractory acute GVHD. Patient Prefer Adherence. 2015;9:105–11.
36. Perfetti P, Carlier P, Strada P, Gualandi F, Occhini D, Van Lint MT, et al. Extracorporeal photopheresis for the treatment of steroid refractory acute GVHD. Bone Marrow Transplant. 2008;42(9):609–17.
37. Budde H, Kolb S, Salinas Tejedor L, Wulf G, Reichardt HM, Riggert J, et al. Modified extracorporeal photopheresis with cells from a healthy donor for acute graft-versus-host disease in a mouse model. PLoS One. 2014;9(8):e105896.
38. Taylor PA, Lees CJ, Blazar BR. The infusion of ex vivo activated and expanded CD4(+)CD25(+) immune regulatory cells inhibits graft-versus-host disease lethality. Blood. 2002;99(10):3493–9.
39. Trzonkowski P, Bieniaszewska M, Juścińska J, Dobyszuk A, Krzystyniak A, Marek N, et al. First-in-man clinical results of the treatment of patients with graft versus host disease with human ex vivo expanded CD4+CD25+CD127- T regulatory cells. Clin Immunol. 2009;133(1):22–6.
40. Brunstein CG, Miller JS, Cao Q, McKenna DH, Hippen KL, Curtsinger J, et al. Infusion of ex vivo expanded T regulatory cells in adults transplanted with umbilical cord blood: safety profile and detection kinetics. Blood. 2011;117(3):1061–70.
41. Ohnuma K, Ishii T, Iwata S, Hosono O, Kawasaki H, Uchiyama M, et al. G1/S cell cycle arrest provoked in human T cells by antibody to CD26. Immunology. 2002;107(3):325–33.
42. Bacigalupo A, Corte G, Ramarli D, van Lint MT, Frassoni F, Marmont A. Intravenous monoclonal antibody (BT 5/9) for the treatment of acute graft-versus-host disease. Acta Haematol. 1985;73(3):185–6.
43. Dominietto A. CD26, ANTI-CD26 and GVHD 1. Lecture presented at XII Congresso Nazionale SIES 2012 Simposio GITMO, 2012, Rome.
44. Arai S, Margolis J, Zahurak M, Anders V, Vogelsang GB. Poor outcome in steroid-refractory graft-versus-host disease with antithymocyte globulin treatment. Biol Blood Marrow Transplant. 2002;8(3):155–60.
45. Nishimoto M, Nakamae H, Koh H, Nakamae M, Hirose A, Hayashi Y, et al. Response-guided therapy for steroid-refractory acute GVHD starting with very-low-dose antithymocyte globulin. Exp Hematol. 2015;43(3):177–9.
46. Martin PJ, Schoch G, Fisher L, Byers V, Anasetti C, Appelbaum FR, et al. A retrospective analysis of therapy for acute graft-versus-host disease: initial treatment. Blood. 1990;76(8):1464–72.
47. Kitajima T, Imamura S. Graft-versus-host reaction enhanced by ultraviolet radiation. Arch Dermatol Res. 1993;285(8):499–501.
48. Weisdorf D, Haake R, Blazar B, Miller W, McGlave P, Ramsay N, et al. Treatment of moderate/severe acute graft-versus-host disease after allogeneic bone marrow transplantation: an analysis of clinical risk features and outcome. Blood. 1990;75(4):1024–30.
49. MacMillan ML, Weisdorf DJ, Wagner JE, DeFor TE, Burns LJ, Ramsay NK, et al. Response of 443 patients to steroids as primary therapy for acute graft-versus-host disease: comparison of grading systems. Biol Blood Marrow Transplant. 2002;8(7):387–94.
50. Mielcarek M, Storer BE, Boeckh M, Carpenter PA, McDonald GB, Deeg HJ, et al. Initial therapy of acute graft-versus-host disease with low-dose prednisone does not compromise patient outcomes. Blood. 2009;113(13):2888–94.
51. Benito AI, Storer BE, Boeckh M, Carpenter PA, McDonald GB, Deeg HJ, Nash RA, et al. Sirolimus (rapamycin) for the treatment of steroid-refractory acute graft-versus-host disease. Transplantation. 2001;72(12):1924–9.
52. Hoda D, Pidala J, Salgado-Vila N, Kim J, Perkins J, Bookout R, Field T, et al. Sirolimus for treatment of steroid-refractory acute graft-versus-host disease. Bone Marrow Transplant. 2010;45(8): 1347–51.
53. Pidala J, Kim J, Anasetti C. Sirolimus as primary treatment of acute graft-versus-host disease following allogeneic hematopoietic cell transplantation. Biol Blood Marrow Transplant. 2009;15(7): 881–5.
54. Ghez D, Rubio MT, Maillard N, Suarez F, Chandesris MO, Delarue R, et al. Rapamycin for refractory acute graft-versus-host disease. Transplantation. 2009;88(9):1081–7.
55. MacMillan ML et al. Early antithymocyte globulin therapy improves survival in patients with steroid-resistant acute graft-versus-host disease. Biol Blood Marrow Transplant. 2002;8(1): 40–6.
56. Khoury H, Weisdorf DJ, Davies SM, DeFor TE, Burns LJ, Ramsay NK, et al. Treatment of steroid-resistant acute graft-versus-host disease with anti-thymocyte globulin. Bone Marrow Transplant. 2001;27(10):1059–64.
57. Cragg L, Blazar BR, Defor T, Kolatker N, Miller W, Kersey J, et al. A randomized trial comparing prednisone with antithymocyte globulin/prednisone as an initial systemic therapy for moderately severe acute graft-versus-host disease. Biol Blood Marrow Transplant. 2000;6(4A):441–7.
58. Basara N, Blau WI, Römer E, Rudolphi M, Bischoff M, Kirsten D, et al. Mycophenolate mofetil for the treatment of acute and chronic GVHD in bone marrow transplant patients. Bone Marrow Transplant. 1998;22(1):61–5.
59. Furlong T, Martin P, Flowers ME, Carnevale-Schianca F, Yatscoff R, Chauncey T, et al. Therapy with mycophenolate mofetil for refractory acute and chronic GVHD. Bone Marrow Transplant. 2009;44(11):739–48.
60. Krejci M, Doubek M, Buchler T, Brychtova Y, Vorlicek J, Mayer J, et al. Mycophenolate mofetil for the treatment of acute and chronic steroid-refractory graft-versus-host disease. Ann Hematol. 2005;84(10):681–5.
61. Alousi AM, Weisdorf DJ, Logan BR, Bolaños-Meade J, Carter S, Difronzo N, et al. Etanercept, mycophenolate, denileukin, or pentostatin plus corticosteroids for acute graft-versus-host disease: a randomized phase 2 trial from the blood and marrow transplant clinical trials network. Blood. 2009;114(3):511–7.
62. Pidala J, Kim J, Perkins J, Field T, Fernandez H, Perez L, et al. Mycophenolate mofetil for the management of steroid-refractory acute graft vs host disease. Bone Marrow Transplant. 2010;45(5): 919–24.
63. Bolanos-Meade J, Logan BR, Alousi AM, Antin JH, Barowski K, Carter SL, et al. Phase 3 clinical trial of steroids/mycophenolate mofetil vs steroids/placebo as therapy for acute GVHD: BMT CTN 0802. Blood 2014;124(22):3221–3227; quiz 3335.
64. de Lavallade H, Mohty M, Faucher C, Fürst S, El-Cheikh J, Blaise D, et al. Low-dose methotrexate as salvage therapy for refractory graft-versus-host disease after reduced-intensity conditioning allogeneic stem cell transplantation. Haematologica. 2006;91(10): 1438–40.
65. Huang XJ, Jiang Q, Chen H, Xu L, Liu D, Chen Y, et al. Low-dose methotrexate for the treatment of graft-versus-host disease after allogeneic hematopoietic stem cell transplantation. Bone Marrow Transplant. 2005;36(4):343–8.
66. Wang Y, LP X, Liu KY, Liu DH, Wang J, Chen H, et al. Low-dose MTX combined with low-dose methylprednisolone as a first-line therapy for the treatment of acute GVHD: safety and feasibility. Bone Marrow Transplant. 2011;46(6):892–8.
67. Inagaki J, Nagatoshi Y, Hatano M, Isomura N, Sakiyama M, Okamura J, Low-dose MTX. for the treatment of acute and chronic graft-versus-host disease in children. Bone Marrow Transplant. 2008;41(6):571–7.
68. Couriel DR, Saliba R, de Lima M, Giralt S, Andersson B, Khouri I, Hosing C, et al. A phase III study of infliximab and corticosteroids for the initial treatment of acute graft-versus-host disease. Biol Blood Marrow Transplant. 2009;15(12):1555–62.

69. Gomez-Almaguer D, Ruiz-Argüelles GJ, del Carmen Tarín-Arzaga L, González-Llano O, Gutiérrez-Aguirre H, Cantú-Rodríguez O, et al. Alemtuzumab for the treatment of steroid-refractory acute graft-versus-host disease. Biol Blood Marrow Transplant. 2008; 14(1):10–5.
70. Schub N, Günther A, Schrauder A, Claviez A, Ehlert C, Gramatzki M, et al. Therapy of steroid-refractory acute GVHD with CD52 antibody alemtuzumab is effective. Bone Marrow Transplant. 2011;46(1):143–7.
71. Schnitzler M, Hasskarl J, Egger M, Bertz H, Finke J. Successful treatment of severe acute intestinal graft-versus-host resistant to systemic and topical steroids with alemtuzumab. Biol Blood Marrow Transplant. 2009;15(8):910–8.
72. Ho VT, Zahrieh D, Hochberg E, Micale E, Levin J, Reynolds C, et al. Safety and efficacy of denileukin diftitox in patients with steroid-refractory acute graft-versus-host disease after allogeneic hematopoietic stem cell transplantation. Blood. 2004;104(4):1224–6.
73. Shaughnessy PJ, Bachier C, Grimley M, Freytes CO, Callander NS, Essell JH, et al. Denileukin diftitox for the treatment of steroid-resistant acute graft-versus-host disease. Biol Blood Marrow Transplant. 2005;11(3):188–93.
74. Massenkeil G, Rackwitz S, Genvresse I, Rosen O, Dörken B, Arnold R. Basiliximab is well tolerated and effective in the treatment of steroid-refractory acute graft-versus-host disease after allogeneic stem cell transplantation. Bone Marrow Transplant. 2002; 30(12):899–903.
75. Schmidt-Hieber M, Fietz T, Knauf W, Uharek L, Hopfenmüller W, Thiel E, et al. Efficacy of the interleukin-2 receptor antagonist basiliximab in steroid-refractory acute graft-versus-host disease. Br J Haematol. 2005;130(4):568–74.
76. Wang JZ, Liu KY, LP X, Liu DH, Han W, Chen H, et al. Basiliximab for the treatment of steroid-refractory acute graft-versus-host disease after unmanipulated HLA-mismatched/haploidentical hematopoietic stem cell transplantation. Transplant Proc. 2011;43(5): 1928–33.
77. Levine JE, Paczesny S, Mineishi S, Braun T, Choi SW, Hutchinson RJ, et al. Etanercept plus methylprednisolone as initial therapy for acute graft-versus-host disease. Blood. 2008;111(4):2470–5.

Clinical Presentation of Nonsclerotic Epidermal Chronic Graft-Versus-Host Disease and Hair and Nail Changes

7

Sarah S. Pinney, Amin M. Alousi, and Sharon R. Hymes

Allogeneic hematopoietic stem cell transplantation (HSCT) is a potentially curative therapy for a wide variety of malignant and nonmalignant conditions, but the development of graft-versus-host disease after transplantation may cause significant morbidity and mortality. The updated National Institutes of Health Consensus Development Project on Criteria for Clinical Trials in Chronic Graft-versus-Host Disease (cGVHD) [1] clarified and built upon the 2005 NIH Consensus Conference criteria for diagnosing and scoring the severity of chronic GVHD [2]. The purpose of these guidelines is to create uniformity in clinical trials, to guide treatment, and to facilitate biomarker studies.

Chronic GVHD of the skin may affect the epidermis, dermis, or subcutaneous layers, and often impacts all three. Organ-specific scoring of cutaneous GVHD separates the clinical findings into predominantly sclerotic and predominantly nonsclerotic variants. The nonsclerotic variants often have a prominent epidermal component, the focus of this chapter.

S.S. Pinney (✉)
Department of Dermatology, University of Texas Houston Medical School, 6655 Travis Street, Suite 980, Houston, TX 77030, USA
e-mail: Sarah.A.Sweeney@uth.tmc.edu

A.M. Alousi
Department of Stem Cell Transplantation and Cellular Therapies, University of Texas M. D. Anderson Cancer Center, 1515 Holcombe Boulevard, #853, Houston, TX 77030, USA
e-mail: aalousi@mdanderson.org

S.R. Hymes
Department of Dermatology, University of Texas M. D. Anderson Cancer Center, 1515 Holcombe Boulevard, Unit 1452, Houston, TX 77030, USA
e-mail: srhymes@mdanderson.org

Diagnosing and Scoring Chronic GVHD

Certain clinical features in the skin are considered diagnostic, meaning that no further testing is needed to establish the presence of cutaneous cGVHD. Others are considered distinctive; these are not sufficient alone to establish the diagnosis of cGVHD without additional testing such as a skin biopsy [1]. In patients with epidermal GVHD without sclerosis, only the findings of poikiloderma, lichen planus–like features; and lichen sclerosus–like features are considered diagnostic. Distinctive features include depigmentation and papulosquamous lesions. The new onset of ichthyosis, keratosis pilaris, hair changes, hyperpigmentation, and hypopigmentation are considered nonspecific, and are not used to establish the initial diagnosis (Table 7.1). The maculopapular or papulosquamous rash, erythema, lichen planus–like features, ichthyosis, and keratosis pilaris–like lesions are scored by the percentage of body surface area (BSA) involved. The clinical findings of dyspigmentation, poikiloderma, hair and nail involvement, and pruritus are recognized and noted, but are not quantified (Table 7.2) [1].

Nail changes, including dystrophy, longitudinal ridging, onycholysis, pterygium, and anychia (loss of the nail entirely) are also considered distinctive features [1]. Hair loss may be associated with cGVHD, but evaluating alopecia in the setting of HSCT is challenging, and the etiology is often multifactorial. Skin pathology can be helpful in determining the etiology and guiding the treatment.

The skin is the organ most commonly involved at the time of initial cGVHD diagnosis. The purpose of this chapter is to better acquaint the medical team with the nonsclerotic epidermal manifestations of cutaneous cGVHD, in the hope that early recognition and uniformity in grading of these clinical features will aid in diagnosis, treatment, and research.

J.A. Cotliar (ed.), *Atlas of Graft-versus-Host Disease*, DOI 10.1007/978-3-319-46952-2_7

Table 7.1 Signs and symptoms of chronic GVHD

Organ or site	Diagnostic (sufficient to establish the diagnosis of chronic GVHD)	Distinctive (seen in chronic GVHD, but insufficient alone to establish a diagnosis)	Other features or unclassified entities
Skin	Poikiloderma Lichen planus–like features Sclerotic features Morphea-like features Lichen sclerosus–like features	Depigmentation Papulosquamous lesions	Sweat impairment Ichthyosis Keratosis pilaris Hypopigmentation Hyperpigmentation
Nails		Dystrophy Longitudinal ridging, splitting, or brittle features Onycholysis Pterygium unguis Nail loss (usually symmetric, affects most nails)	
Scalp and body hair		New onset of scarring or nonscarring scalp alopecia (after recovery from chemoradiotherapy) Loss of body hair Scaling	Thinning scalp hair, typically patchy, coarse, or dull (nor explained by endocrine or other causes) Premature gray hair

Adapted from Jagasia et al. [1]

Table 7.2 Skin scoring of chronic graft-versus-host disease (cGVHD)

	Score 0	Score 1	Score 2	Score 3
GVHD features to be scored by BSA:	No BSA involved	1–18 % BSA	19–50 % BSA	>50 % BSA
Check all that apply: Maculopapular rash/erythema Lichen planus–like features Sclerotic features Papulosquamous lesions or ichthyosis Keratosis pilaris–like GVHD				
Skin features score: *Other skin GVHD features (NOT scored by BSA)* *Check all that apply:* Hyperpigmentation Hypopigmentation Poikiloderma Severe or generalized pruritus Hair involvement Nail involvement	No sclerotic features	Superficial sclerotic features "Not hidebound" (able to pinch)		*Check all that apply*: Deep sclerotic features "Hidebound" (unable to pinch) Impaired mobility Ulceration
Abnormality present but explained entirely by non-GVHD documented cause (specify): ________________				

Adapted from Jagasia et al. [1]
BSA body surface area

Clinical Manifestations of cGVHD

Diagnostic Features

Diagnostic features for cGVHD (requiring no further testing to establish the presence of cutaneous cGVHD) include lichen planus–like lesions, lichen sclerosus, and poikilodermatous skin changes [1]. Each diagnostic feature may be seen alone, but they often appear in combination, along with other epidermal or sclerotic features of cutaneous GVHD.

Lichen Planus–like GVHD

Lichen planus is characterized by purple-hued, polygonal papules and plaques, sometimes with a fine white scale and an overlying network of white lines (Wickham striae). Lichen planus of the hair follicle is termed *lichen planopilaris* (Figs. 7.1, 7.2, 7.3, 7.4, 7.5, 7.6, 7.7, 7.8, 7.9, 7.10 and 7.11).

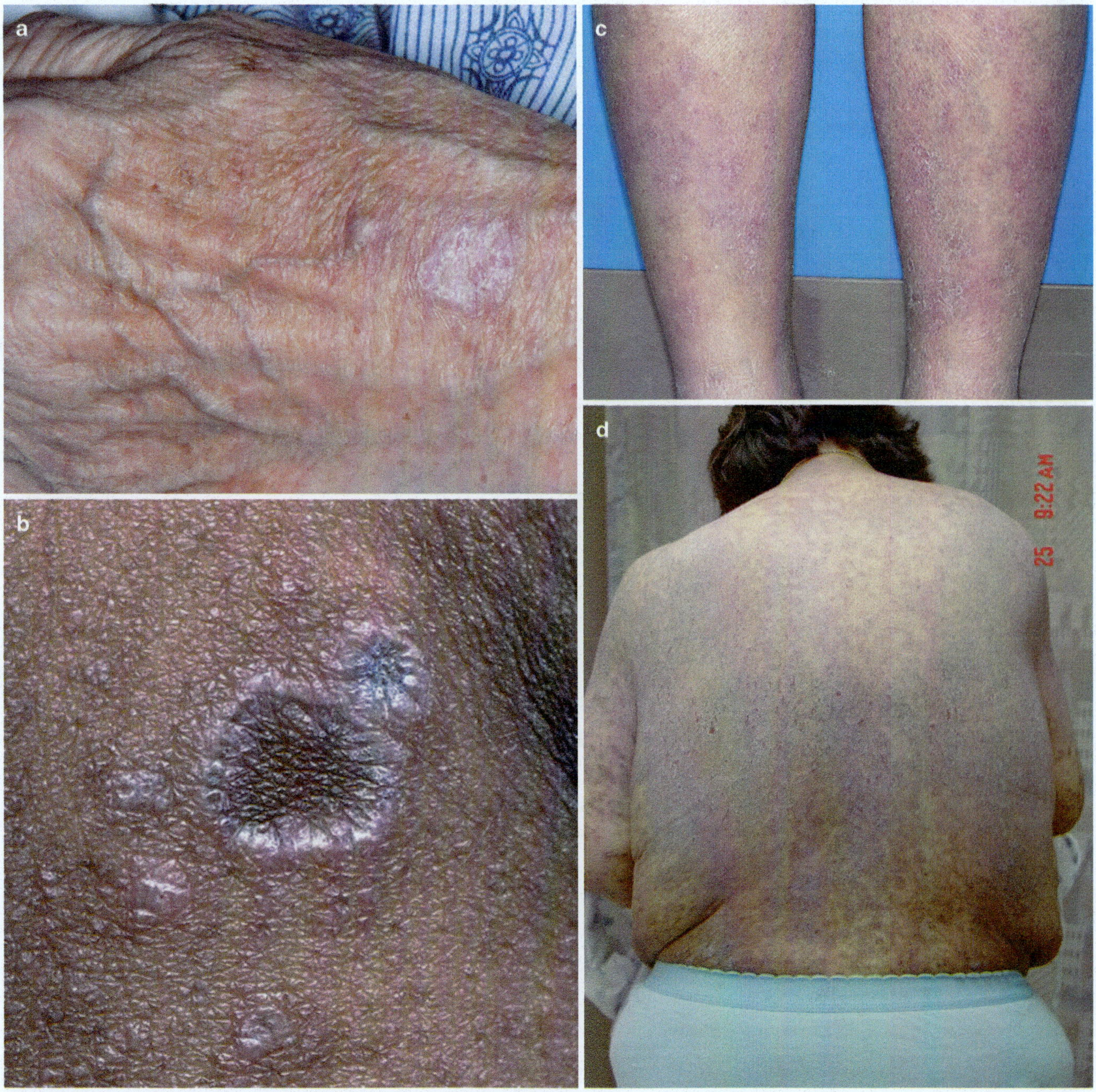

Fig. 7.1 The purple, polygonal lichen planus–like papules and plaques may be solitary (**a**, **b**) or may become confluent (**c**, **d**)

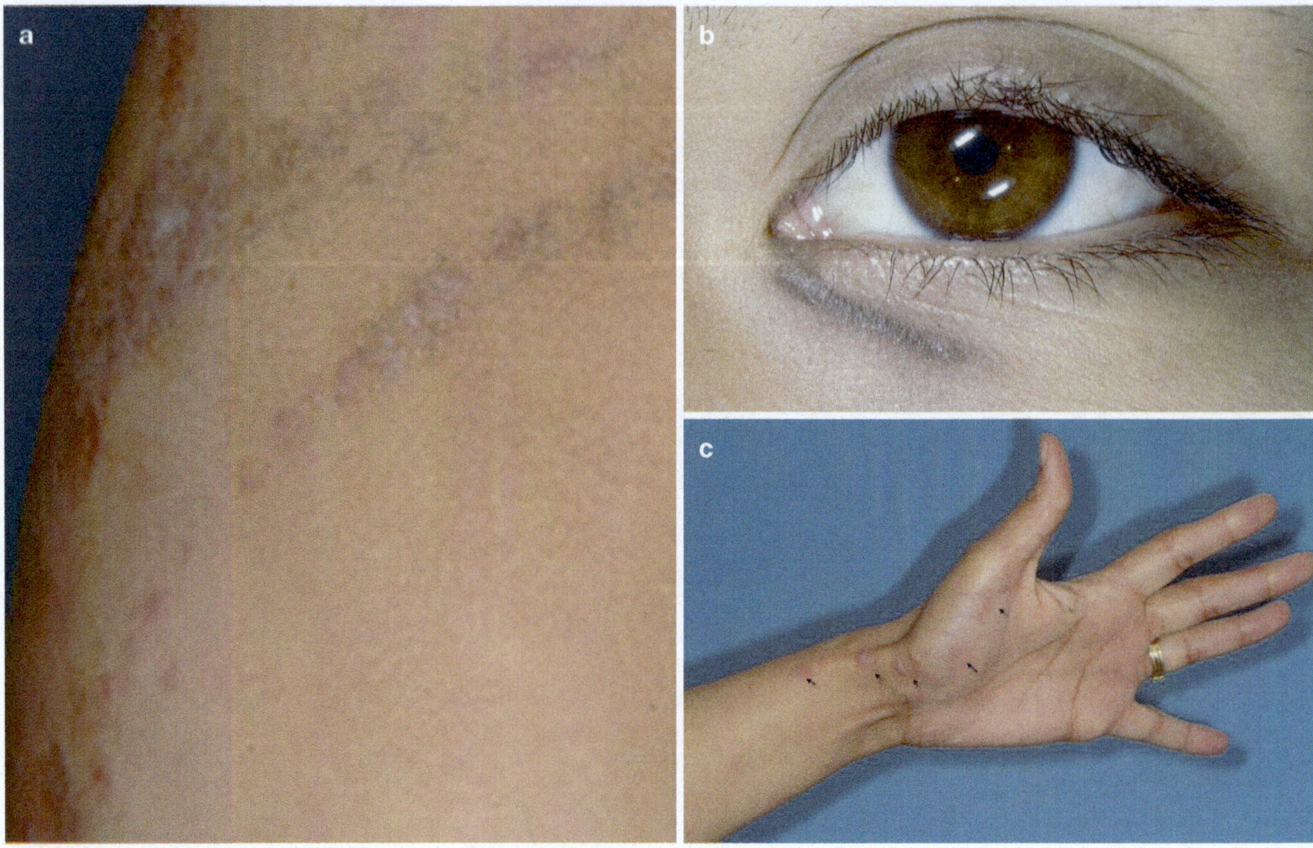

Fig. 7.2 (**a**, **b**) Lichen planus-like GVHD may koebnerize, following lines of pressure or trauma. (**c**) An unusual sporotrichoid pattern (*arrows*) is present without known antecedent. Trauma

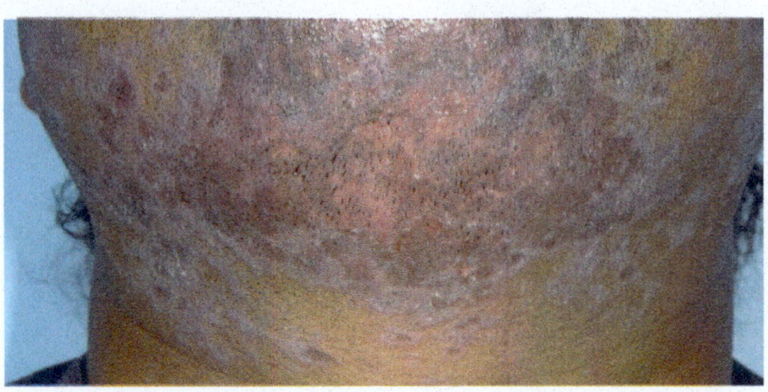

Fig. 7.3 Inflammation may lead to significant postinflammatory pigment changes, including the hypopigmentation and hyperpigmentation seen in the beard area of this patient

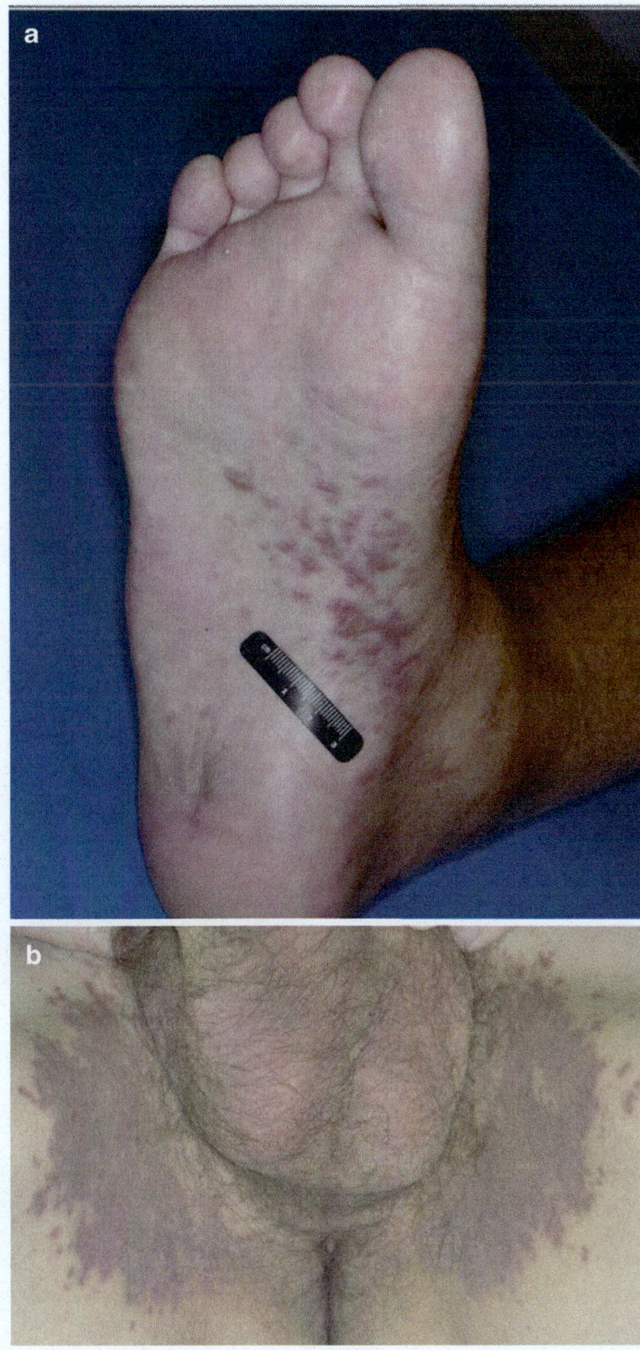

Fig. 7.4 Unusual presentations of lichen planus–like GVHD may occur, including prominent lesions in distribution that may mimic tinea pedis (**a**) and tinea cruris (**b**). This patient had been treated with topical antifungal agents

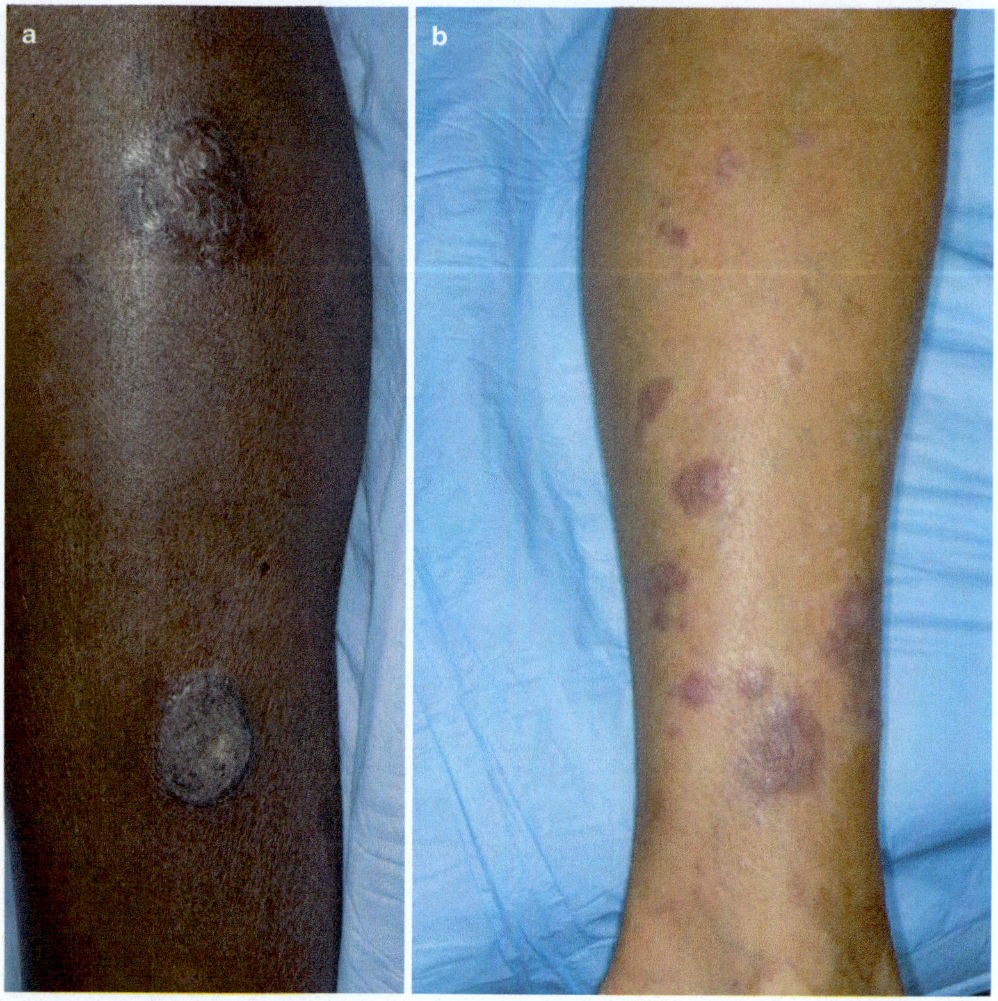

Fig. 7.5 (**a**, **b**) Lichen planus–like GVHD may become hypertrophic, mimicking prurigo nodularis or squamous cell carcinoma

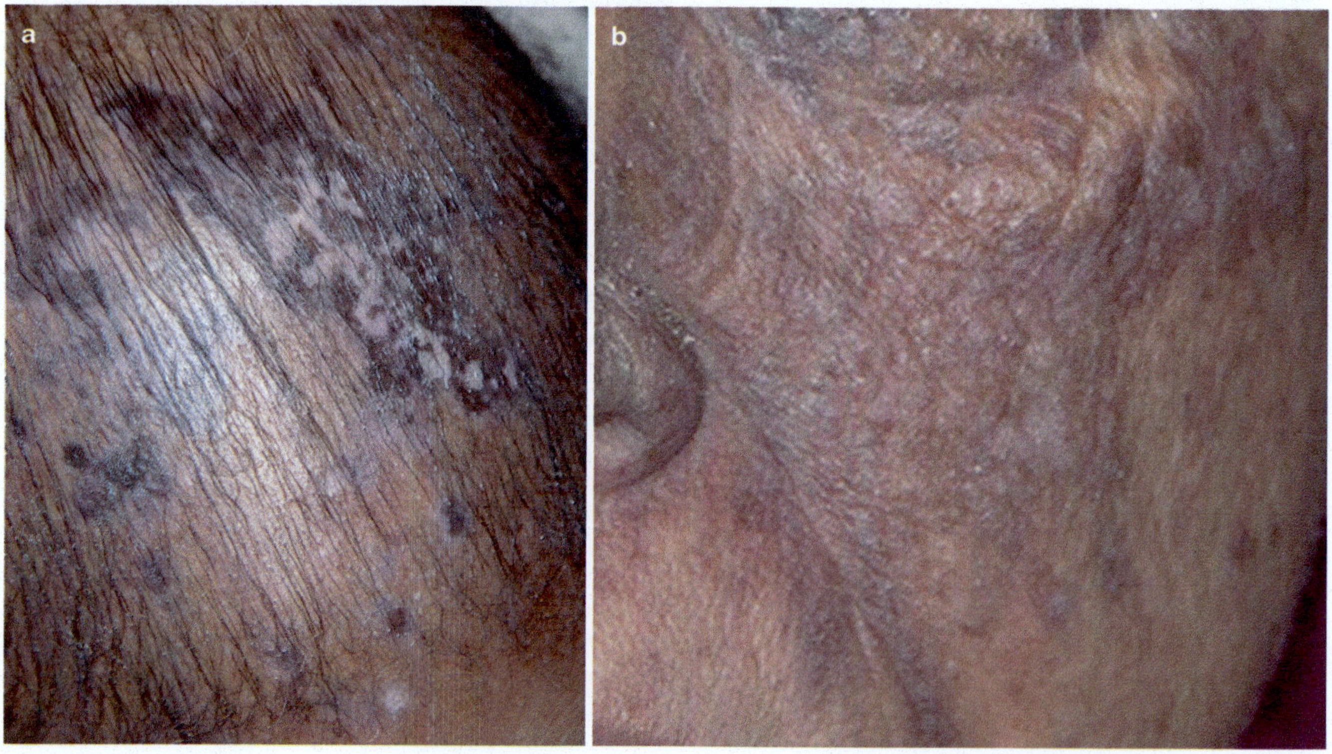

Fig. 7.6 Lichen planus–like changes may cause scarring. These scalp (**a**) and facial (**b**) lesions are difficult to distinguish from those of chronic cutaneous lupus

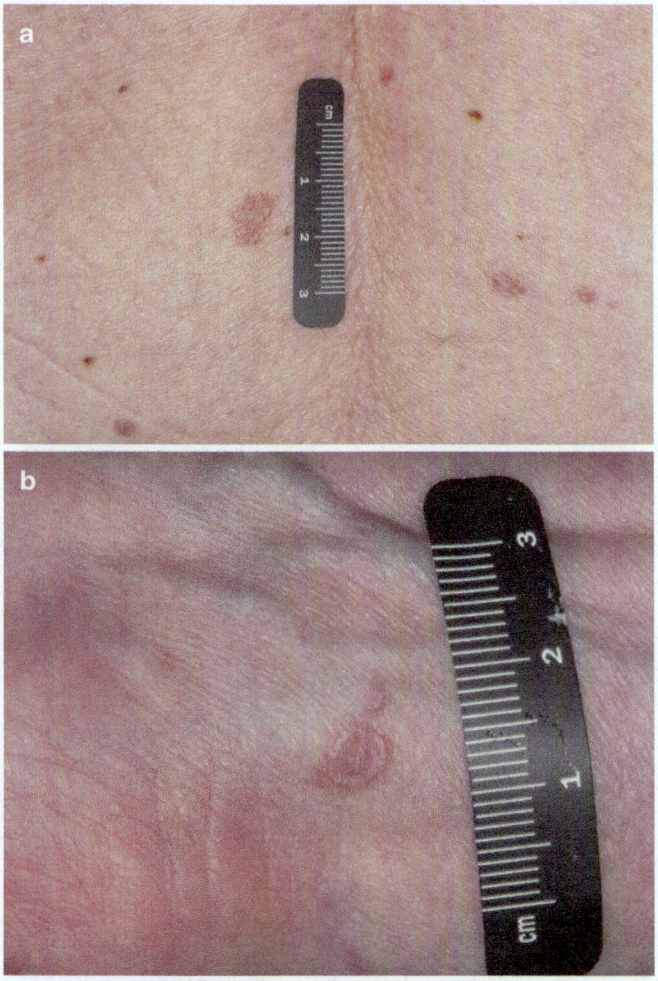

Fig. 7.7 (**a**, **b**) Lichen planus–like cGHVD may not present with the classic purple hue. These scattered, shiny, flat-topped papules showed classic pathologic findings of lichen planus–like GVHD

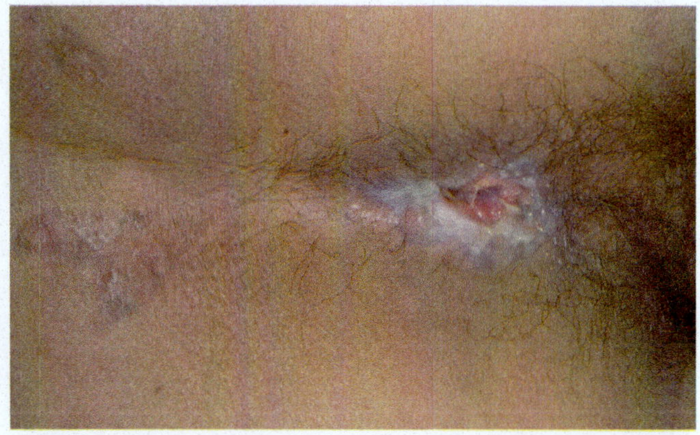

Fig. 7.8 Erosive lichen planus–like GVHD around the anus was associated with erosive oral GVHD in this patient. Patients with pain in the perineum, including the vaginal area, should be carefully examined

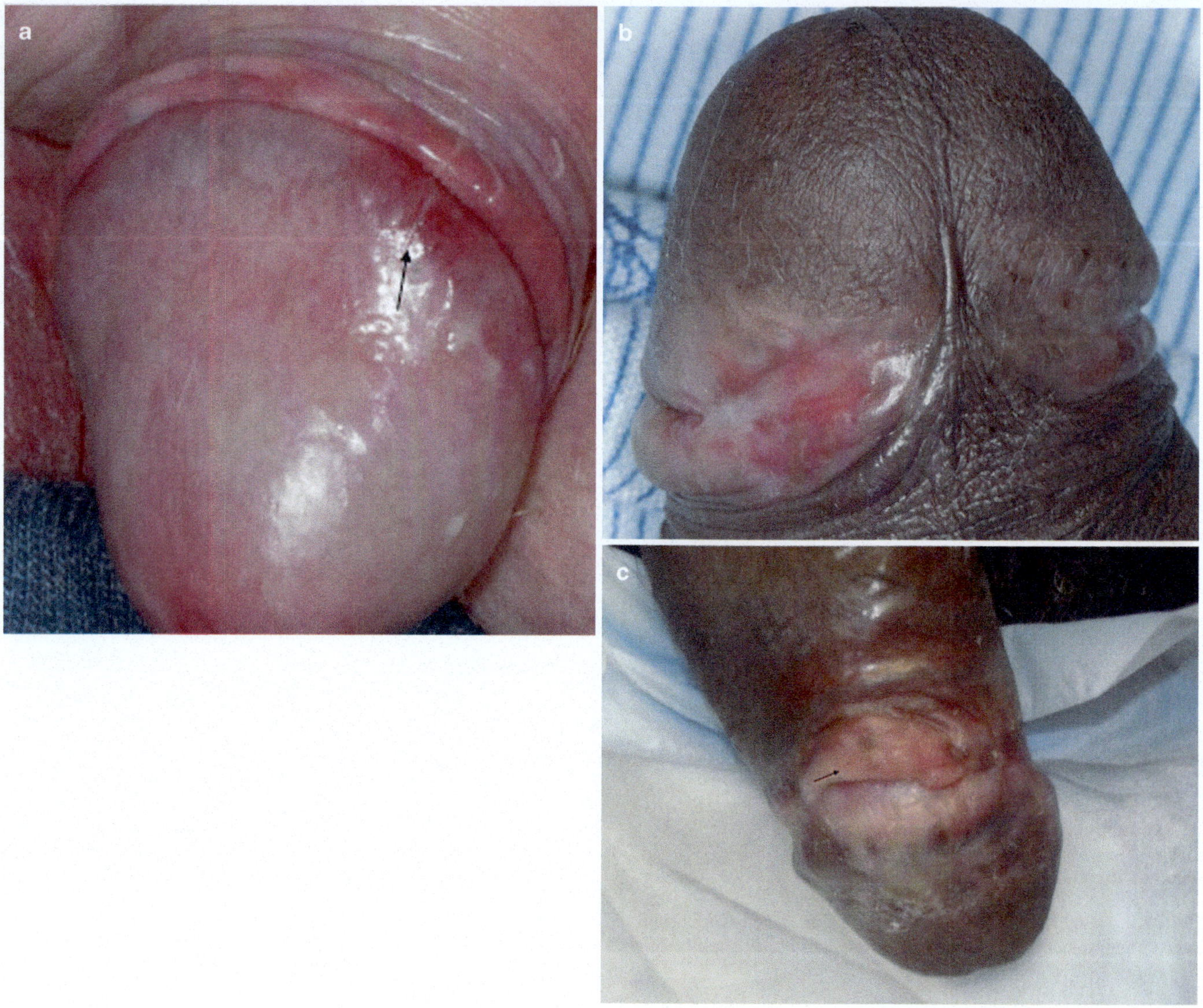

Fig. 7.9 (**a**) Involvement of the penis may present with subtle erosions on the glans (*arrow*). (**b**) Lesions may be more prominent, such as these hypertrophic eroded plaques. These findings need to be distinguished from other etiologies of balanitis. (**c**) This patient has biopsy-proven GVHD, but later developed a biopsy-proven squamous-cell carcinoma (*arrow*)

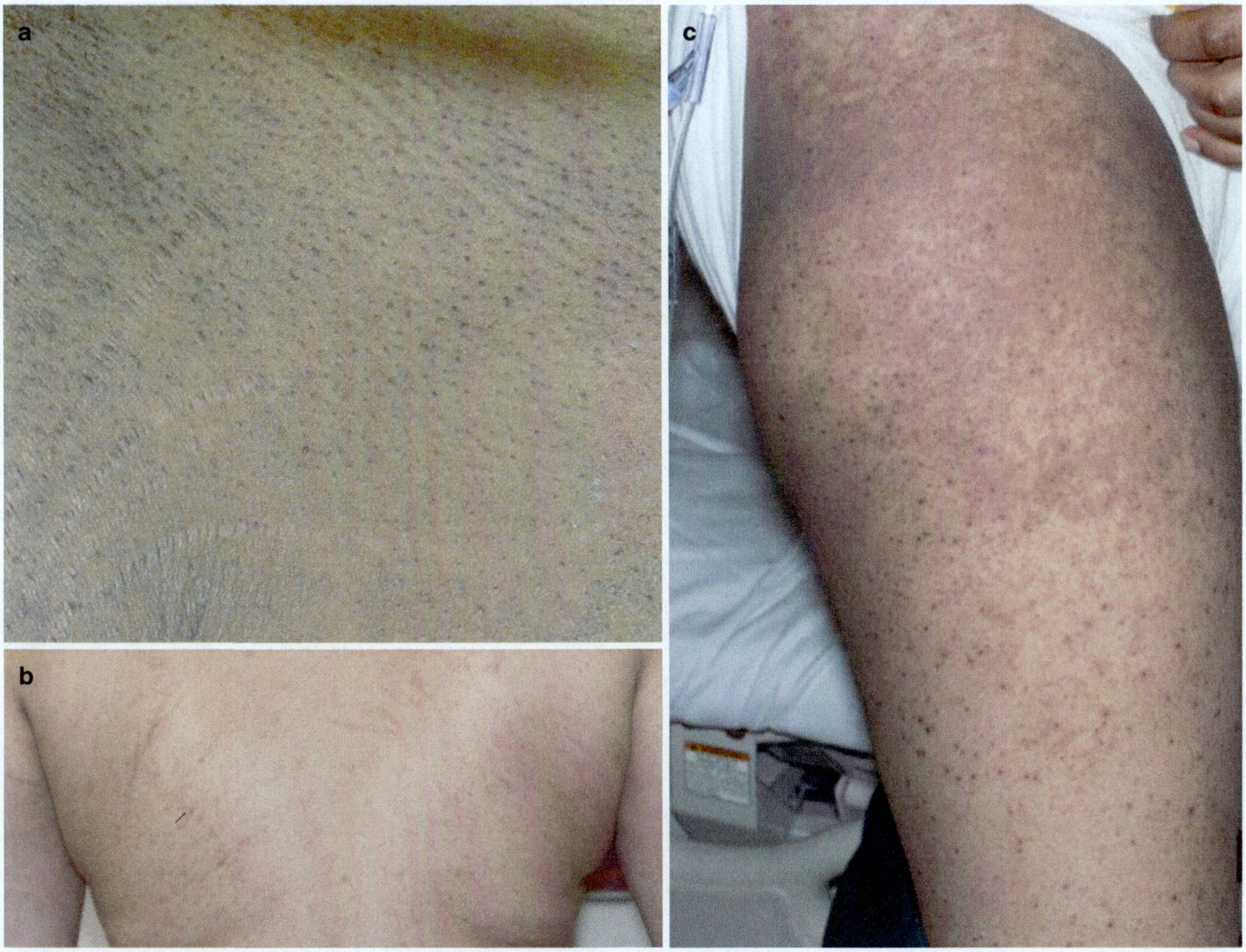

Fig. 7.10 (**a**, **b**), Both patients demonstrate subtle folliculocentric purple papules (*arrow in* **b**), which were biopsy-proven lichen planopilaris. The flagellate lines in *B* developed after bleomycin administration before transplantation. (**c**) This patient has lichen planopilaris-like cGVHD on the lower arm and confluent lichen planus-like cGVHD on the upper arm

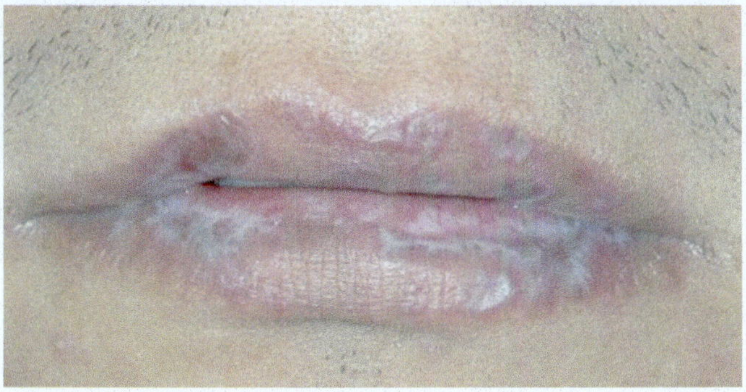

Fig. 7.11 Wickham striae, characterized by lacy reticulated lines, are seen on the lips of this patient

Lichen Sclerosus–like GVHD

Lesions of lichen sclerosus show marked epidermal thinning with an ivory color and wrinkled surface (Figs. 7.12, 7.13 and 7.14).

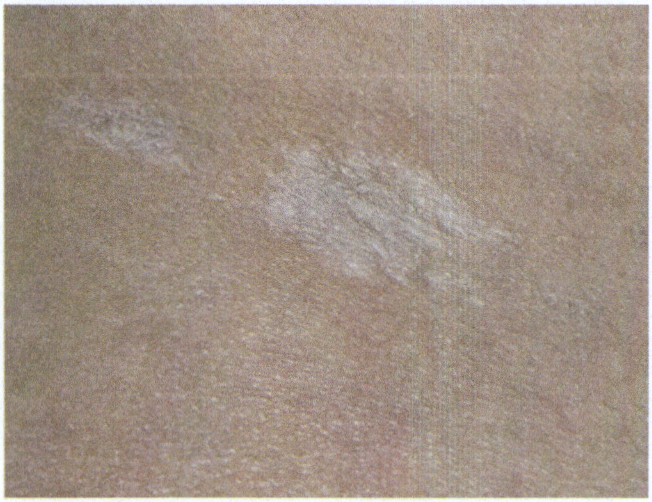

Fig. 7.12 These well demarcated lesions show the characteristic features of hypopigmentation with marked epidermal atrophy in cases of lichen sclerosus-like cGVHD

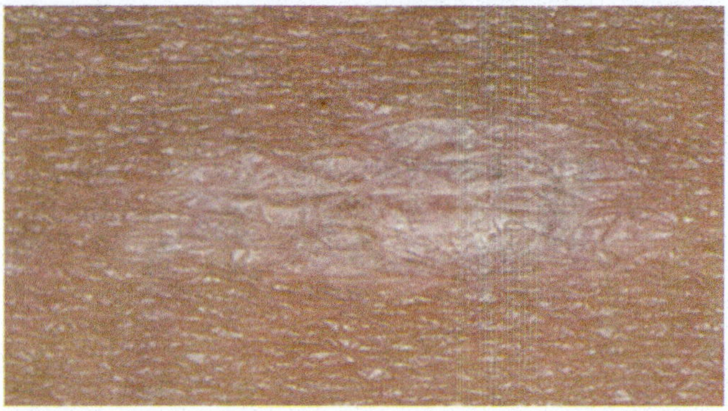

Fig. 7.13 "Cigarette paper wrinkling" on the surface of these lesions is characteristic of epidermal atrophy and changes in the dermal collagen in patients with lichen sclerosus-like cGVHD

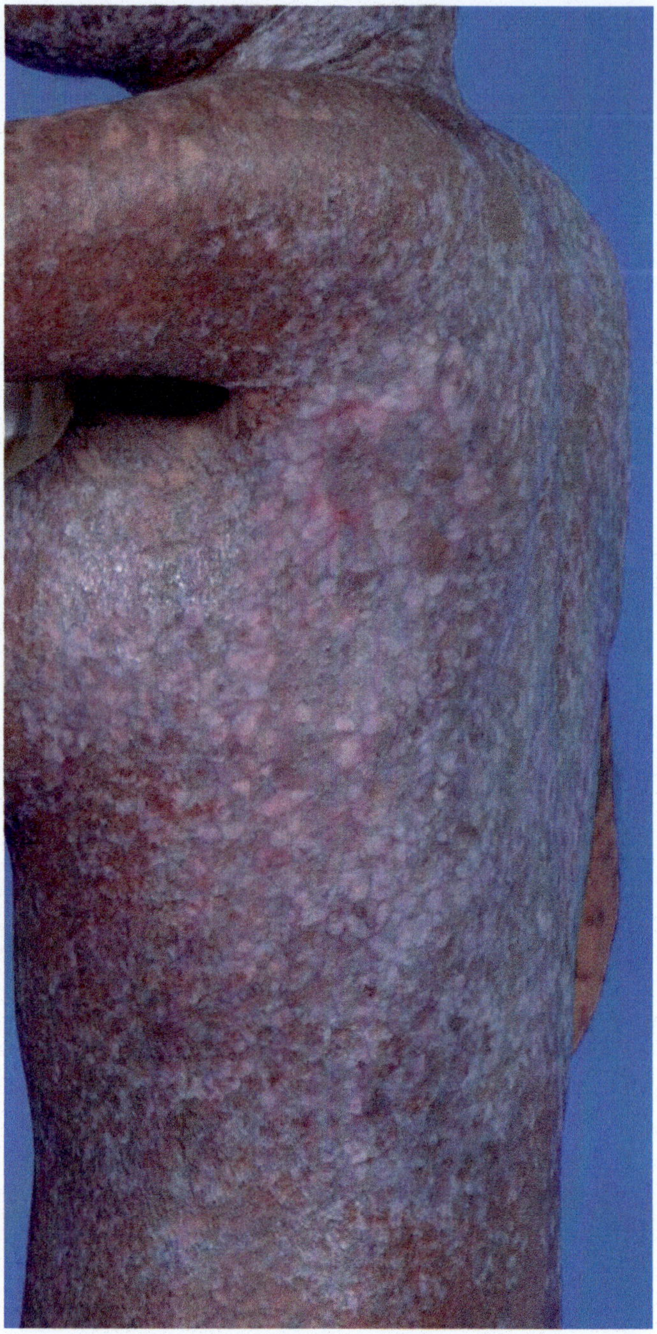

Fig. 7.14 This patient has extensive, confluent lichen sclerosus–like GVHD, as well as lichen planus–like changes

Poikiloderma

Poikilodermatous changes include hypopigmentation, hyperpigmentation, telangiectasia, and atrophy (Figs. 7.15 and 7.16).

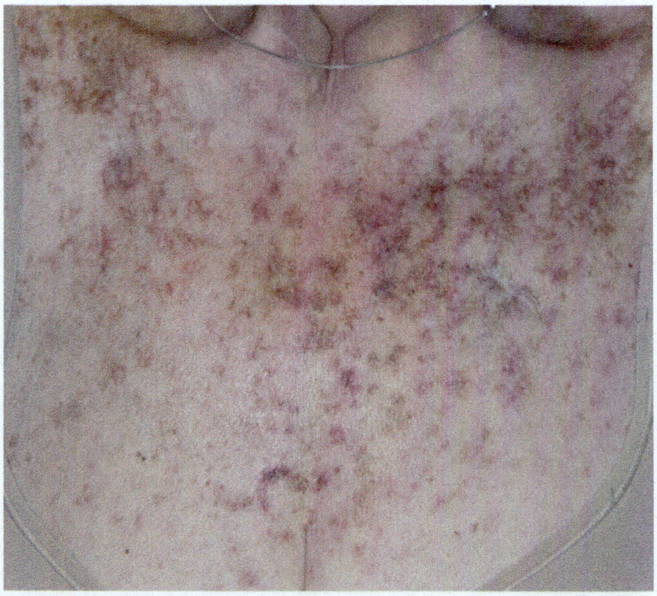

Fig. 7.15 In the setting of GVHD, poikilodermatous changes are characterized clinically by hypopigmentation, hyperpigmentation, telangiectasia and atrophy, along with histologic changes of GVHD. This patient developed new-onset poikiloderma, followed by fasciitis and sclerotic cGVHD

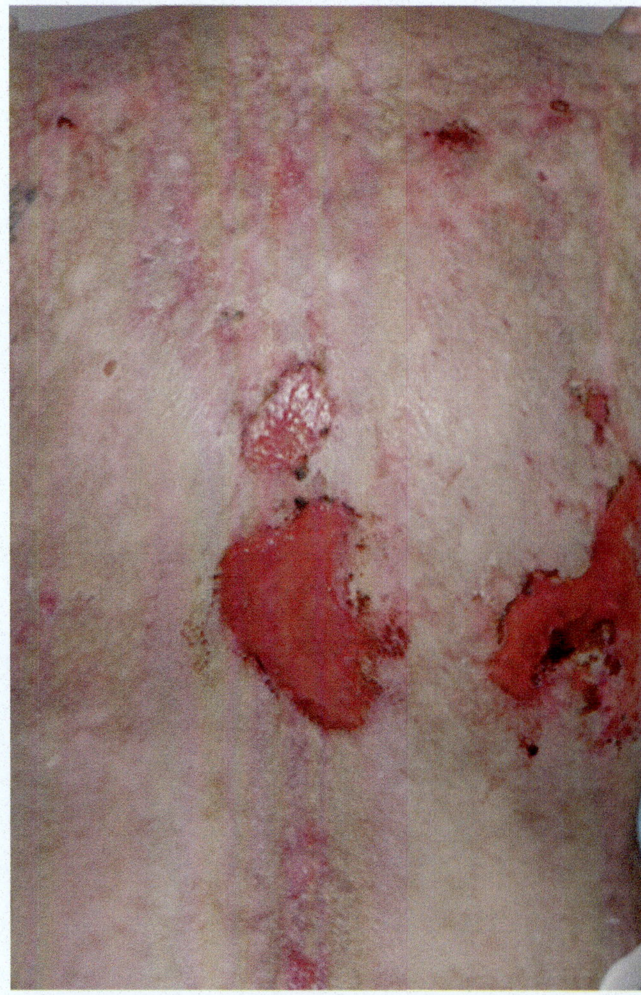

Fig. 7.16 The atrophy seen in the setting of poikiloderma may cause non-healing erosions in areas of friction

Distinctive Features

Distinctive features (not sufficient alone to establish the diagnosis of cGVHD without additional testing) include papulosquamous eruptions such as maculopapular (morbilliform), psoriasiform, or pityriasiform (maculopapular lesions with fine branny or powdery scale) skin changes, as well cutaneous depigmentation [1].

Papulosquamous Eruptions

The morphology of these may be variable. While sometimes morbilliform, these lesions may also be pityriasiform or resemble psoriasis or eczema (Figs. 7.17, 7.18, 7.19, 7.20, 7.21 and 7.22). Pathology is often helpful for diagnosis and treatment, as the differential diagnosis may include drug-induced or virus-induced rashes.

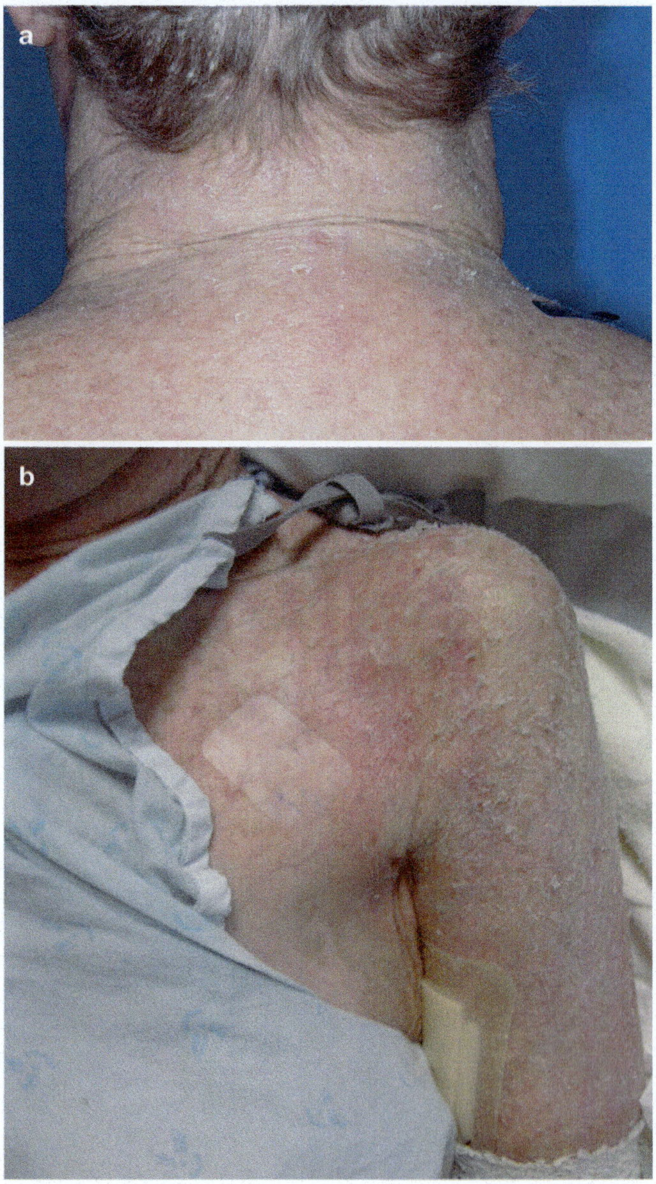

Fig. 7.17 (**a**) This patient has a morbilliform rash on the upper back and neck, with abundant scale in the scalp and neck. (**b**) This patient has a more prominent erythematous component and is becoming erythrodermic

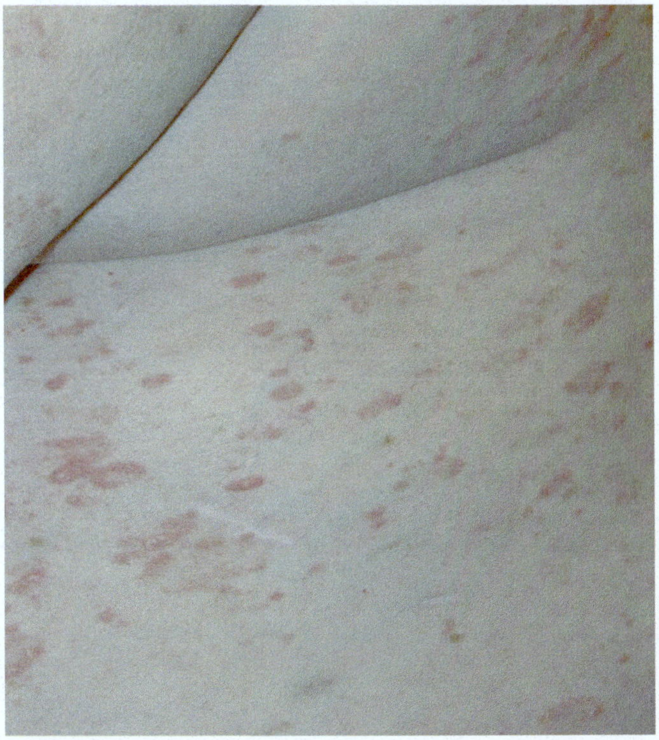

Fig. 7.18 Pityriasis rosea–like rash in a patient with biopsy-proven cutaneous GVHD

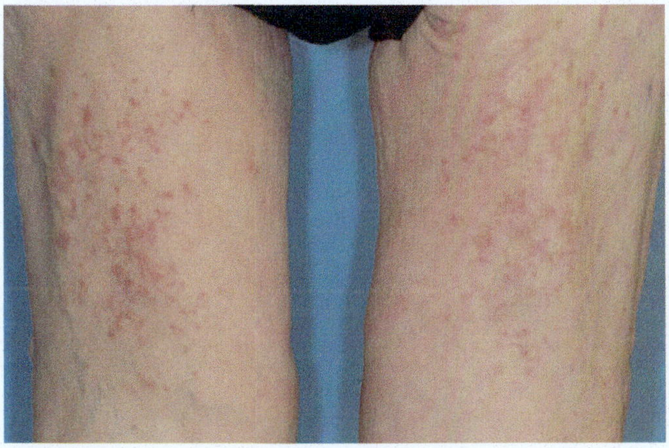

Fig. 7.19 Biopsy-proven cGVHD presenting as a morbilliform eruption with less scale. These lesions are sometimes difficult to distinguish from a morbilliform drug eruption

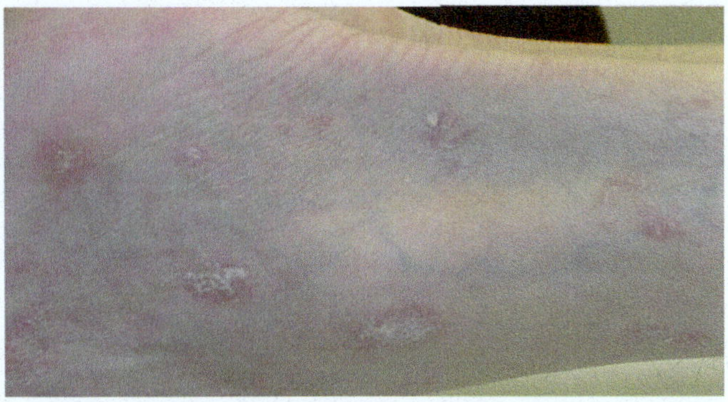

Fig. 7.20 These well-circumscribed psoriatic-appearing plaques proved to be GVHD by pathology

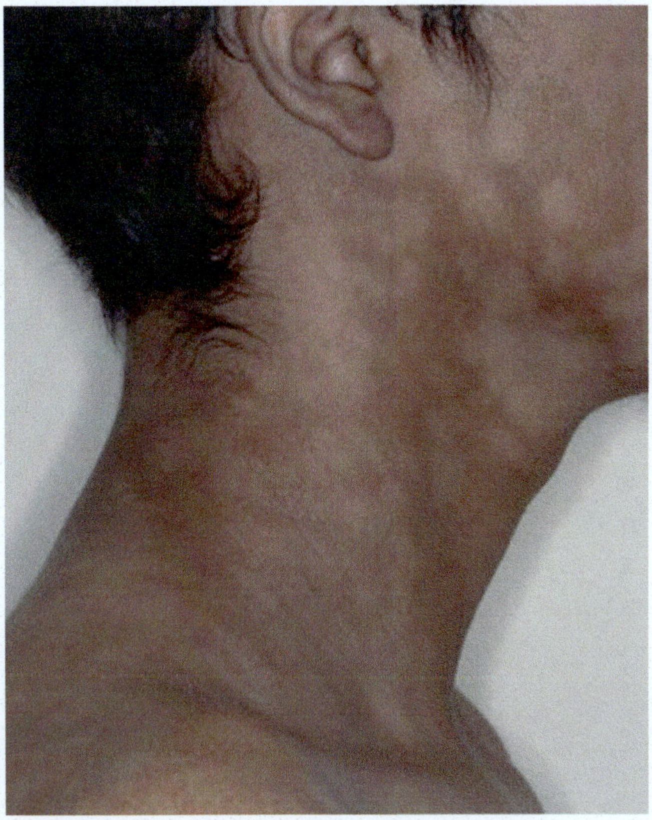

Fig. 7.21 The hypopigmented, slightly scaly areas on the neck appear to be pityriasis alba, but were proven to be GVHD by biopsy

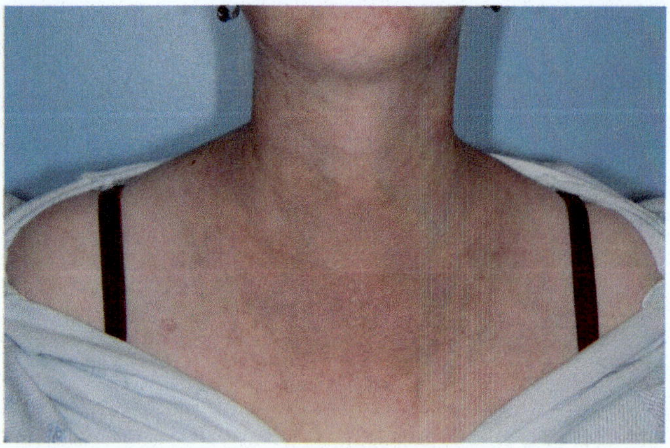

Fig. 7.22 The papulosquamous lesions may be more prominent in sun-exposed areas. The differential diagnosis includes a photo-induced drug rash or connective tissue disease

Depigmentation

In patients with no previous inflammatory skin lesions, the onset of depigmentation after HSCT is considered to be a distinctive feature of cGVHD. Biopsy is consistent with loss of melanocytes, which cannot be distinguished from vitiligo (Fig. 7.23).

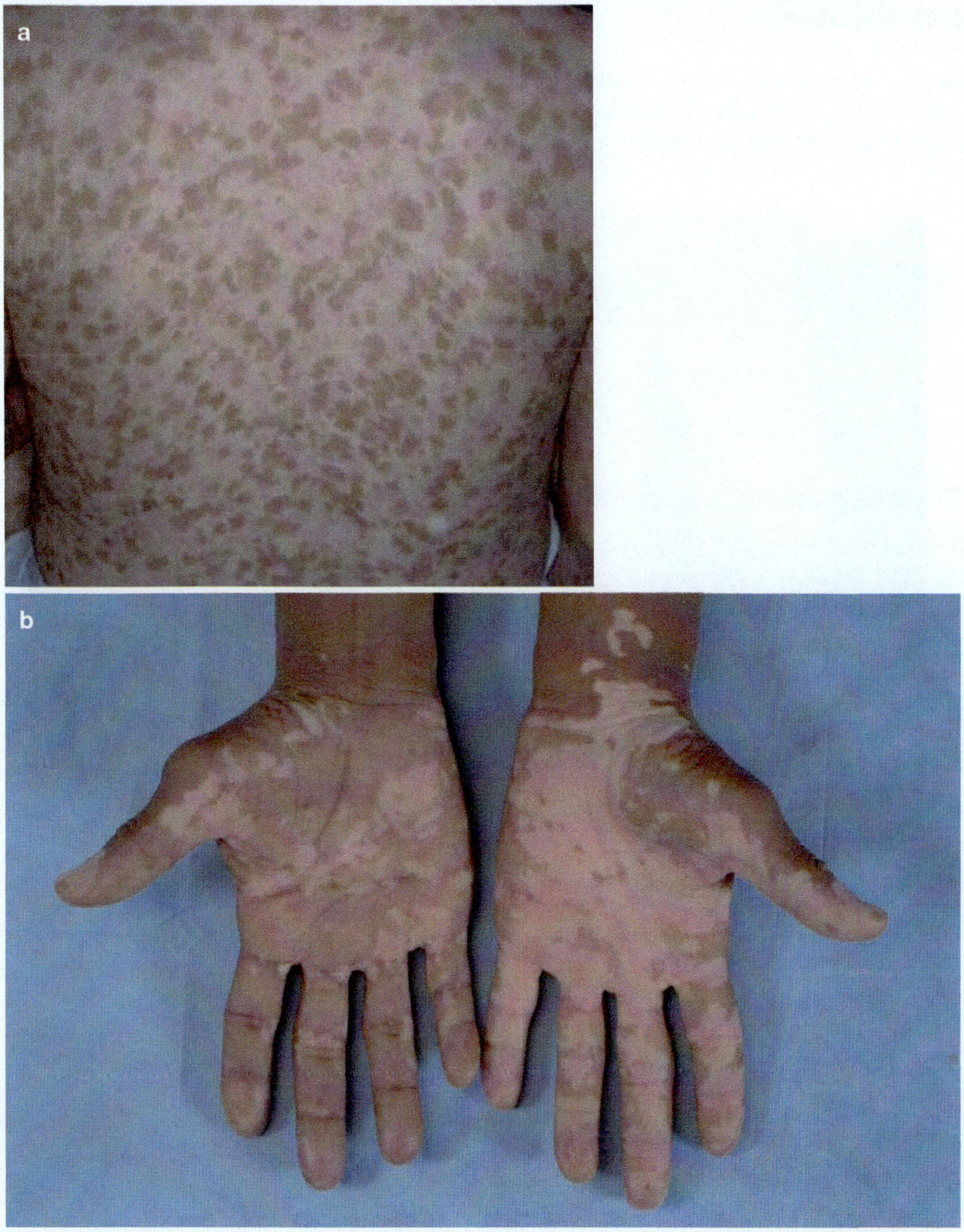

Fig. 7.23 Depigmentation. (**a**, **b**) This patient developed depigmented patches on the trunk and extremities after stem cell transplantation. Biopsy confirmed cGVHD

Additional Manifestations

Other features seen in, but not specific to, cGVHD include new-onset ichthyosis (Fig. 7.24), keratosis pilaris (Fig. 7.25), reactive erythema (Fig. 7.26), and acral erythema

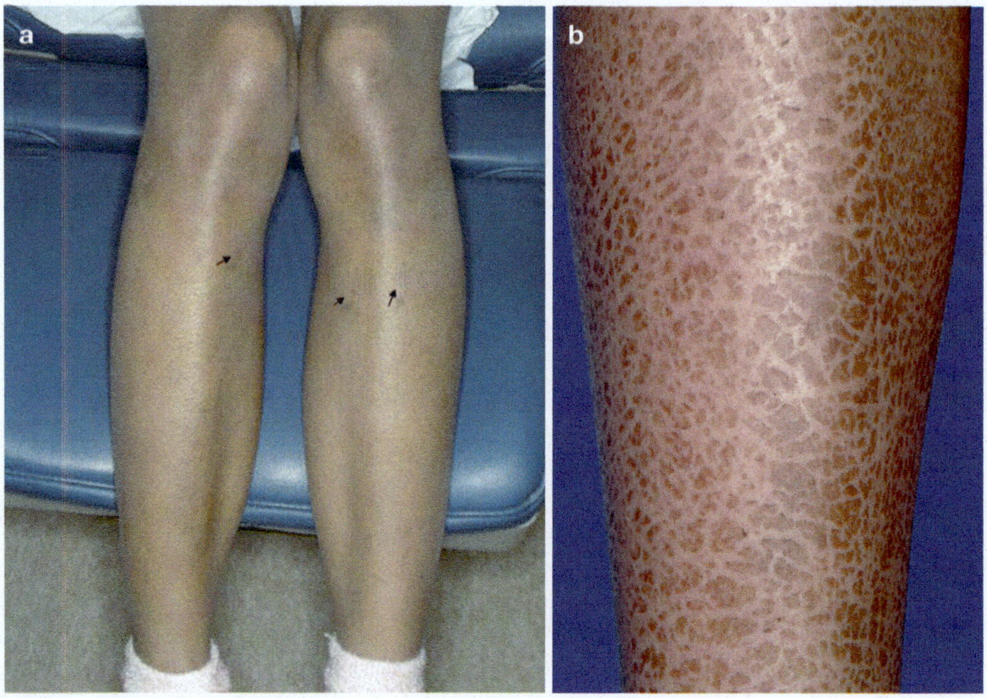

Fig. 7.24 Ichthyosis. The sudden onset of icthyosis should alert the clinician to the possibility of cGHVD. (**a**) The patient was noted to have scaly, dermatitic-appearing plaques on the legs (*arrows*). (**b**) Six weeks later, she developed widespread ichthyosis, along with other systemic manifestations of cGVHD

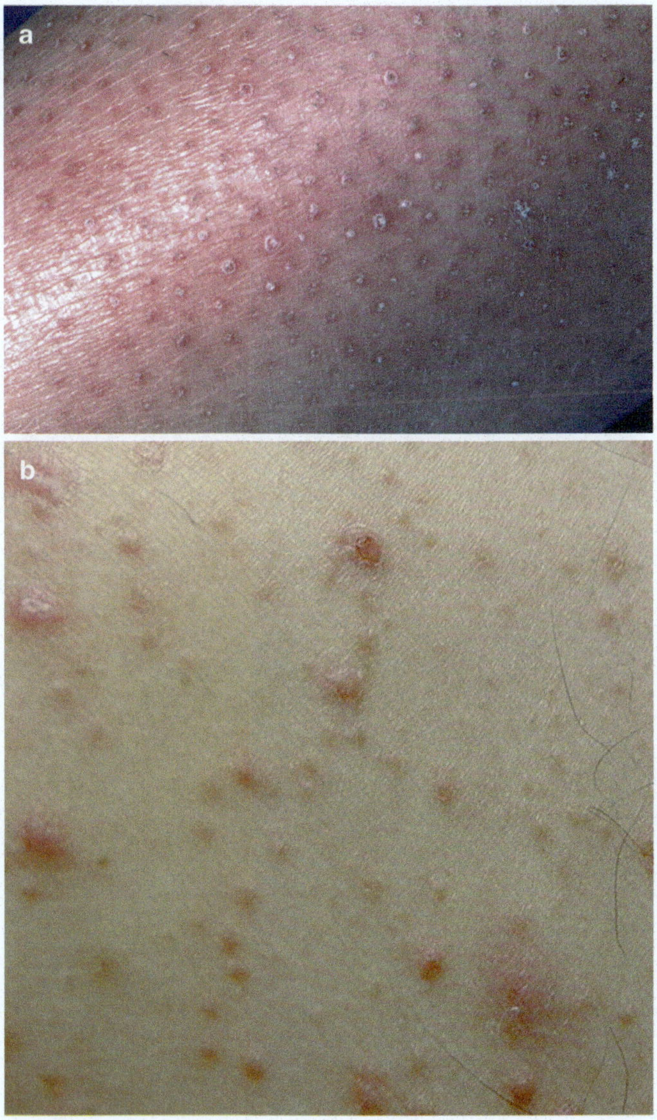

Fig. 7.25 Keratosis pilaris. (**a**) These keratotic papules with central adherent scale may appear suddenly and clinically differ from classic keratosis pilaris in distribution. (**b**) The patient may also present with erythematous follicular papules, resembling inflamed keratosis pilaris

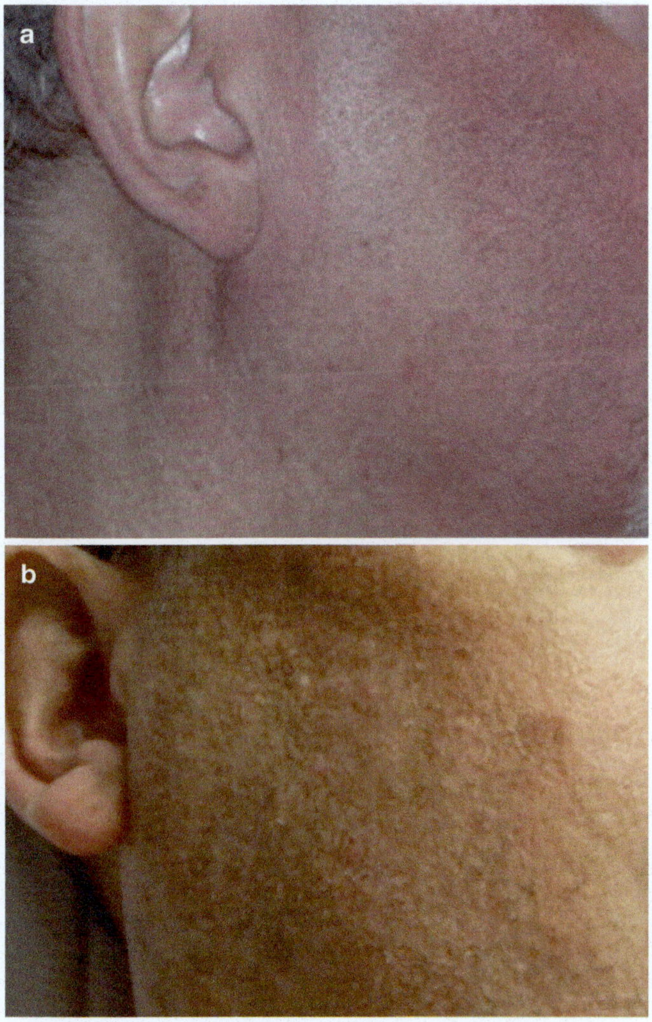

Fig. 7.26 (**a**) Reactive erythema including diffuse erythema may signal the onset of skin cGVHD. (**b**) After resolution, pitting scarring may result, possibly from follicular involvement

Other Morphologies

Other reactive erythemas, including urticarial or erythema multiforme–like lesions may occur (Fig. 7.27). Lesions of the hands and feet may be mistaken for eczema (Fig. 7.28).

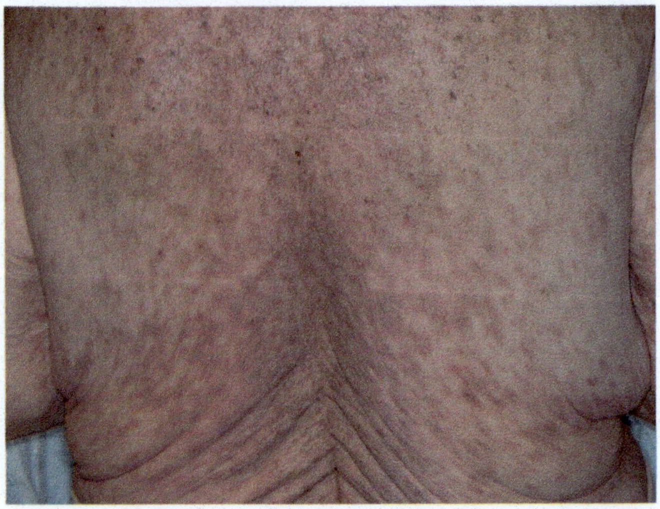

Fig. 7.27 This patient has changes of poikiloderma on the upper back, and erythema multiforme on the lower back. She later developed fasciitis

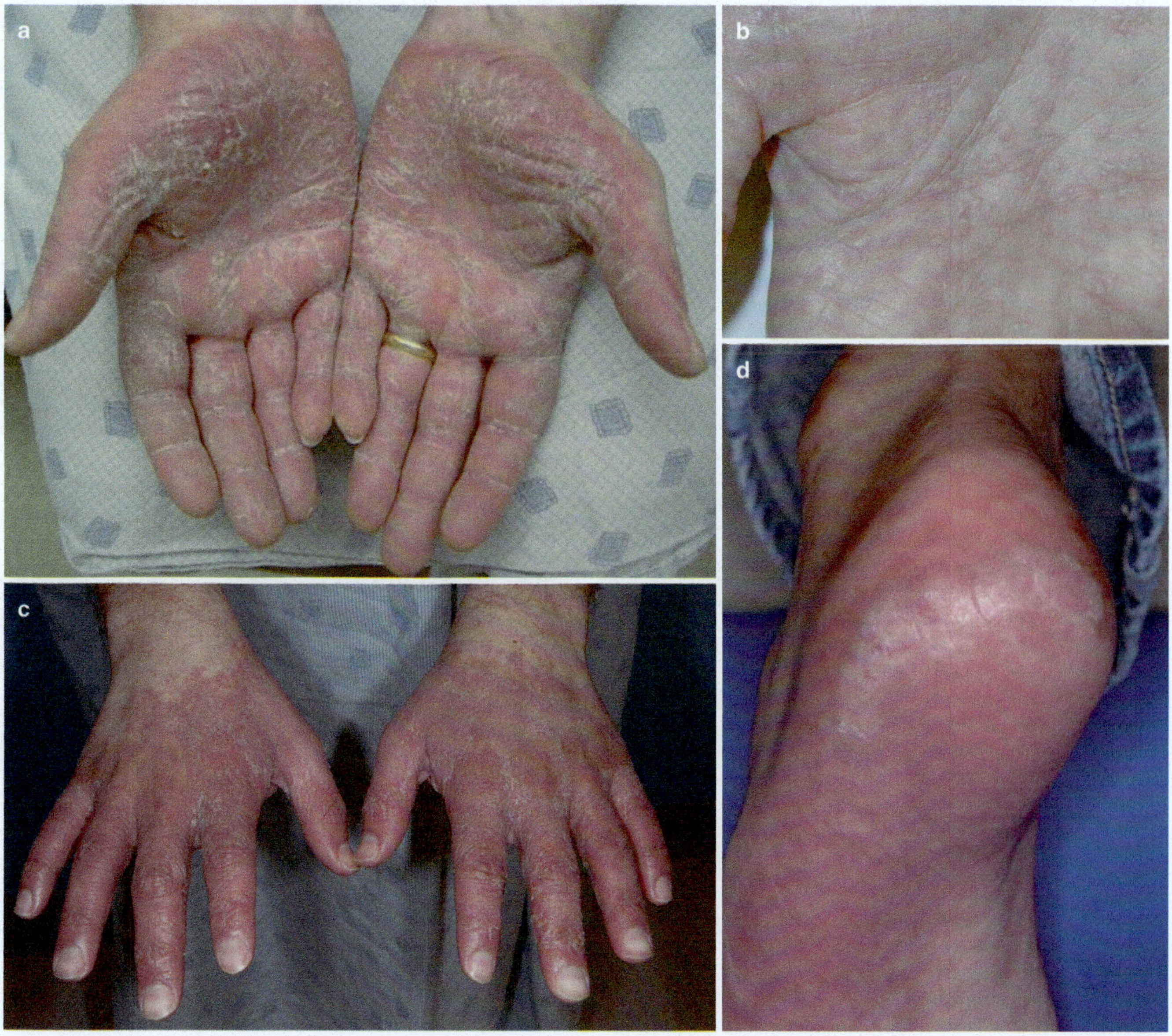

Fig. 7.28 (**a**) This patient was thought to have recalcitrant hand eczema, until biopsy confirmed that GVHD. (**b**) This patient has cGVHD of the palms, with the formation of vesicles. (**c**, **d**) The dorsal hands and feet may also be affected

Hair (Alopecia)

The etiology of alopecia is often multifactorial in transplant patients. Pathology may be helpful in furthering determining the etiology (Figs. 7.29, 7.30 and 7.31).

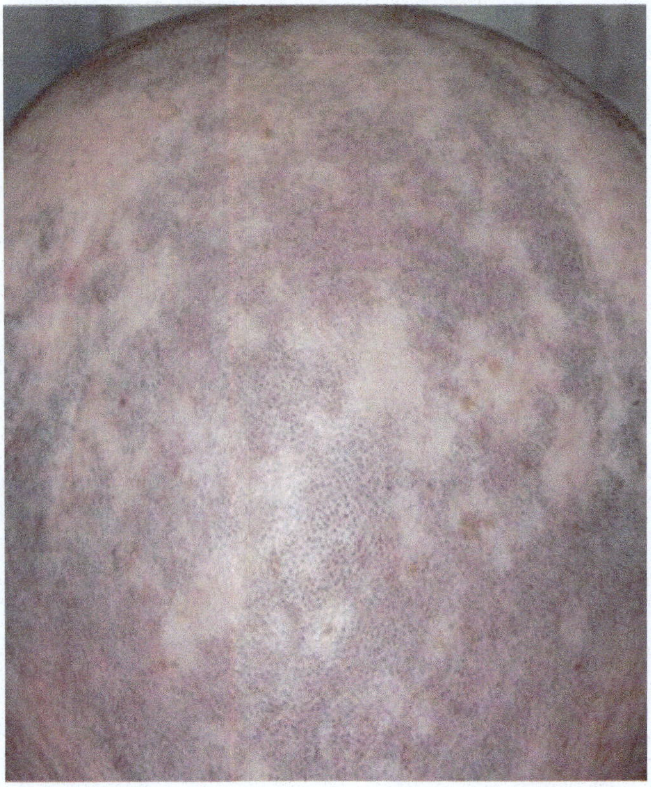

Fig. 7.29 Lichen planopilaris–like cGVHD leading to patchy alopecia

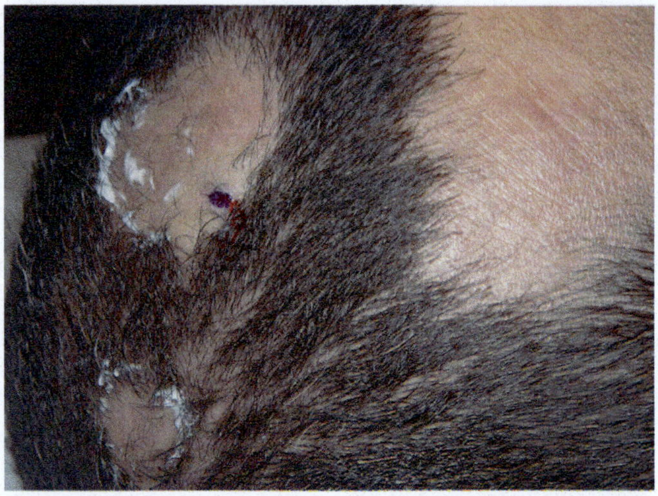

Fig. 7.30 *De novo* alopecia areata in a patient with active papulosquamous cutaneous cGVHD on the trunk. The white cream was applied for anesthesia prior to biopsy

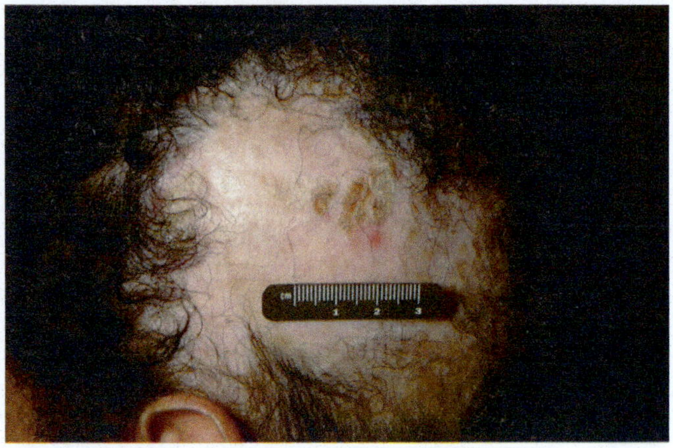

Fig. 7.31 Sclerosis of the dermis leads to destruction of the hair apparatus and alopecia

Nail Changes

Nail changes in GVHD may be relatively nonspecific, but some changes are more characteristic (Figs. 7.32 and 7.33).

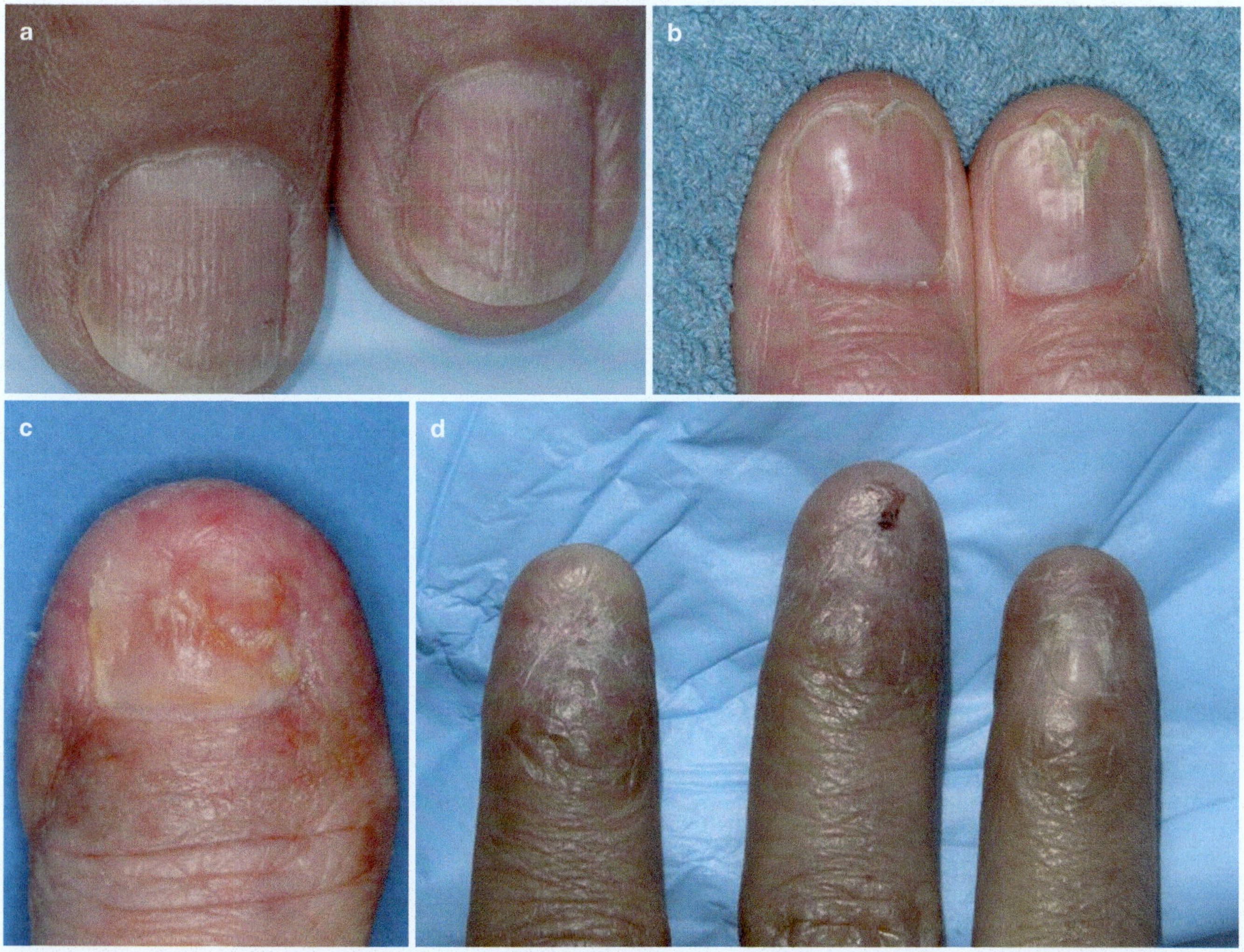

Fig. 7.32 Nail GVHD may be characterized by relatively nonspecific changes of longitudinal ridging, brittle nails, dystrophy (**a**) or onycholysis (**b**). More characteristic changes include pterygium unguis (**c**) or complete loss of the nail (**d**)

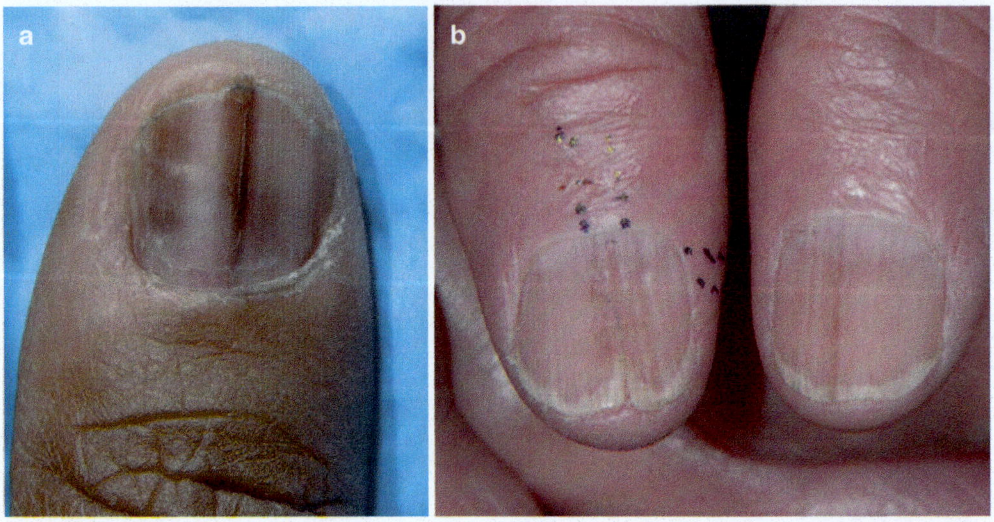

Fig. 7.33 An interesting nail change is melanonychia striata, which may occur from the localized nail bed, especially in darker-skinned individuals (**a**) and sometimes in multiple nails (**b**)

Conclusion

The new onset of sclerotic skin, lichen planus, poikiloderma, and lichen sclerosus after allogeneic HSCT are sufficient to establish the diagnosis of chronic cutaneous GVHD. Epidermal cGVHD may present with a myriad of different and subtle phenotypes, however, mimicking relatively banal and otherwise common dermatologic conditions such as xerosis, keratosis pilaris, ichthyosis, and eczema. When these findings appear *de novo* in the right clinical setting, the clinician should consider the possibility that they represent cutaneous cGVHD.

Sometimes the distribution is atypical, as in keratosis pilaris–like GVHD, not always confined to extensor surfaces. Often there are other, more definitive signs of GVHD that appear at the same time, or there is history of a triggering factor, such as changes in the immunosuppressive regimen, an infection, or sunburn. Pathology is often helpful in diagnosis.

From a treatment perspective, cutaneous epidermal cGVHD is more amenable than sclerotic cutaneous cGVHD to topical modalities of therapy, including corticosteroids, calcineurin inhibitors, and phototherapy. Complete skin examinations, mapping and documentation of skin findings, close follow-up, and pathology all contribute to the early recognition of epidermal cGVHD.

References

1. Jagasia MH, Greinix HT, Arora M, Williams KM, Wolff D, Cowen EW, et al. National Institutes of Health Consensus Development Project on Criteria for Clinical Trials in Chronic Graft-versus-Host Disease: I. The 2014 Diagnosis and Staging Working Group Report. Biol Blood Marrow Transplant. 2015;21:389–401. e1
2. Filipovich AH, Weisdorf D, Pavletic S, Socie G, Wingard JR, Lee SJ, et al. National Institutes of Health consensus development project on criteria for clinical trials in chronic graft-versus-host disease: I. Diagnosis and Staging Working Group report. Biol Blood Marrow Transplant. 2005;11:945–56.

8 Dermal and Subcutaneous Chronic Graft-Versus-Host Disease

Benjamin H. Kaffenberger and Samantha M. Jaglowski

Dermal and subcutaneous chronic graft-versus-host disease (cGVHD) is a severely restricting form of cGVHD, which may begin insidiously before progressing to ulcerations, limb movement limitations, and even restrictive lung disease. Multiple studies have demonstrated the use of total body irradiation and mobilized stem cells as risks for this form of cGVHD. As more peripheral blood-based hematopoietic stem cell transplants (HSCT) are performed, the incidence of this form of cGVHD is likely to increase. Several unique clinical signs can help to identify early disease.

Treatments are often cumbersome, expensive, and/or experimental. The ideal treatment would be able to target both active immune disease, including fibroblastic growth signals, and inactive fibrosis. There is support for photochemotherapy and narrow-band UVB phototherapy, as well as other skin-directed treatments and systemic immunomodulators. Clinical trials are necessary to ascertain the ideal treatment regimen.

Clinical Presentation

Chronic graft-versus-host disease (cGVHD) in its myriad forms occurs in about 50 % of patients after HSCT, but it varies widely based on many factors, including human leukocyte antigen (HLA) match, GVHD prophylaxis, age, donor sex, and the disease being treated with the transplant [1, 2]. Dermal and subcutaneous cGVHD may present differently depending on the depth and degree of involvement. Pedagogically, the different morphologies are most easily remembered by considering their non-GVHD autoimmune counterpart. For superficial dermal sclerotic disease, the counterpart is lichen sclerosus. For more extensive and deeper dermal sclerotic disease, it is morphea. Deeper than the dermis is the subcutaneous fat, where the presentation can resemble lupus panniculitis. The deepest disease, occurring at the fascial interface and fibrous connective tissue, is clinically analogous to eosinophilic fasciitis. Although there are different morphologies, there are no data separating the prognosis of these entities. It is best to group them as sclerotic-type cGVHD, as there is often coexisting fibrosis of the dermis, subcutaneous fat, and fascia.

The sclerosis is commonly called sclerodermoid, but there are substantial differences between systemic sclerosis and cGVHD, so it is better to recognize this disease as sclerotic-type cGVHD [3]. Sclerotic-type cGVHD tends to occur in about 20 % of patients who develop any form of cGVHD, with a higher incidence in patients who have received peripherally mobilized stem cell transplants and higher doses of total body irradiation [4]. The development of sclerotic-type cGVHD is also associated with prolonged immunosuppression following HSCT [4], which may be a surrogate for having an earlier subtype of GVHD. Other forms of cGVHD (for example, the lichenoid form) often evolve over time into a dermal and subcutaneous cGVHD, but the reverse does not happen. Additional clinical findings associated with the sclerosing dermal and fascial forms of cGVHD include elevated platelet counts, higher levels of C3 complement, and diminished pulmonary function tests [5].

The morphologies and associated signs are listed below, in order from superficial to deep. There is substantial variation, however, and often sclerotic-type cGVHD will have overlapping depths of involvement.

B.H. Kaffenberger (✉)
Division of Dermatology, The Ohio State University Wexner Medical Center, 2012 Kenny Road, 2nd Floor, Columbus, OH 43214, USA
e-mail: Benjamin.Kaffenberger@osumc.edu

S.M. Jaglowski
Department of Internal Medicine, Division of Hematology, The Ohio State University Wexner Medical Center, 400 West 10th Avenue, Columbus, OH 43220, USA
e-mail: Samantha.jaglowski@osumc.edu

J.A. Cotliar (ed.), *Atlas of Graft-versus-Host Disease*, DOI 10.1007/978-3-319-46952-2_8

Superficial Dermis: Lichen Sclerosus Type

The most superficial form is lichen sclerosus–like disease. These hypopigmented, thin patches and plaques often have a slight cigarette-paper epidermal atrophy that can be observed on close inspection. Follicular plugging may also be noted. The lesions tend to develop within interflexural areas of the body, including the neck, axilla, popliteal fossa, antecubital fossa, breast, and gluteal folds. There often are peripheral skip plaques surrounding a larger plaque, which will eventually coalesce if treatment is not commenced. Based on the tension on these interflexural areas, they also have a tendency to develop into highly painful ulcerations, which heal poorly. When they finally do heal, the result is further scarring and worsened mobility of the underlying joint (Fig. 8.1).

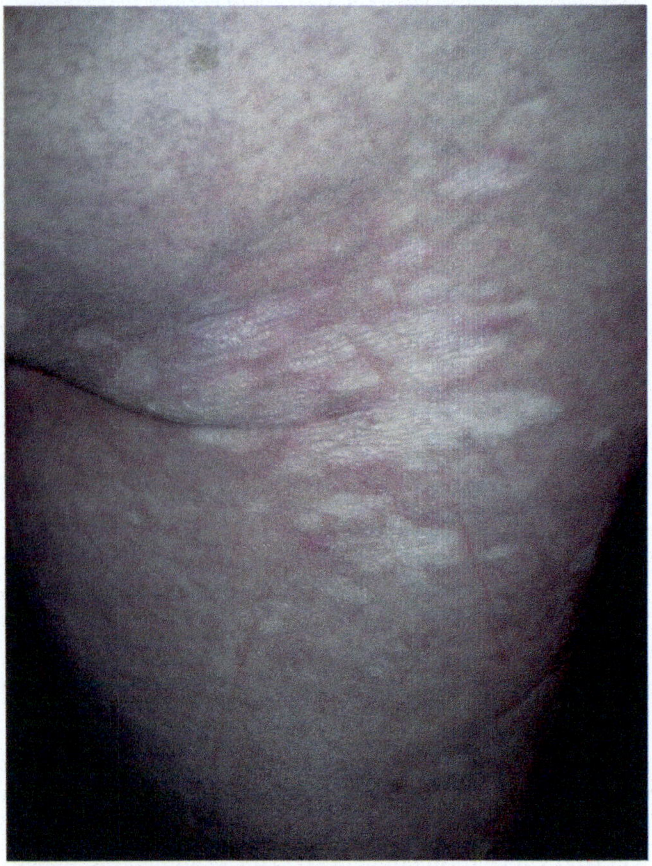

Fig. 8.1 Shiny, hypopigmented plaques with satellite plaques over the gluteal fold, representing superficial dermal chronic graft-versus-host disease (cGVHD) of the lichen sclerosus type

Deep Dermis: Morpheaform Type

The classic sclerotic-type (morpheaform) cGVHD tends to occur deeper in the dermis and thus does not result in the superficial hypopigmentation or cigarette-paper atrophy (Fig. 8.2). However, both superficial and deep forms of these entities may coexist. It tends to occur *de novo* in areas of pressure and chronic friction, such as the waistband (Fig. 8.3), the axilla, and areas of chronic edema, such as the lower extremity. Other than areas of edema and chronic pressure, there are also many reports of the isotopic and isomorphic development within areas of trauma or preexisting cutaneous damage, such as herpess zoster (Fig. 8.4), port sites, or previous needle-sticks [6, 7]. The similarities to morphea are very interesting, as there are also many reports of morphea developing within areas of localized cutaneous radiotherapy [8]. A specific entity that tends to develop out of morpheaform cGVHD is the angiomatosis phenomenon (Fig. 8.5) [9]. These patients present with long-standing sclerosis with superimposed vascular patches or even nodules that may look like dense telangiectasias to very large pyogenic granulomas.

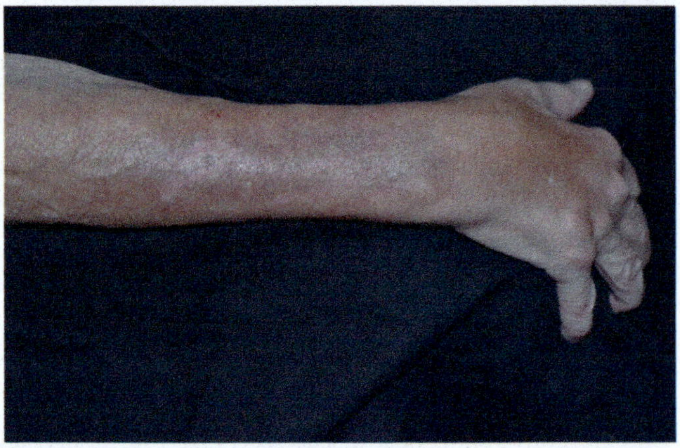

Fig. 8.2 The right forearm of a patient with extensive induration over the dorsal arms, representing deeper dermal involvement; superficial hypopigmentation is no longer visible

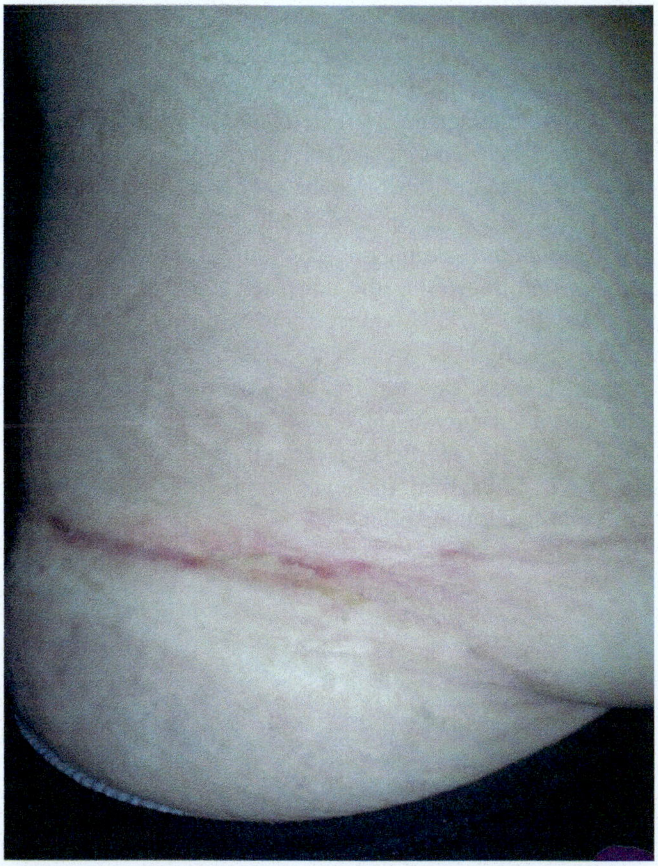

Fig. 8.3 Sclerotic-type cGVHD developing at the site of the waistband, representing chronic friction, with features of both morpheaform and lichen sclerosus morphologies, as well as a central ulceration

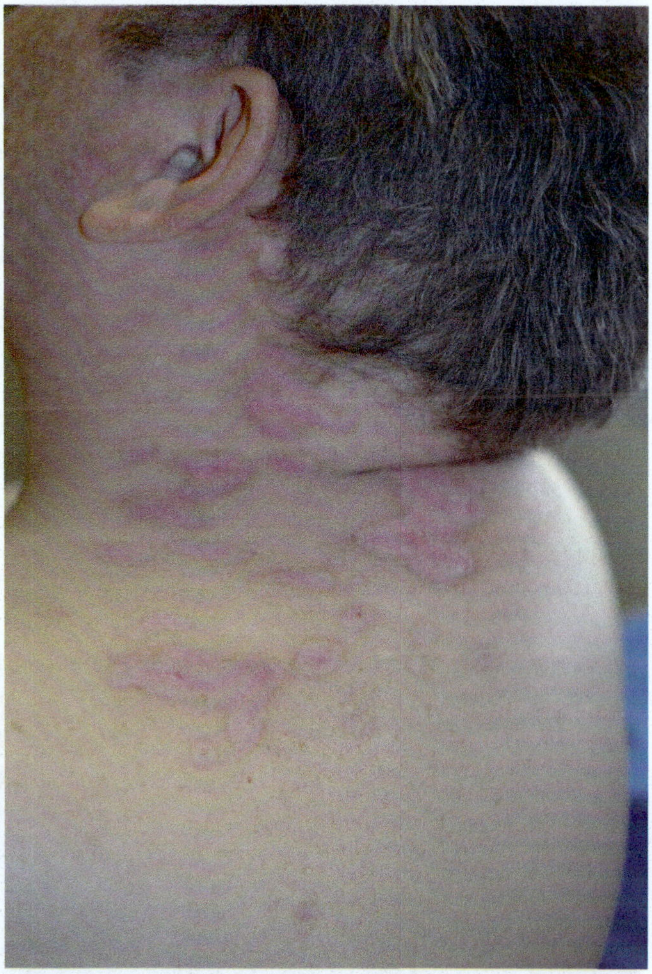

Fig. 8.4 Infiltrated hypopigmented plaques developing at the site of previous herpes zoster

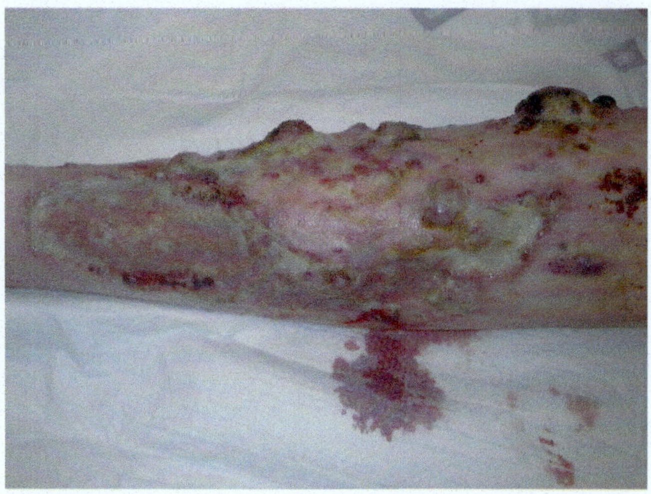

Fig. 8.5 Extensive vascular plaques and tumors developing over the lower extremity, interspersed with large ulcerations at the site of previous plaques, occurring within long-standing sclerotic-type cGVHD and representing the GVHD-angiomatosis phenomenon

Subcutaneous Fat (Panniculitic) cGVHD

The next layer of the integument is the subcutaneous fat or the panniculus. The typical autoimmune or autoinflammatory diseases that affect this area are called panniculitis, with examples such as erythema nodosum, lupus panniculitis, or erythema induratum. Subcutaneous involvement of cGVHD typically has an appearance that would best fit a severe form of lupus panniculitis. The evanescent erythema and indurated patches typical for erythema nodosum are not present; instead, the skin has normal coloration with extensive underlying rippling, resembling a cobblestone appearance or accentuated cellulite. The architecture of the subcutaneous fat consists of numerous lobules that are held in place by fibrous septae that encompass the lobules and provide structure. cGVHD in this setting appears to thicken the septae, resulting in a regularly spaced fat herniations surrounded by tethered septae (Fig. 8.6).

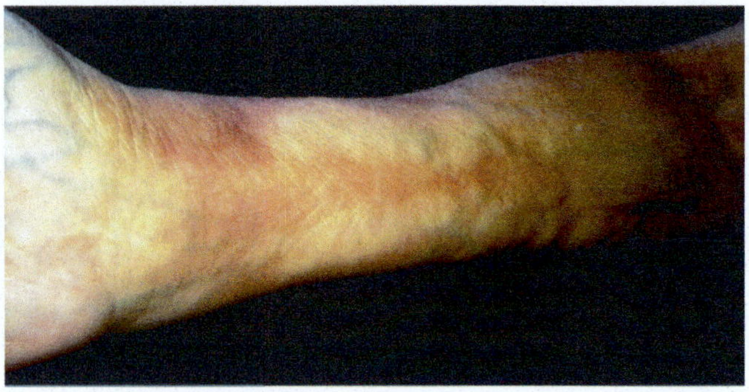

Fig. 8.6 Infiltrated plaques diffusely over the distal arm, with the proximal arm developing a cobblestoning or "pseudocellulite" appearance from the involvement of the subcutaneous fat

Fascial cGVHD

Although the fascia is of musculoskeletal derivation and is not part of the integument, there is often fibrosis adherent to this layer. The prototype autoimmune disease of this level is eosinophilic fasciitis or Shulman syndrome. The fascial disease in cGVHD does not have an age or sex predilection, and the findings may be unnoticed initially except for a subtle groove sign, indicating the tethering of the skin along the tendons (Fig. 8.7). The other signs of involvement include the restricted prayer sign (Fig. 8.8) and the pipestem deformity (Fig. 8.9). This last finding tends to indicate that the disease has progressed to involve not only fascia but full-thickness to the superficial layers of the dermis. At this point, the skin is diffusely infiltrated and immobile from the underlying muscle or bone.

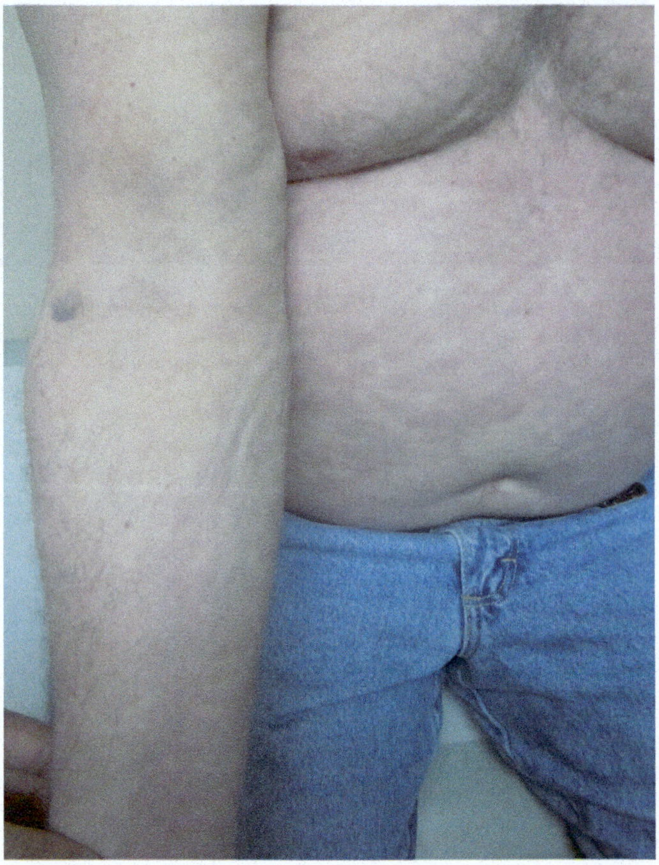

Fig. 8.7 Linear groove over the right forearm flexors, forming the "groove sign" of fascial involvement of sclerotic-type cGVHD

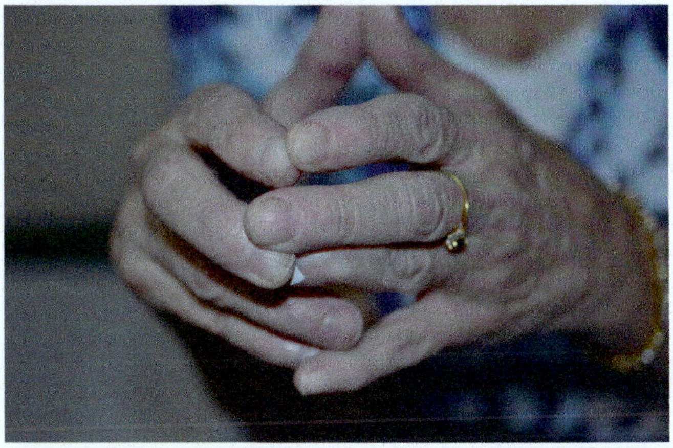

Fig. 8.8 The impaired "prayer sign" preventing the patient from flatly apposing her hands, indicating fascial disease of her forearms

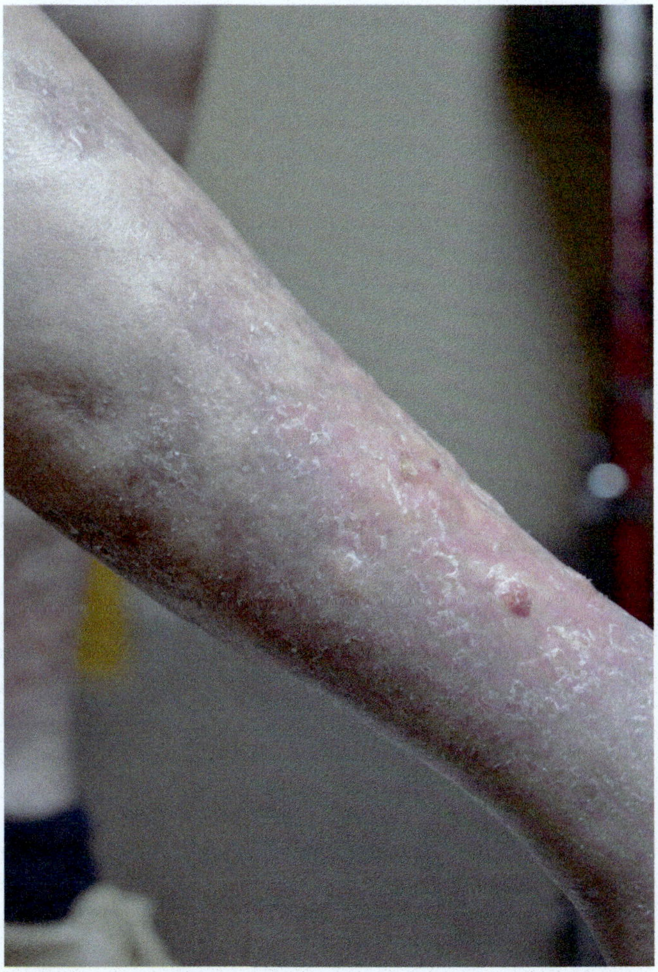

Fig. 8.9 Diffuse involvement over lower extremity from the superficial dermis to the subcutaneous fat and fascia, resulting in the "pipestem" deformity. This patient also has an incidental findings of GVHD angiomatosis

Prognosis

When comparing patients with all forms of cGVHD to those without cGVHD, there is reduced overall and nonrelapse survival [10–12], although mild disease does not appear to impact survival. Consistently, higher mortality has been shown in patients with all types of cGVHD, when comparing severe to mild [13]. When looking at the impact of body surface area involvement in patients with sclerotic-type cGVHD, mortality is higher for those with more extensive sclerotic disease [5].

Although there is an impaired survival rate in patients with moderate or severe sclerotic-type cGVHD, another significant issue is the loss of quality of life (QOL) from associated lung disease, contractures, immobility, pruritus, ulcerations, and pain. Patients with cGVHD have been shown to have an overall QOL similar to patients with other severe autoimmune diseases such as multiple sclerosis, systemic sclerosis, and systemic lupus erythematosus [14]. Studies have shown that about 40 % of patients who develop cGVHD will be on disability or medical leave because of their illness [13]. Specifically, patients with sclerotic-type cGVHD tend to complain of more restriction of movement, loss of grip strength, skin color changes, skin ulcerations, itching, and joint stiffness than patients with other forms of GVHD [5].

Treatment

Treatments can be subdivided into those that are skin-directed and those that are systemic. The ultimate treatment decision will depend on more than just cutaneous involvement, especially if higher-risk organs such as the GI tract, lungs, and liver are also involved. Patients with mild disease may not need treatment; they may be benefiting from some graft-versus-leukemia effect at that stage [15].

Scoring Systems to Determine the Effect of Treatment

One of the difficulties in assessing the prognosis and QOL features is that cGVHD is a multiorgan disease. It is difficult to assess sclerotic-type skin disease alone without the effect of oral, genital, ocular, or lung disease. However, the discussion of treatment efficacy will attempt to focus on studies using cutaneous endpoints.

The most commonly used validation system is the National Institutes of Health (NIH) consensus conference criteria, based on a simple four-point scale to assess a patient for no involvement or mild, moderate, or severe involvement [15]. This system was initially created on the basis of expert opinion, and although it appears very simplistic, developing stronger, organ-specific staging methods has not proved better in predicting disease mortality [16]. As no scales have yet surpassed this system, it is usually used for clinical trials, often supplemented with QOL measurements. The QOL tools typically used are the Lee symptom scale, a validated rating specifically for patients with cGVHD [13], and the SF-36 Short Form Health Survey, among others.

Skin-Directed Therapeutics

Topical Corticosteroids, Vitamin D Analogues, Calcineurin Inhibitors

There are very limited data on topical immune modulators (which have indications for psoriasis and atopic dermatitis), and their expected benefit for patients with deep dermal disease is low, but they do offer the benefit of being inexpensive and generally low-risk. In a case series of 18 patients with cGVHD, 13 of the 18 found a benefit from topical tacrolimus in terms of scaling, pain, or "tightness," but validated response scales were not used and the patients did not necessarily have the sclerotic disease [17]. For patients with superficial dermal disease (*ie*, lichen sclerosus–like disease) topical corticosteroids and calcineurin inhibitors may have a particular benefit. Topical corticosteroids and calcineurin inhibitors are the standard of care for patients with lichen sclerosus. A typical treatment consists of a super-high-potency corticosteroid such as augmented betamethasone dipropionate 0.05 % or clobetasol 0.05 % cream/ointment applied twice daily to the affected area, then transitioning to tacrolimus 0.1 % ointment as the patient improves. The transition to tacrolimus ointment is important, to prevent concerns such as worsening of dermal atrophy, telangiectasias, and development of striae. One should be wary of occluding the tacrolimus ointment for long periods of time or over large surface areas, as systemic absorption has occurred in patients with cGVHD. Using lichen sclerosus as a model, it appears very reasonable to treat patients with superficial cutaneous cGVHD initially with topical immunomodulators. For patients with deeper disease, one can try to use topical immunomodulator to manage the associated pruritus.

Phototherapy

Based on the action spectrum of available phototherapy wavelengths, ultraviolet A (UVA) spectrum with the longer wavelengths (320–400 nm) would appear more effective for deeper disease. To maximize the strength of the UVA and minimize the amount of required time for patients, patients may ingest 8-methoxypsoralen (psoralen + UVA = PUVA or photochemotherapy) or have the same compounded into a 1 % topical ointment to be applied 30–60 min prior to the phototherapy. The other commonly used light spectrum is narrow-band ultraviolet B (nbUVB, 311–313 nm). The advantage of this wavelength is that it is shorter, with a decreased risk of melanoma and nonmelanoma skin cancers. With the shorter wavelength, however, it is generally considered less able to treat deep skin disease. Both treatments work through inactivation of antigen-presenting cells and activated T cells, while building antigen tolerance over time. One side benefit from instituting phototherapy is the reduction in itch, although it generally takes about 2 months for improvement. A systematic review has suggested a benefit from both UVA1 and PUVA for patients being treated for sclerotic-type cGVHD as well as for the prototype diseases—lichen sclerosus, morphea, and eosinophilic fasciitis [18].

Narrow-Band UVB

Studies in cGVHD are only case series, but there is a report of two patients with sclerotic-type cGVHD who noticed a substantial improvement in pruritus and dryness of their skin after 30–40 treatments using nbUVB, without benefit to their deep sclerosis [19]. Conversely, recent reports suggest that at least one patient with sclerotic-type cGVHD has shown improvement from the use of nbUVB, but the cumulative dose energy was twice as much as the previous report [20]. At this time, there is sparse evidence to suggest a benefit for patients with sclerotic forms of cGVHD, but given the low cost, minimal adverse effects, and clear benefit in patients with acute and overlap forms of GVHD, a trial for 2–3 months may be reasonable.

Photochemotherapy/PUVA

The active medicine with this technique is 8-methoxypsoralen, the same chemical used in extracorporeal photopheresis. As mentioned previously, UVA with a longer wavelength penetrates well into the dermis. In patients who had the lichen sclerosus subtype, using PUVA in combination with multiple systemic therapies resulted in some improvement in two patients and significant improvement in three patients treated with 20–160 treatments [21]. Another three patients showed significant objective improvement by depth of fibrosis using PUVA, as did one patient with nbUVB and one with UVA1 [22]. PUVA appears effective for some patients, but even if a strong response is generated, these patients should ensure a follow-up with dermatology at least once yearly, as there is an increased risk of melanoma and nonmelanoma skin cancer.

UVA1

UVA1 is a mid-range wavelength that is administered for sclerotic diseases without concomitant ingestion or application of psoralen. It is used primarily for patients with sclerotic disease such as morphea. The greatest limitation to its use is finding dermatologists who have the device, which tends to be very expensive and requires long treatment sessions. Several single-patient case reports suggest efficacy in highly pretreated patients [22, 23]. Studies have shown complete remission in three of five patients with sclerotic-type cGVHD and partial improvement in two of five patients in an average of 21 sessions [24]. Another study showed that in patients with sclerotic-type disease, all three patients had a partial response to UVA1 treatments, with all being able to reduce their immunosuppression [25].

Non–skin-directed Systemic Therapeutics

Systemic therapeutics are used to suppress graft activity, although the ideal treatment would be one that results in modulation of graft-versus-host activity without loss of the graft-versus-leukemia/lymphoma effect.

Conventional Immunosuppression, Corticosteroids, Steroid-Sparing Immunosuppressants, Calcineurin Inhibitors

High-dose (1 mg/kg) oral corticosteroids and steroid-sparing agents such as mycophenolate mofetil make up the first-line standard of care for patients with moderate or severe cGVHD. If patients improve, then the corticosteroids are weaned. In practice, if the patient's GVHD is skin-predominant, utilizing a skin-directed therapy such as PUVA or UVA1 or an immunomodulator such as extracorporeal photopheresis (ECP) is a reasonable option to help wean systemic corticosteroids. If steroids fail, there is no clear evidence-based escalation. Although steroid-sparing options such as mycophenolate mofetil and cyclosporine are available, studies have shown no treatment benefit for the latter [26] and actually decreased survival for the former [27].

Tacrolimus tends to be the default immunosuppression after transplantation. Its dose is titrated to effect based on whether acute or overlap GVHD develops, but there are reports that sirolimus may be an effective additive. In the initial paper, 8 of 11 patients with sclerotic involvement of their skin responded to therapy with low-therapeutic dosing of sirolimus in combination with their typical immunosuppression [28]. Similarly, in follow-up studies, 70–94 % of patients with sclerotic cGVHD demonstrated some improvement with immunosuppressant regimens inclusive of sirolimus [29, 30]. However, drug interactions, acute kidney injury, and edema may limit its use [31].

Extracorporeal Photopheresis

Extracorporeal photopheresis (ECP) utilizes the same technique as cutaneous photochemotherapy, except that it is performed *ex vivo*. 8-MOP is incubated with the patient's leukocytes prior to UVA irradiation, with the end result of increasing graft tolerance and T-cell regulation systemically.

In patients with severe cGVHD, including 20 with extensive cutaneous lichenoid or sclerotic involvement, a 53 % improvement in scoring measurements was seen, and over 80 % of patients were able to decrease their concomitant immunosuppression [32]. Patients with sclerotic-type cGVHD actually may have a slightly higher response rate to ECP (71 %) when compared with all patients with cutaneous cGVHD (59 %) [33]. In a prospective study, patients were able to decrease their standard immunosuppression and showed significant skin improvement in the nonblinded analysis [34].

Rituximab

There is also evidence for the use of rituximab, a monoclonal CD20 chimeric antibody typically reserved for lymphomas, leukemias, rheumatoid arthritis, and autoimmune blistering diseases. It is dosed in the lymphoma protocol, at 375 mg/m^2 × 4 weeks, a regimen that can be repeated after 3 months. In early studies of eight patients with sclerotic-type cGVHD, clinical improvement was noted in four, including improvement in pulmonary function testing from loosening of the chest wall [35]. Further prospective studies on cutaneous sclerosis have demonstrated a significant clinical response in 27 % of patients, no higher than patients treated with imatinib [36]. Of note, the study used different validated scoring methods than most cGVHD studies. A meta-analysis of rituximab in this setting asserted that cutaneous response rates vary between 0 % and 83 %, but small study sizes and variable outcome measures prevent clear interpretation [37].

Imatinib

Imatinib, a tyrosine kinase inhibitor targeted to the Philadelphia chromosome, has shown abilities to modulate transforming growth factor–β and platelet-derived growth factor. It is typically dosed at 400 mg daily in adults. Although it demonstrated substantial cutaneous improvement in several early case series, it demonstrated only 30–35 % partial response in larger case series of patients with sclerotic-type cGVHD [38, 39]. When compared prospectively with rituximab, the rate of a significant clinical response in the skin was only 26 % [36].

Ruxolitinib

Ruxolitinib, a selective JAK1/JAK2 inhibitor approved for use in myelofibrosis and polycythemia vera, has recently become a new agent for cGVHD treatment. Overall, the data are sparse. An early preclinical study [40] led to a prospective trial demonstrating an 85 % overall response rate [41], but the response rate differed from rates in previous studies and was based on the ability to taper steroids and systemic immunosuppression by 50 %. No clear specifics were given on the form of cutaneous cGVHD treated.

Low-Dose Interleukin-2

There is evidence for increased immune tolerance to decrease the activity of cGVHD through the use of low-dose interleukin-2 infusions [42, 43]. In the studies, slightly under 50 % demonstrated some improvement in their skin, subcutaneous tissue, and underlying fascia [44]. Unfortunately, this treatment is very expensive and time-consuming for patients.

Ibrutinib

Ibrutinib is an oral medication that is a first-in-class inhibitor of bruton tyrosine kinase (BTK) and IL-2–inducible T-cell kinase (ITK). It has showed efficacy in multiple preclinical studies [45, 46]. Clinical trials are currently under way to asses its efficacy for cGVHD.

Pathology

Histopathology

For the diagnosis of sclerotic-type cGVHD, tissue confirmation is not typically necessary. The disease is most often a late finding associated with previous forms of GVHD, and the clinical findings at this stage are almost pathognomonic in this setting. If histopathology is performed, thickening of collagen bundles throughout the superficial, deep, or entire dermis; panniculitis (inflammation of subcutaneous fat); and fibrous thickening of the fascia with surrounding inflammation of fat and septae are all considered specific criteria for sclerotic-type cGVHD [47]. Follicular plugging and some vacuolar degeneration of the basal keratinocytes may still be present, particularly in the lichen sclerosus variant [48].

In this setting of sclerotic disease, the GVHD-angiomatosis phenomenon may occur within sclerotic plaques. A biopsy in this case would demonstrate an extensive endothelial proliferation with surrounding fibrosis, sometimes with an associated lobular endothelial protrusion and a surrounding epithelial collarette. Intravascular papillary endothelial hyperplasia and thromboses may be seen within dilated channels [9] (Fig. 8.10).

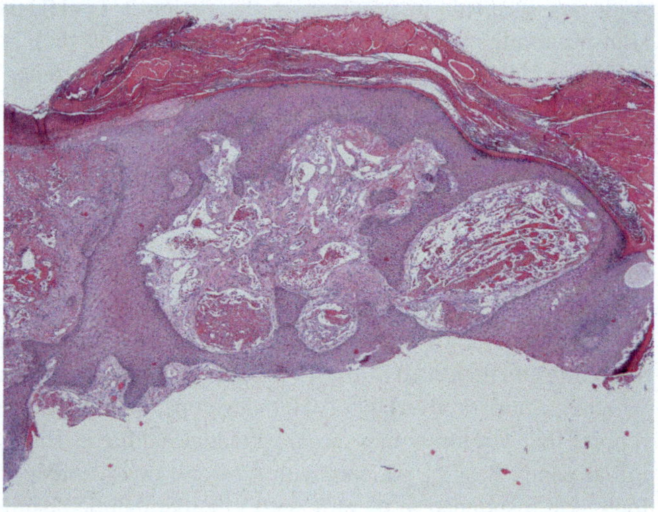

Fig. 8.10 Low-power pathology of a GVHD-angiomatosis finding on the lower extremity, demonstrating extensive endothelial proliferation and vessels of varying sizes, with a surrounding collarette of epidermis and an overlying serum crust (H&E, 40×)

Immunophenotype and Molecular Findings

There usually is a sparse infiltrate with extensive collagen deposition. The sclerotic form appears to be driven by a Th1 phenotype with additional upregulation of interferon-γ, CXCR9, CXCL10, and CCL5 [49].

The endothelial cells typical of this type of sclerosis tend to demonstrate a full component of normal endothelial surface expression markers [46]. Chimerism has been shown within the epidermal, endothelial, and fibroblast cells, with a substantial proportion donor-derived [50, 51]. In patients with GVHD angiomatosis, it does appear that the endothelial proliferation is of donor origin [52] (Fig. 8.11).

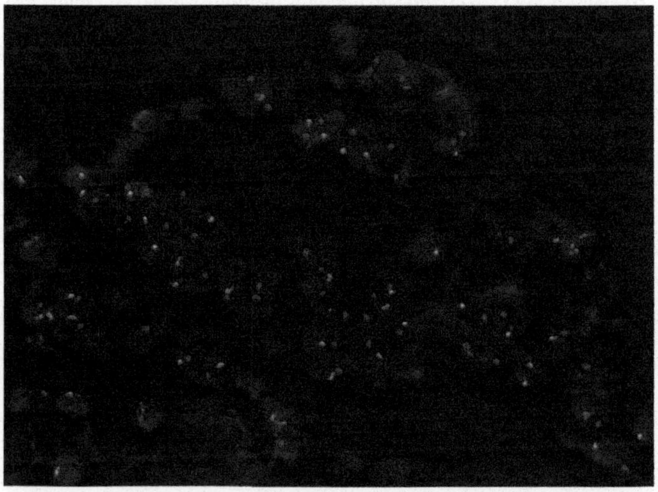

Fig. 8.11 High-power fluorescence in situ hybridization (FISH) demonstrating anastomosing endothelial cells underlying the epidermis with a Y chromosome (*red*) in a female patient with GVHD angiomatosis and a sex-mismatched donor. The X chromosome is green (400×).

Differential Diagnosis

The diagnosis is based on clinical presentation, previous history of GVHD, and rarely a biopsy. The most important features are recognizing that the patient had an allogeneic HSCT with the onset of the skin induration. The deep forms of sclerosis are very easy to recognize. The superficial stage sometimes can require looking at other specific features, including follicular plugging, locations such as flexural surfaces on the body, or involvement in areas of low-grade trauma or friction.

Lichen Sclerosus, Morphea, Systemic Sclerosis, Lupus Panniculitis, Eosinophilic Fasciitis

As mentioned above, sclerotic-type cGVHD can mimic all these prototype autoimmune skin diseases. With that being said, if these diseases occur after transplantation, they would be recognized as clinical variants of cGVHD.

Nephrogenic Systemic Fibrosis

It is possible that a toxic exposure can result in similar sclerotic findings. Nephrogenic systemic fibrosis occurs from gadolinium deposition when patients undergo a contrast MRI in the setting of acute or chronic kidney disease, but it is now seen much less often because of aggressive screening for kidney disease in patients receiving MRIs. The disease typically presents with varying degrees of superficial to deep infiltration, ranging from superficial *peau-d'orange*–like plaques over the extremities to the deep cobblestoning of subcutaneous involvement. Contractures and an impaired prayer sign may also occur, just as in sclerotic-type cGVHD. Over time, the skin develops a firmer, "woody" induration of the area. Gadolinium is detectable in skin biopsy specimens, by scanning electron micrograph, or by mass spectroscopy [53]. The most critical differentiating factor, however, is the presence of renal failure in combination with a contrast MRI.

Toxic Oil Syndromes

Toxic oil syndromes have occurred unpredictably throughout the past century, involving substances such as jet aircraft oil in the 1950s, contaminated rice oil in the 1960s, and contaminated rapeseed oil in the 1980s. All these epidemics contained different contaminants and may have been presented as typical food oils [54]. When these syndromes occur, patients may notice a rapid onset of myalgias, dyspnea, and a striking eosinophilia with an abrupt development that would be atypical for cGVHD. Over time, fascial tightening and sclerosis are noted, which can be similar to cGVHD. These diseases are extremely unlikely but might be reasonable to consider in the setting of a rapid onset of myalgias and marked eosinophilia.

Vascular Tumors

The GVHD-angiomatosis phenomenon may be confused for pyogenic granulomas, cavernous hemangiomas, and atypical vascular lesions that following radiation exposure. However, GVHD angiomatosis develops solely within areas of preexisting sclerotic-type cGVHD. Otherwise, without proper clinical context, biopsy specimens could very well be read as a pyogenic granuloma, cavernous hemangioma, or another endothelial growth [9]. If a biopsy is performed, no endothelial cell atypia is found, which should rule out atypical vascular lesions and angiosarcomas [55].

Conclusion

This case highlights the late onset of acute GVHD, the insidious development of sclerotic-type cGVHD, difficulty in treating patients with cGVHD, and the development of GVHD angiomatosis within the areas of sclerosis. Unfortunately, patients will often notice a nonspecific edema prior to the development of the sclerotic findings. In this treatment setting, there is no clear second-line therapeutic option behind corticosteroids. After the failure of steroids and steroid-sparing agents, ECP and rituximab also failed. Sirolimus did appear to result in disease stability, but she already had extensive cGVHD of the skin. Based on this patient and many others like her, better therapeutic options are needed. The ideal treatment would not only arrest the development of further cGVHD but also target the inactive fibrosis that is the hallmark of the deep cutaneous forms of cGVHD.

References

1. Carlens S, Ringdén O, Remberger M, Lönnqvist B, Hägglund H, Klaesson S, et al. Risk factors for chronic graft-versus-host disease after bone marrow transplantation: a retrospective single centre analysis. Bone Marrow Transplant. 1998;22:755–61.
2. Atkinson BK, Horowitz MM, Gale RP, Bekkum DW, Van GE, RA G, et al. Risk factors for chronic graft-versus-host disease after HLA-identical sibling bone marrow transplantation. Blood. 1990;75:2459–64.
3. Hymes SR, Alousi AM, Cowen EW. Graft-versus-host disease: part I. Pathogenesis and clinical manifestations of graft-versus-host disease. J Am Acad Dermatol 2012;66:515.e1–18.
4. Inamoto Y, Storer BE, Petersdorf EW, Nelson JL, Lee SJ, Carpenter PA, et al. Incidence, risk factors, and outcomes of sclerosis in patients with chronic graft-versus-host disease. Blood. 2013;121:5098–103.
5. Martires KJ, Baird K, Steinberg SM, Grkovic L, Joe GO, Williams KM, et al. Sclerotic-type chronic GVHD of the skin: clinical risk factors, laboratory markers, and burden of disease. Blood. 2011;118:4250–7.
6. Martires KJ, Baird K, Citrin DE, Hakim FT, Pavletic SZ, Cowen EW. Localization of sclerotic-type chronic graft-vs-host disease to sites of skin injury. Arch Dermatol. 2011;147:1081–6.
7. Mehra T, Metzler G, Bauer J, Köberle M, Garbe C. Isotopic response of graft versus host disease following herpes zoster infection: case report and review of the literature. Acta Derm Venereol. 2012;92:383–4.
8. Spalek M, Jonska-Gmyrek J, Gałecki J. Radiation-induced morphea – a literature review. J Eur Acad Dermatol Venereol. 2015;29:197–202.
9. Kaffenberger BH, Zuo RC, Gru A, Plotner AN, Sweeney SA, Devine SM, et al. Graft-versus-host disease-associated angiomatosis: a clinicopathologically distinct entity. J Am Acad Dermatol. 2014;71:745–53.
10. Jacobsohn D, Kurland BF, Pidala J, Inamoto Y, Chai X, Palmer JM, et al. Correlation between NIH composite skin score, patient-reported skin score, and outcome: results from the chronic GVHD consortium. Blood. 2012;120:2545–52.
11. Lee SJ. Severity of chronic graft-versus-host disease: association with treatment-related mortality and relapse. Blood. 2002;100:406–14.
12. Pidala J, Kim J, Anasetti C, Nishihori T, Betts B, Field T, et al. The global severity of chronic graft-versus-host disease, determined by National Institutes of Health consensus criteria, is associated with overall survival and non-relapse mortality. Haematologica. 2011;96:1678–84.
13. Lee SK, Cook EF, Soiffer R, Antin JH. Development and validation of a scale to measure symptoms of chronic graft-versus-host disease. Biol Blood Marrow Transplant. 2002;8:444–52.
14. Pidala J, Kurland B, Chai X, Majhail N, Weisdorf DJ, Pavletic S, et al. Patient-reported quality of life is associated with severity of chronic graft-versus-host disease as measured by NIH criteria: report on baseline data from the chronic GVHD consortium. Blood. 2011;117:4651–7.
15. Filipovich AH, Weisdorf D, Pavletic S, Socie G, Wingard JR, Lee SJ, et al. National Institutes of Health consensus development project on criteria for clinical trials in chronic graft-versus-host disease: I. Diagnosis and staging working group report. Biol Blood Marrow Transplant. 2005;11:945–56.
16. Inamoto Y, Martin PJ, Storer BE, Palmer J, Weisdorf DJ, Pidala J, et al. Association of severity of organ involvement with mortality and recurrent malignancy in patients with chronic graft-versus-host disease. Haematologica. 2014;99:1618–23.
17. Choi CJ, Nghiem P. Tacrolimus ointment in the treatment of chronic cutaneous graft-vs-host disease: a case series of 18 patients. Arch Dermatol. 2001;137:1202–6.
18. Breuckmann F, Gambichler T, Altmeyer P, Kreuter AUVA. UVA1 phototherapy and PUVA photochemotherapy in connective tissue diseases and related disorders: a research based review. BMC Dermatol. 2004;4:11.
19. Enk CD, Elad S, Vexler A, Kapelushnik J, Gorodetsky R, Kirschbaum M. Chronic graft-versus-host disease treated with UVB phototherapy. Bone Marrow Transplant. 1998;22:1179–83.
20. Sorenson E, McAndrew R, Patel V, Logan AC, Koo J, Levin E. Narrowband UV-B phototherapy for steroid-refractory sclerotic chronic cutaneous graft-vs-host disease. JAMA Dermatol. 2015;151:635.
21. Schaffer JV, McNiff JM, Seropian S, Cooper DL, Bolognia JL. Lichen sclerosus and eosinophilic fasciitis as manifestations of chronic graft-versus-host disease: Expanding the sclerodermoid spectrum. J Am Acad Dermatol. 2005;53:591–601.
22. Gottlöber P, Leiter U, Friedrich W, Bunjes D, Schulz A, Kerscher M, Peter RU. Chronic cutaneous sclerodermoid graft-versus-host

disease: evaluation by 20-MHz sonography. J Eur Acad Dermatol Venereol. 2003;17:402–7.
23. Grundmann-Kollmann M, Behrens S, Gruss C, Gottlöber P, Peter R, Kerscher M. Chronic sclerodermic graft-versus-host disease refractory to immunosuppressive treatment responds to UVA1 phototherapy. J Am Acad Dermatol. 2000;42:134–6.
24. Pinton P, Porta F, Izzi T, Venturini M, Capezzera R, Zane C, et al. Prospects for ultraviolet A1 phototherapy as a treatment for chronic cutaneous graft-versus-host disease. Haematologica. 2003;88:1169–75.
25. Wetzig T, Sticherling M, Simon JC, Hegenbart U, Niederwieser D, Al-Ali HK. Medium dose long-wavelength ultraviolet A (UVA1) phototherapy for the treatment of acute and chronic graft-versus-host disease of the skin. Bone Marrow Transplant. 2005;35:515–9.
26. Koc S, Leisenring W, Flowers ME, Anasetti C, Deeg HJ, Nash RA, et al. Therapy for chronic graft-versus-host disease: a randomized trial comparing cyclosporine plus prednisone versus prednisone alone. Blood. 2002;100:48–51.
27. Martin P, Storer B, Rowley S, Flowers M, Lee S, Carpenter P, et al. Evaluation of mycophenolate mofetil for initial treatment of chronic graft-versus-host disease. Blood. 2009;113:5074–82.
28. Couriel DR, Saliba R, Escalón MP, Hsu Y, Ghosh S, Ippoliti C, et al. Sirolimus in combination with tacrolimus and corticosteroids for the treatment of resistant chronic graft-versus-host disease. Br J Haematol. 2005;130:409–17.
29. Jurado M, Vallejo C, Pérez-Simón J, Brunet S, Ferra C, Balsalobre P, et al. Sirolimus as part of immunosuppressive therapy for refractory chronic graft-versus-host disease. Biol Blood Marrow Transplant. 2007;13:701–6.
30. Jedlickova Z, Burlakova I, Bug G, Baurmann H, Schwerdtfeger R, Schleuning M. Therapy of sclerodermatous chronic graft-versus-host disease with mammalian target of rapamycin inhibitors. Biol Blood Marrow Transplant. 2011;17:657–63.
31. Johnston LJ, Brown J, Shizuru JA, Stockerl-Goldstein KE, Stuart MJ, Blume KG, et al. Rapamycin (sirolimus) for treatment of chronic graft-versus-host disease. Biol Blood Marrow Transplant. 2005;11:47–55.
32. Seaton ED, Szydlo RM, Kanfer E, Apperley JF, Russell-Jones R. Influence of extracorporeal photopheresis on clinical and laboratory parameters in chronic graft-versus-host disease and analysis of predictors of response. Blood. 2003;102:1217–23.
33. Couriel DR, Hosing C, Saliba R, Shpall EJ, Anderlini P, Rhodes B, et al. Extracorporeal photochemotherapy for the treatment of steroid-resistant chronic GVHD. Blood. 2006;107:3074–80.
34. Flowers ME, Apperley JF, van Besien K, Elmaagacli A, Grigg A, Reddy V, et al. A multicenter prospective phase 2 randomized study of extracorporeal photopheresis for treatment of chronic graft-versus-host disease. Blood. 2008;112:2667–74.
35. Ratanatharathorn V, Ayash L, Reynolds C, Silver S, Reddy P, Becker M, et al. Treatment of chronic graft-versus-host disease with anti-CD20 chimeric monoclonal antibody. Biol Blood Marrow Transplant. 2003;9:505–11.
36. Arai S, Pidala J, Pusic I, Chai X, Jaglowski S, Khera N, et al. A randomized phase II crossover study of imatinib or rituximab for cutaneous sclerosis after hematopoietic cell transplantation. Clin Cancer Res. 2016;22:319–27.
37. Kharfan-Dabaja MA, Mhaskar AR, Djulbegovic B, Cutler C, Mohty M, Kumar A. Efficacy of rituximab in the setting of steroid-refractory chronic graft-versus-host disease: a systematic review and meta-analysis. Biol Blood Marrow Transplant. 2009;15:1005–13.
38. Baird K, Comis LE, Joe GO, Steinberg SM, Hakim FT, Rose JJ, et al. Imatinib mesylate for the treatment of steroid-refractory sclerotic-type cutaneous chronic graft-versus-host disease. Biol Blood Marrow Transplant. 2015;21:1083–90.
39. de Masson A, Bouaziz JD, Peffault de Latour R, Wittnebel S, Ribaud P, Rubio MT, et al. Limited efficacy and tolerance of imatinib mesylate in steroid-refractory sclerodermatous chronic GVHD. Blood. 2012;120:5089–90.
40. Choi J, Cooper ML, Alahmari B, Ritchey J, Collins L, Holt M, et al. Pharmacologic blockade of JAK1/JAK2 reduces GvHD and preserves the graft-versus-leukemia effect. PLoS One. 2014;9:e109799.
41. Zeiser R, Burchert A, Lengerke C, Verbeek M, Maas-Bauer K, Metzelder SK, et al. Ruxolitinib in corticosteroid-refractory graft-versus-host disease after allogeneic stem cell transplantation: a multicenter survey. Leukemia. 2015;29:2062–8.
42. Matsuoka K, Koreth J, Kim HT, Bascug G, McDonough S, Kawano Y, et al. Low-dose interleukin-2 therapy restores regulatory T cell homeostasis in patients with chronic graft-versus-host disease. Sci Transl Med. 2013;5:179ra43.
43. Koreth J, Matsuoka K, Kim HT, McDonough SM, Bindra B, Alyea EP 3rd, et al. Interleukin-2 and regulatory T cells in graft-versus-host disease. N Engl J Med 2011;365(22):2055–2066.
44. Svensson LG, Ph D, Tuzcu EM, Webb JG, Fontana GP, Makkar RR, et al. Interleukin-2 and regulatory T cells in graft-versus-host disease. N Engl J Med. 2011;365:2055–66.
45. Dubovsky JA, Flynn R, Du J, Harrington BK, Zhong Y, Kaffenberger B, et al. Ibrutinib treatment ameliorates murine chronic graft-versus-host disease. J Clin Invest. 2014;124:4867–76.
46. Schutt SD, Fu J, Nguyen H, Bastian D, Heinrichs J, Wu Y, et al. Inhibition of BTK and ITK with ibrutinib is effective in the prevention of chronic graft- versus-host disease in mice. PLoS One. 2015;10:e0137641.
47. Shulman HM, Kleiner D, Lee SJ, Morton T, Pavletic SZ, Farmer E, et al. Histopathologic diagnosis of chronic graft-versus-host disease: National Institutes of Health consensus development project on criteria for clinical trials in chronic graft-versus-host disease: II. Pathology working group report. Biol Blood Marrow Transplant. 2006;12:31–47.
48. Penas PF, Jones-Caballero M, Aragues M, Fernandez-Herrera J, Fraga J, Garcia-Diez A. Sclerodermatous graft-vs-host disease. Arch Dermatol. 2002;138:924–34.
49. Bruggen MC, Klein I, Greinix H, Bauer W, Kuzmina Z, Rabitsch W, et al. Diverse T-cell responses characterize the different manifestations of cutaneous graft-versus-host disease. Blood. 2014;123:290–9.
50. Willemze AJ, Bakker AC, von dem Borne PA, Bajema IM, Vossen JM. The effect of graft-versus-host disease on skin endothelial and epithelial cell chimerism in stem-cell transplant recipients. Transplantation. 2009;87:1096–101.
51. Ogawa Y, Kodama H, Kameyama K, Yamazaki K, Yasuoka H, Okamoto S, et al. Donor fibroblast chimerism in the pathogenic fibrotic lesion of human chronic graft-versus-host disease. Investig Ophthalmol Vis Sci. 2005;46:4519–27.
52. Kaffenberger BH, Zhang E, Duncan JR, Jaglowski S, Klisovic RB, Devine SM, et al. Endothelial chimerism in chronic sclerotic-type chronic graft-versus-host disease and GVHD-associated angiomatosis. Br J Dermatol 2016. doi:10.1111/bjd.14484 [Epub ahead of print].
53. High WA, Ayers RA, Chandler J, Zito G, Cowper SE. Gadolinium is detectable within the tissue of patients with nephrogenic systemic fibrosis. J Am Acad Dermatol. 2007;56:21–6.
54. Posada de la Paz M, Philen RM, Borda AI. Toxic oil syndrome: the perspective after 20 years. Epidemiol Rev. 2001;23:231–47.
55. Lucas DR. Angiosarcoma, radiation-associated angiosarcoma, and atypical vascular lesion. Arch Pathol Lab Med. 2009;133:1804–9.

9 Pediatric Graft-Versus-Host Disease

Valerie Carlberg, Emily Simons, Sophia Delano, and Jennifer T. Huang

Children undergo hematopoietic stem cell transplantation (HSCT) for a variety of reasons: hematologic malignancies, select visceral organ malignancies, bone marrow failures, immunodeficiencies, metabolic disorders, autoimmune disorders, and other life-threatening conditions [1, 2]. In 2013, 13 % of HSCT patients in the United States were younger than 21 years of age [3]. As in adults, acute and chronic graft-versus-host disease (GVHD) are among the most important causes of nonrelapse mortality in children after HSCT. Most GVHD literature focuses on adult patients, however, and is not universally applicable to pediatric patients. This chapter focuses on unique characteristics of acute and chronic GVHD in children, highlighting both what is known and what is yet to be understood about these complex diseases.

V. Carlberg
Department of Dermatology, School of Medicine, Oregon Health and Science University, 3181 SW Sam Jackson Park Road, Portland, OR, USA
e-mail: carlbergv@ohsu.edu

E. Simons
Dermatology Program, Boston Children's Hospital, 300 Longwood Avenue, Boston, MA, USA
e-mail: emily.simons@hms.harvard.edu

S. Delano
Division of Dermatology, Department of Medicine, University of Massachusetts Medical School, 55 North Lake Avenue, Worcester, MA, USA
e-mail: sophia.delano@umassmed.edu

J.T. Huang (✉)
Department of Dermatology, Harvard Medical School, Dermatology Program, Boston Children's Hospital, Fegan 6, Dermatology Program, 300 Longwood Avenue, Boston, MA, USA
e-mail: jennifer.huang@childrens.harvard.edu

Acute Graft-Versus-Host Disease in Pediatric Patients

Introduction to Acute GVHD

Acute GVHD is one of the most common and serious complications following HSCT in pediatric patients; it primarily affects the skin, liver, and gastrointestinal tract. There are many similarities between pediatric and adult GVHD, but several variables in pediatric patients contribute to unique clinical features, diagnostic criteria, and treatment of pediatric acute GVHD.

Incidence of Acute GVHD

Pediatric patients have a lower incidence of acute GVHD than adults. Decreased incidence may be attributed to more frequent use of cord blood as a stem cell source, nonmalignant indications for transplantation, limited history of prior infections, and overall improved state of health in children [2]. The incidence of grade II–IV acute GVHD ranges from 40 to 85 % depending on the degree of HLA mismatch in children receiving unrelated bone marrow transplantation, and is about 27 % in those receiving grafts from HLA-identical siblings [4–7]. There is greater tolerance of the same degree of HLA mismatch in cord blood transplants over bone marrow transplants, with the reported incidence of acute GVHD ranging from 19 to 41 % [2, 8, 9]. T-cell–depleted grafts also decrease the incidence of acute GVHD, with an incidence of 19 % in one study [8].

J.A. Cotliar (ed.), *Atlas of Graft-versus-Host Disease*, DOI 10.1007/978-3-319-46952-2_9

Risk Factors for Acute GVHD

As in adults, the most significant risk factor for acute GVHD in pediatric patients is HLA mismatch between donor and recipient. Additional clinical, genetic, and biomarker-based risk factors have been postulated in both patient populations (Table 9.1).

Table 9.1 Potential risk factors for acute GVHD in pediatric patients

Host variables
Recipient age <1 or >10 years [10]
Malignancy as indication for transplant, as well as features of more advanced disease (WBC >50 × 10^9/L and cytogenetic abnormalities t(4;11), t(9;22), and hypodiploidy) [2, 6, 10–12]
Prior damage to gut (viral illness, prolonged fasting) [12]
Donor or graft variables
HLA mismatch [2]
Use of unrelated donor [2]
ABO blood group mismatch [2]
Older donor age (>8) [11, 13, 14]
Female multiparous donor to male recipient [11, 13]
Graft stem cell source (PBSC > BM > UCB) [4, 11]
Graft with high CD34+ cell dose or low regulatory T-cell content [12]
Other variables
Conditioning with total body irradiation [2, 6, 11, 12]
Single-agent GVHD prophylaxis [12, 14]
Genetic polymorphisms within genes encoding for innate immunity, or inflammatory/immunoregulatory proteins in either donor or host [12]

BM bone marrow, *GVHD* graft-versus-host disease, *HLA* human leukocyte antigen, *PBSC* peripheral blood stem cell, *UCB* unrelated cord blood, *WBC* white blood cell

Clinical Features of Acute GVHD

Although acute GVHD most often occurs within 1–2 months after HSCT [6, 15], the diagnosis can be made at any point after transplantation. Because time-based criteria are currently less emphasized, there is a greater emphasis on clinical features in making the diagnosis of acute GVHD [10, 15, 16].

Acute GVHD most commonly targets the skin, liver, and gastrointestinal tract [1, 17]. The skin is the most frequently affected organ and is often the first involved [15]. The classic rash is pruritic, may be painful, and is characterized by erythematous macules and papules coalescing on the trunk and extremities (often sparing the scalp), resembling the morbilliform rash of measles (Fig. 9.1). Acral involvement is common (Figs. 9.2 and 9.3). In severe GVHD, bullae and desquamation may develop, and with extensive involvement, may resemble toxic epidermal necrolysis (TEN) (Figs. 9.4 and 9.5). Gastrointestinal symptoms include nausea, vomiting, anorexia, abdominal pain, and diarrhea [15].

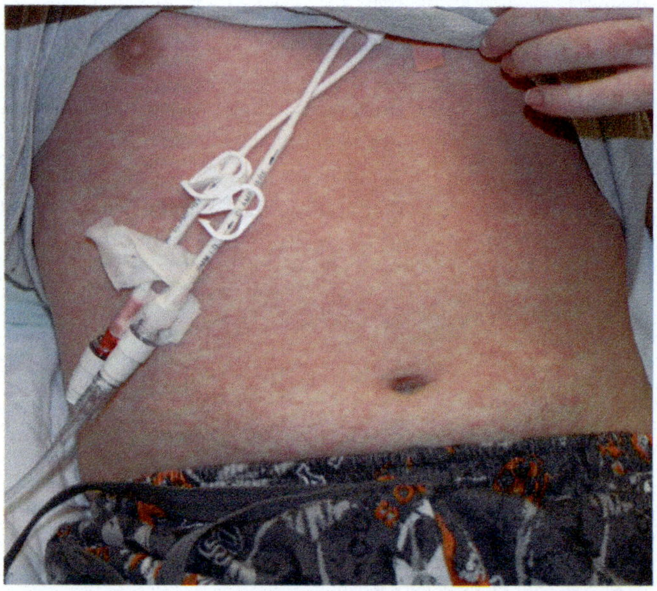

Fig. 9.1 Acute GVHD presenting as a morbilliform skin eruption

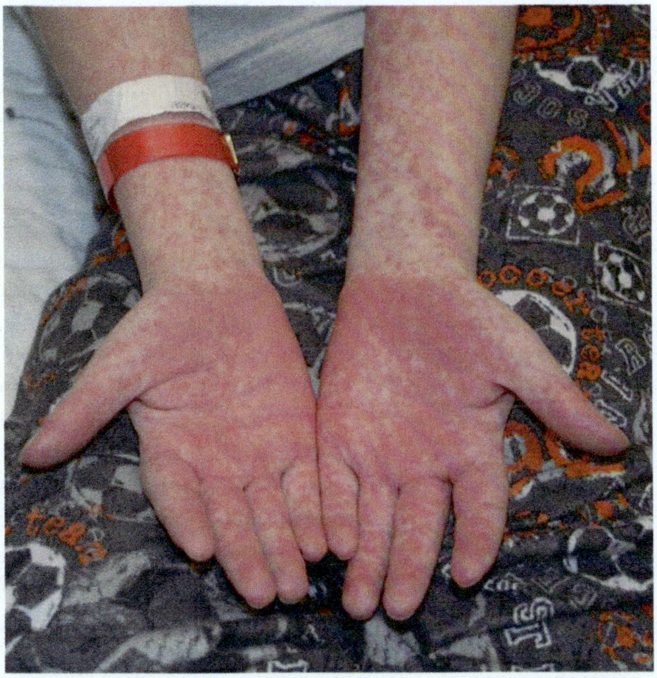

Fig. 9.2 Acral involvement in acute GVHD

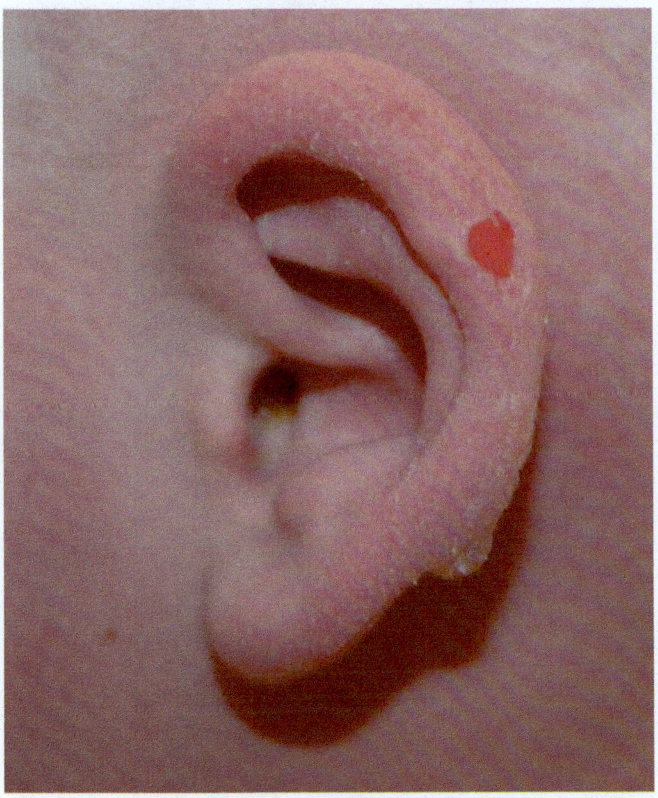

Fig. 9.3 Acral involvement (ear) in acute GVHD

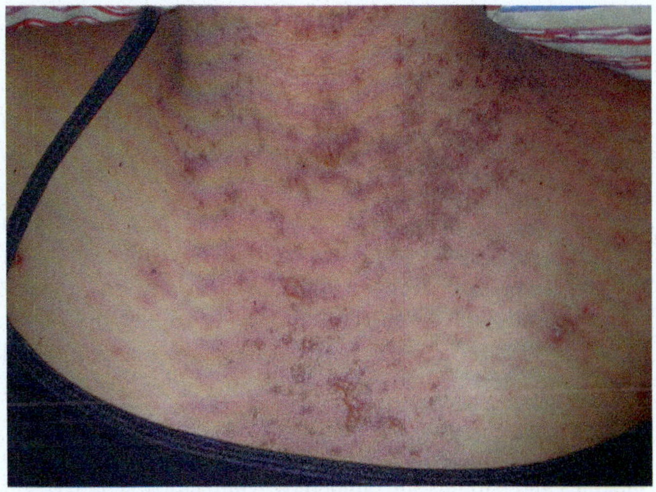

Fig. 9.4 Bullous lesions are a poor prognostic sign in acute GVHD

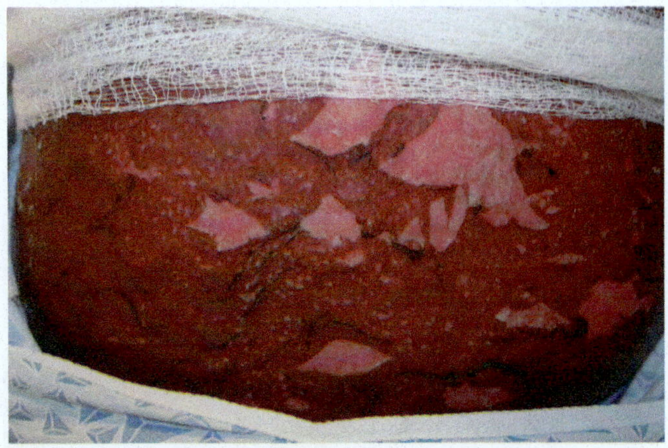

Fig. 9.5 Toxic epidermal necrolysis–like acute GVHD

Differential Diagnosis for Acute GVHD

The differential diagnosis for acute GVHD includes bacterial/viral exanthem, engraftment syndrome, toxic erythema of chemotherapy, drug hypersensitivity reaction, and radiation recall dermatitis [1, 2].

Infectious exanthema occur more commonly in children [18] and solid-organ transplant and HSCT recipients are at increased risk for HHV6 and HHV7 reactivation, making infectious etiologies important to consider. Signs and symptoms of infection typically accompany the classic childhood exanthems, and the distribution and evolution of the rash may be helpful in differentiating these from acute GVHD. The viral exanthem of HHV6 is characterized by erythematous macules and papules surrounded by white halos, which begin on the trunk and spread to the neck and proximal extremities. It is accompanied by high fever (101–106 °F) and resolves over several days [18].

Engraftment syndrome occurs within days of granulocyte recovery and is characterized by fever >38.3 °C without a source of infection, rash over more than 25 % of body surface area that is not attributable to medication, and pulmonary edema [19]. Toxic erythema of chemotherapy (TEC) is a spectrum of cutaneous reactions to chemotherapeutic agents, most commonly presenting with erythema and tenderness of the palms, soles, and flexural regions including the axillae and groin (Fig. 9.6) [20]. There may be an increased incidence of TEC with conditioning regimens composed of busulfan and fludarabine, with a median onset of 22 days after dose administration [21].

Drug hypersensitivity reactions to non-chemotherapeutic agents should also be considered, although they tend to occur more in adults. Drug reactions typically occur within 1–14 days of initiating a drug, manifesting as a morbilliform rash on the trunk, which spreads to the extremities and less commonly involves the face, palms, or soles. Radiation recall dermatitis should also be considered in the setting of total body irradiation or recent history of sunburn followed by methotrexate for GVHD prophylaxis (Fig. 9.7).

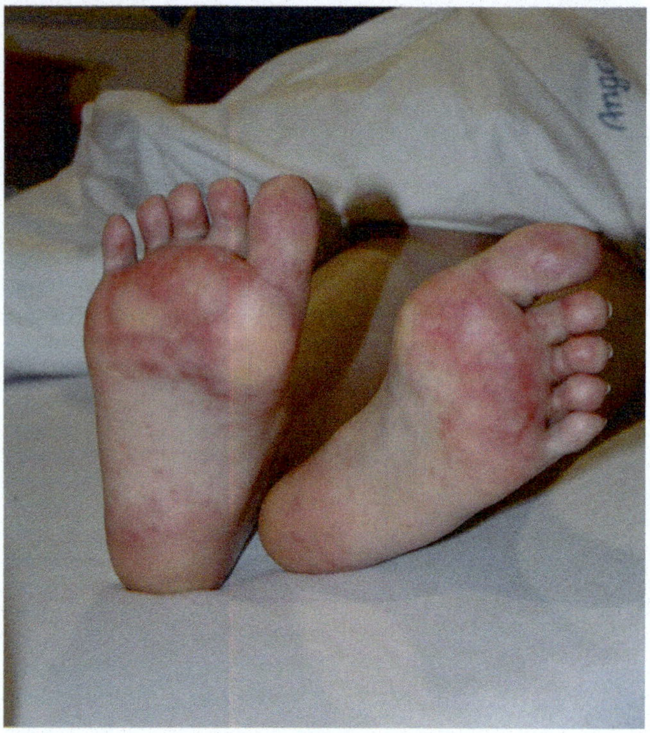

Fig. 9.6 Toxic erythema of chemotherapy presenting as tender, erythematous nodules on acral surfaces

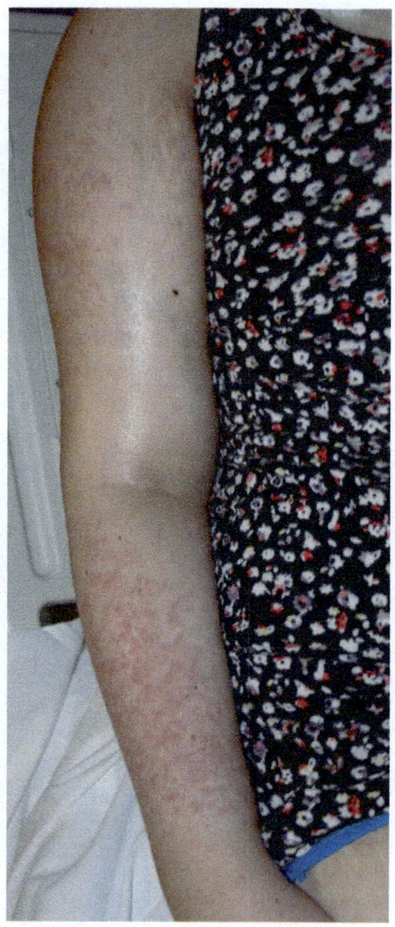

Fig. 9.7 Radiation recall dermatitis in a child with prior history of sunburn folowed by methotrexate for GVHD prophylaxis

Histopathology and Laboratory Evaluation of Acute GVHD

Though skin biopsies may confirm a diagnosis of acute GVHD if clinical suspicion is high, the histologic findings are nonspecific. Histologic findings include sparse lymphocytic interface and perivascular inflammation with variable degrees of adnexal extension. Dyskeratosis, spongiosis, lymphocytic exocytosis, and satellitosis may also be present. In addition to lymphocytic infiltration, eosinophils may be noted, making it difficult to distinguish acute GVHD from drug hypersensitivity reactions. In more severe acute GVHD, subepidermal clefting and full-thickness epidermal necrosis may be seen, mimicking toxic epidermal necrolysis [22, 23]. Many of the differential diagnoses show similar features, making biopsy unhelpful or misleading if wrongly interpreted [24–29]. Thus, clinical observation is key in making an accurate diagnosis, with close attention paid to time course, evolution of disease, and response to withdrawal of a potential offending agent.

Laboratory evaluation shows hyperbilirubinemia and may show transaminitis [15]. Viral serologies may be helpful for suspected viral exanthema [18].

Classification of Acute GVHD

Proper classification of acute GVHD is important, as this largely directs therapy. In 1974, Glucksberg devised the original staging system for acute GVHD, which was later modified during the Keystone Conference in 1994 [30]. The Keystone staging attempted to classify acute GVHD based upon the extent of skin, liver, and gut involvement, but the staging of pediatric gut GVHD was not discussed during the Keystone Conference, and stool output varies considerably between children and adults. The current proposal set forth by the University of Michigan and now utilized by the Mount Sinai Acute GVHD International Consortium redefines the Keystone criteria based on volume of diarrhea per kilogram of body weight, rather than absolute volume (Table 9.2) [32]. An additional consideration when staging pediatric acute GVHD is the difference in the distribution of body surface area between adults and children, as children have larger heads and smaller extremities than adults.

Table 9.2 Staging and grading of acute GVHD in children

Stage	Skin	Liver (bilirubin)	Upper GI	Lower GI (stool output per day)
0	No GVHD rash	<2 mg/dL	No or intermittent nausea, vomiting, or anorexia	<10 mL/kg/day or <4 episodes/day
1	Rash <25 % BSA	2–3 mg/dL	Persistent nausea, vomiting, or anorexia	10–19.9 mL/kg/day or 4–6 episodes/day
2	Rash 25–50 % BSA	3.1–6 mg/dL		20–30 mL/kg/day or 7–10 episodes/day
3	Rash >50 % BSA	6.1–15 mg/dL		>30 mL/kg/day or >10 episodes/day
4	Generalized erythroderma + bullae	>15 mg/dL		Severe abdominal pain ± ileus or grossly bloody stool (regardless of stool volume)
Grade[a]				
0	None	None	None	None
I	Stages 1–2	None	None	None
II	Stage 3	Stage 1	Stage 1	Stage 1
III	Stage 0–3	Stage 2–3	Stage 0–1	Stages 2–3
IV	Stage 4 or	Stage 4 or	Stage 0–1	Stage 4

Adapted from Harris et al. [31]; *with permission*

BSA body surface area, *GI* gastrointestinal

[a]Grade is based on most severe target organ, regardless of presence/absence of other organ involvement

Treatment of Acute GVHD

Because of the difficulty in treating acute GVHD, there is a significant emphasis on prevention. Prophylactic regimens typically consist of one or a combination of the following agents: prednisone, cyclosporine, tacrolimus, sirolimus, methotrexate, mycophenolate mofetil, antithymocyte globulin, or alemtuzumab [2].

Once acute GVHD occurs, the prophylactic regimen can be adjusted and additional treatment may be considered, based on the grade of disease. Grade I acute GVHD, which is limited to the skin, usually has a favorable course and can be treated with topical corticosteroids and calcineurin inhibitors or narrow-band ultraviolet B phototherapy (nbUVB). For moderate to severe (grade II–IV) acute GVHD, high-dose systemic corticosteroids are employed as the first line of therapy [2, 33]. Unfortunately, only about half of patients are responsive to steroids [15, 32]. If there is no response to systemic corticosteroids after 2–7 days or if there is rapid progression within 48–72 h, second-line therapies should be considered. Table 9.3 outlines treatment agents subject to trials in pediatric patients.

Additional agents, such as cyclophosphamide and thalidomide, have been discussed in case reports and small case series [52, 53], but their efficacy and safety have yet to be demonstrated in larger studies. Some agents with trials in adults have not been studied in children.

Table 9.3 Treatment of moderate to severe (grade II–IV) acute GVHD in pediatric patients

Agent(s)	Study design and references	Patients, *n* (% pediatric)	Population with aGVHD, %	Treatment regimen	Response of aGVHD overall	Response of Skin aGVHD	Survival of patients with aGVHD
First-line therapy							
Prednisone or MPred	Prospective, randomized, controlled, multi-institution trial [34]	95 (34)	100	*Low dose* = 2 mg/kg/day IV MPred; *High dose* = 10 mg/kg/day IV MPred	At 5 days, 65 % of the low-dose treatment group responded and 71 % of the high-dose group responded	Not specified	63 % at 3 years for both treatment groups
	Retrospective, single-institution chart review [35]	443 (40)	100	60 mg/m^2 PO (or MPred IV equivalent, 48 mg/m^2) for 14 days followed by an 8-week taper	At 28 days, 35 % achieved CR, 20 % achieved PR, 40 % achieved NR, and 5 % were NE	Not specified	53 % at 1 year
Second-line therapies (steroid-refractory disease)							
Anti-thymocyte globulin (ATG)	Prospective, randomized, open-label, single-institution trial [36]	100 (46)	100	*ATG + steroids:* 15 mg/kg equine ATG IV + 20 mg/m^2 prednisone twice daily for 5 days followed by 8-week prednisone taper. *Steroids:* 20 mg/m^2 prednisone PO or IV 3 times daily for 7 days followed by 8-week taper. All patients with skin aGVHD also received 0.1 % topical triamcinolone three times daily	No significant difference between groups. At 42 days, 76 % achieved response (CR or PR) and 24 % achieved NR in both treatment groups	No significant difference between groups. At 42 days, 79 % achieved response (CR or PR) in those treated with ATG + steroids	No significant difference between groups. 60 % at 100 days, 48 % at 6 months, and 40 % at 2 years in those treated with ATG + steroids
Daclizumab	Retrospective, single-institution chart review [37]	14 (100)	71	2 mg/kg IV weekly for 8 weeks followed by 1 mg/kg IV weekly for 4 weeks	At 12 weeks, 45 % achieved CR, 18 % achieved PR, 27 % achieved NR, 9 % were NE	At 12 weeks, 50 % achieved CR and 20 % achieved PR	50 % at the time of publication (follow-up time not specified)

(continued)

Table 9.3 (continued)

Agent(s)	Study design and references	Patients, *n* (% pediatric)	Population with aGVHD, %	Treatment regimen	Response of aGVHD overall	Response of Skin aGVHD	Survival of patients with aGVHD
Extracorporeal photopheresis (ECP)	Prospective, nonrandomized, single-institution study [38]	72 (100)	100	Twice weekly for 1 month, then every 2 weeks for 2 months, and then monthly for at least 3 more months, for a total of 22 procedures	At completion of treatment, 72 % achieved CR, 11 % achieved PR, and 17 % achieved NR	At completion of treatment, 78 % achieved CR, 13 % achieved PR, and 9 % achieved NR	71 % at 5 years
	Prospective, nonrandomized, multi-institution study [39]	77 (100)	43	Twice weekly for 1 month, then every 2 weeks for 2 months, and then monthly for at least 3 more months, for a total of 22 procedures	At completion of treatment (range 8–467 days), 54 % achieved CR, 21 % achieved PR, and 24 % achieved NR	At the completion of treatment (range 8–467 days), 76 % achieved CR	69 % for responding patients vs. 12 % for non-responders at 5 years
	Prospective, nonrandomized, single-institution study [40]	73 (100)	68	2–3 times weekly until clinical improvement, then twice weekly for 2 times, then twice weekly every other week for 3 times, and finally twice monthly	At the completion of treatment, 32 % achieved CR, 36 % achieved PR, and 32 % achieved NR	At the completion of treatment, 83 % achieved response (CR or PR)	64 % at 1 year and 46 % at 5 years
	Retrospective, nonrandomized, single-institution study [41]	25 (100)	60	2 consecutive days weekly for 1 month, then every 2 weeks for 2 months, and then monthly for 3 months, for a median total of 12 procedures (range 4–21)	At completion of treatment, 47 % achieved CR, 27 % achieved PR, and 27 % achieved NR	At completion of treatment, 80 % achieved CR	100 % for responding patients *vs.* 15 % for nonresponders at a median of 1.6 years (range 0.8–4)
	Retrospective, single-institution chart review [42]	27 (100)	78	Twice weekly until clinical improvement for a median of 6 procedures (range 2–25)	At median of 167 days (range 4–1816), 52 % achieved CR, 38 % achieved PR, and the rest were NR	At median of 167 days (range 4–1816), 81 % achieved CR	69 % at 1816 days for both acute and chronic GVHD
Etanercept	Prospective, randomized phase II, single-institution trial [43]	160 (19)	100	*Etanercept + steroids:* 0.4 mg/kg etanercept SQ twice weekly for 8 weeks + 2 mg/kg/day IV MPred; *Steroids:* 2 mg/kg/day IV MPred	At 4 weeks, 69 % of etanercept + steroids group achieved CR *vs.* 33 % of the group treated with steroids alone	At 4 weeks, 81 % of the etanercept + steroids group achieved CR *vs.* 47 % of the group treated with steroids alone	No significant difference between groups: 69 % for those treated with etanercept + steroids *vs.* 55 % for those treated with steroids alone
Infliximab	Retrospective, single-institution chart review [44]	10 (100)	100	10 mg/kg IV weekly for 3–4 doses	At a median of 11 days (range 5–17), 80 % achieved CR and 20 % achieved PR	Not specified	40 % at 8–30 months
	Retrospective, multi-institution chart review [45]	24 (100)	75	10 mg/kg IV weekly for a median of 4 doses (range 1–58)	At 56 days, 69 % achieved CR	At 56 days, 86 % achieved CR	67 % at 6 months; 13 % beyond 3 years

Mesenchymal stem cells (MSC)	Retrospective, multi-institution chart review [32]	37 (100)	100	Median dose of 2×10^6 cells/kg (range $0.9–3 \times 10^6$ cells/kg) IV for a median of 2 infusions (range 1–13)	At completion of treatment, 65 % achieved CR, 22 % achieved PR, 14 % achieved NR or had progression	At median of 6 days (range 4–10), 57 % achieved CR, 23 % achieved PR, and 20 % achieved NR	37 % OS at median follow-up of 2.9 years (range 1.7 months–6.7 years); 65 % for those who achieved CR *vs.* 0 % for those who did not
	Prospective, multi-institution pilot study [46]	12 (100)	100	2×10^6 cells/kg IV twice weekly for 4 weeks	At completion of treatment, 58 % achieved CR, 17 % achieved PR, and 25 % achieved MR	At completion of treatment, 100 % achieved CR	58 % at 100 days and 42 % at median follow-up of 611 days (range 427–1111)
	Prospective, open-label, single-arm, multi-institution study [47]	75 (100)	100	2×10^6 cells/kg IV twice weekly for 4 weeks	At 28 days, 61 % achieved response (CR or PR) and 39 % achieved NR (MR, stable, or progressive)	At 28 days, 44 % achieved CR, 32 % achieved PR, 12 % achieved NR, and 12 % were NE	58 % OS at 100 days; 76 % for responders *vs.* 28 % for nonresponders
Mycophenolate mofetil (MMF)	Retrospective, single-institution chart review [48]	14 (100)	100	Median initial dose of 40 mg/kg/day (range 30–74) PO was increased to median maximum dose of 60 mg/kg/day (range, 34–107) PO	At 8 weeks, 79 % achieved CR and 21 % were NE	At 8 weeks, 100 % achieved CR	87 % at median follow-up of 35 months (range 14–86)
Methotrexate (MTX)	Retrospective, single-institution chart review [49]	35 (100)	100	10 mg/m² IV weekly	At 4 weeks, 37 % achieved CR and 9 % achieved PR	At 4 weeks, 52 % achieved CR, 17 % achieved PR, and 9 % progressed	62 % at 6 months
	Retrospective, single-institution chart review [50]	27 (100)	37	3–10 mg/m² IV or PO weekly for a median of 5 doses	At completion of treatment (1–7 weeks), 50 % achieved CR, 20 % achieved PR, 30 % were stable, and none progressed	At completion of treatment (1–7 weeks), 62 % achieved CR, 25 % achieved PR, 13 % were stable, and none progressed	70 % at 6 months and 60 % beyond 14 months
Pentostatin	Prospective, single-institution, phase I trial [51]	23 (22)	100	1.5 mg/m² IV for 3 days for 1–2 cycles	At 28 days, 64 % achieved CR, 14 % achieved PR, 9 % achieved MR, and 13 % progressed	At 28 % days, 81 % achieved CR, 6 % achieved PR, and 12 % achieved NR	25 % at 1 year

aGVHD acute graft versus host disease, *ATG* anti-thymocyte globulin, *CR* complete response, *ECP* extracorporeal photopheresis, *GVHD* graft-versus-host disease, *IV* intravenous, *MMF* mycophenolate mofetil, *MPred* methylprednisolone, *MR* mixed response, *MSC* mesenchymal stem cells, *MTX* methotrexate, *NE* not evaluable, *NR* no response, *OS* overall survival, *PO* per os (by mouth), *PR* partial response, *SQ* subcutaneous

Outcomes of Acute GVHD

Though acute GVHD correlates with increased engraftment and graft-versus-tumor effect [5], unfortunately it does not correlate with survival in pediatric HSCT recipients. In fact, acute GVHD increases the risk of chronic GVHD by 11-fold, and steroid-refractory acute GVHD indicates a poor prognosis [5]. Mortality from acute GVHD ranges from 8 % for mild acute GVHD to 55 % for severe acute GVHD, and is usually due to infection, hepatic failure, or malnutrition [11, 12, 54]. Many of the aforementioned prophylactic and treatment strategies result in some response, but none have been shown to be more effective than the others. Furthermore, no therapies have been shown to decrease mortality or prevent progression to chronic GVHD [12]. As our understanding of the pathogenesis of acute GVHD expands, additional targeted therapies are likely to arise [55]. Until then, additional randomized controlled studies are needed to assess the safety and efficacy of these therapies in children.

Chronic Graft-Versus-Host Disease in Pediatric Patients

Introduction to Chronic GVHD

Chronic GVHD is a major cause of morbidity and mortality for children after HSCT. However, less is known about chronic GVHD in children than in adults because the incidence of HSCT is lower in children, and chronic GVHD occurs half as frequently in pediatric HSCT recipients. Most literature focuses on adult populations, with limited data regarding the spectrum of cutaneous disease, safety and efficacy of treatment, and outcomes in children.

Incidence of Chronic GVHD

In the United States, over 1500 allogeneic HSCTs are reported annually in patients less than 20 years old, and the incidence of chronic GVHD across all types of allogeneic HSCT is about 25 %, suggesting that at least 400 cases of chronic GVHD occur in children annually [56, 57]. This incidence is about one half that of adult populations.

The incidence of chronic GVHD varies widely by risk factors, from as few as 6 % of sibling umbilical cord-blood transplant recipients to 65 % of unmatched peripheral blood stem cell transplant recipients [8, 58, 59]. In cohorts that received HLA-matched bone marrow transplantation, approximately 27–35 % of children developed chronic GVHD, compared with 57–60 % of adults [60–62]. Males are 50 % more likely than females to be affected by chronic GVHD, in part because of the increased risk of chronic GVHD associated with female donor to male recipient transplantation [57].

Risk Factors for Chronic GVHD

The risk factors for chronic GVHD in children are largely the same as for adults and include acute GVHD, female donor to male recipient, peripheral blood stem cell transplant (PBSCT) versus bone marrow or umbilical cord source, increasing patient and donor age, HLA mismatch, non–T--cell-depleted grafts, malignant diagnosis, and history of total body irradiation [57, 61]. Concerns have been raised that increased use in children of PBSCT, which currently accounts for only 3–4 % of transplants in children, compared with 20–40 % of transplants in adults, could substantially increase the incidence of chronic GVHD [4, 56].

Prior acute GVHD is the strongest risk factor for chronic GVHD, and severity of chronic GVHD tends to increase with severity of acute GVHD. Prevention of acute GVHD is critical for chronic GVHD prevention. Chronic GVHD in children can occur, however, in the absence of acute GVHD [61].

Clinical Features of Chronic GVHD

Children tend to develop symptoms of chronic GVHD at a median of 6 months after transplantation [62]. About 40 % of these patients manifest extensive disease; the remainder experience limited involvement of the skin, liver, or both [57]. Skin is the most commonly affected organ, with cutaneous features in 65–80 % of children with chronic GVHD, followed by oral lesions in half, liver disease in a third, and GI involvement in 25–60 % [57, 63]. Lungs and eyes may be less commonly affected by chronic GVHD in children than other organs, though one study reports eye involvement in 50 % of patients [57, 64]. Oral lesions may be erythematous, reticular, or ulcerative; they often are not painful, leading to under-reporting [63].

Clinical features of cutaneous chronic GVHD reported in children can be classified similarly to those in adults [16]. Peripheral edema often precedes chronic GVHD (particularly sclerotic forms) in children (Fig. 9.8) [65]. Dyspigmentation is almost universal and vitiligo is a known, but less common, presentation (Figs. 9.9 and 9.10) [62, 65]. The depth of sclerotic disease ranges from superficial lichen sclerosus–like lesions to dermal fibrosis and myofascial involvement (Figs. 9.11 and 9.12) [65]. Eczematous and ichthyosiform features can be found in sclerotic and non-sclerotic disease and may be more common in children than adults (Fig. 9.13) [65]. The reported incidence of lichenoid lesions varies widely; they may be more common in steroid-refractory chronic GVHD [64–66].

Focal or diffuse alopecia may occur in up to 50 % of children and can be scarring or non-scarring (Fig. 9.14) [62]. Nails are affected in up to 45 % of children, with periungual erythema and/or dystrophy [62, 65]. Pterygium inversum unguis, in which the distal nail bed adheres to the nail plate, is common in severe chronic GVHD and is associated with a higher risk of lung involvement in children (Fig. 9.15) [65].

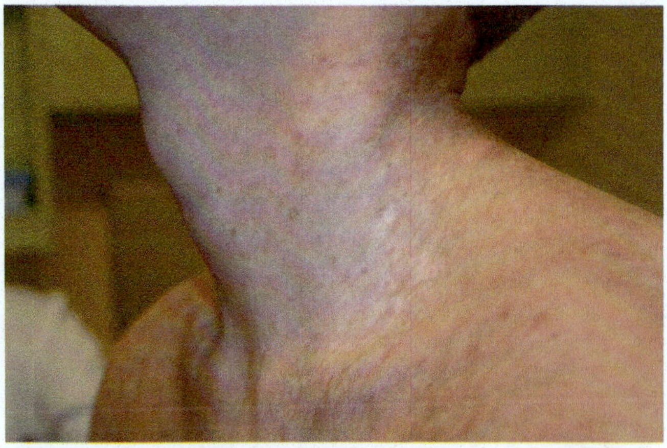

Fig. 9.9 Dyspigmentation (both hyperpigmentation and hypopigmentation) in a child with chronic GVHD

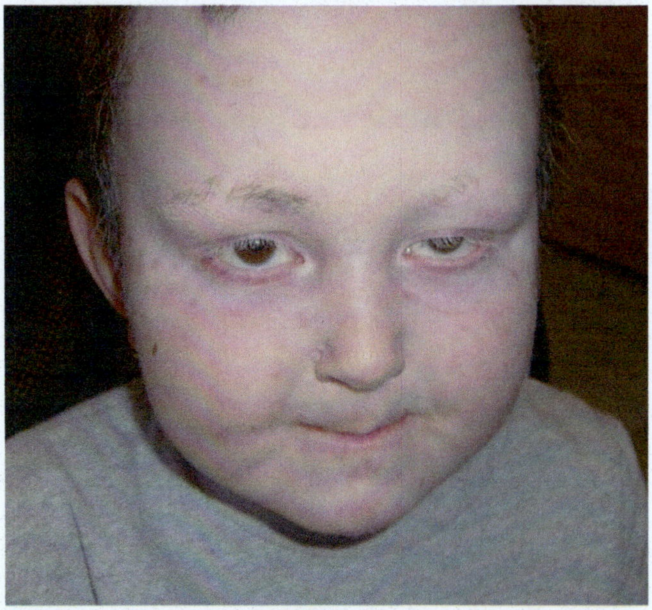

Fig. 9.10 Vitiliginous changes in a child with chronic GVHD of the skin

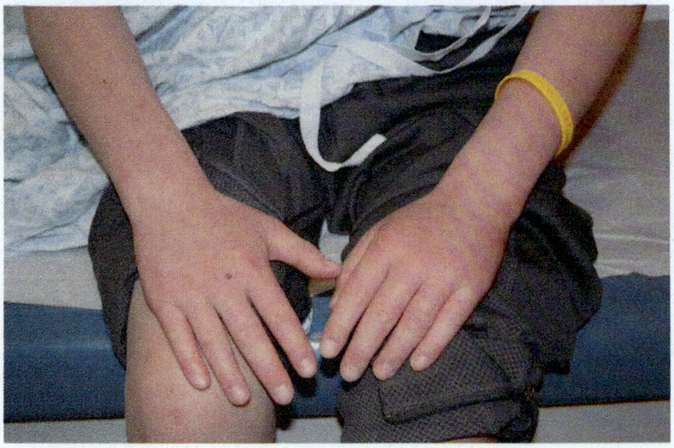

Fig. 9.8 Acral edema as an early sign of sclerotic chronic GVHD

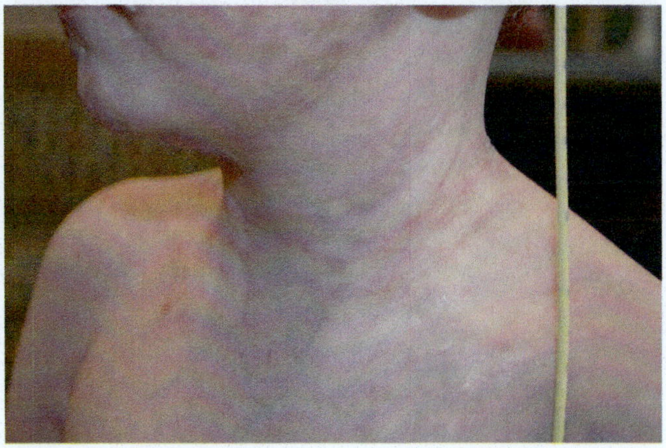

Fig. 9.11 Morpheaform sclerotic chronic GVHD

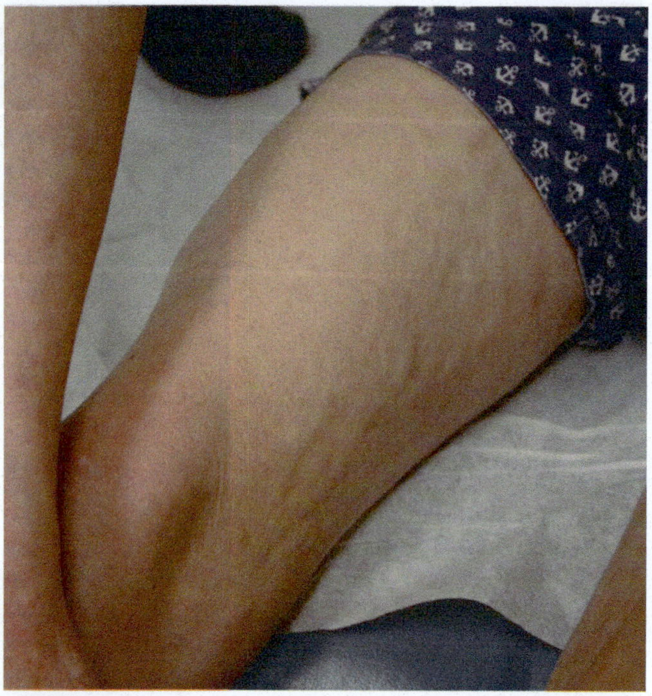

Fig. 9.12 Sclerotic chronic GVHD with myofascial involvement

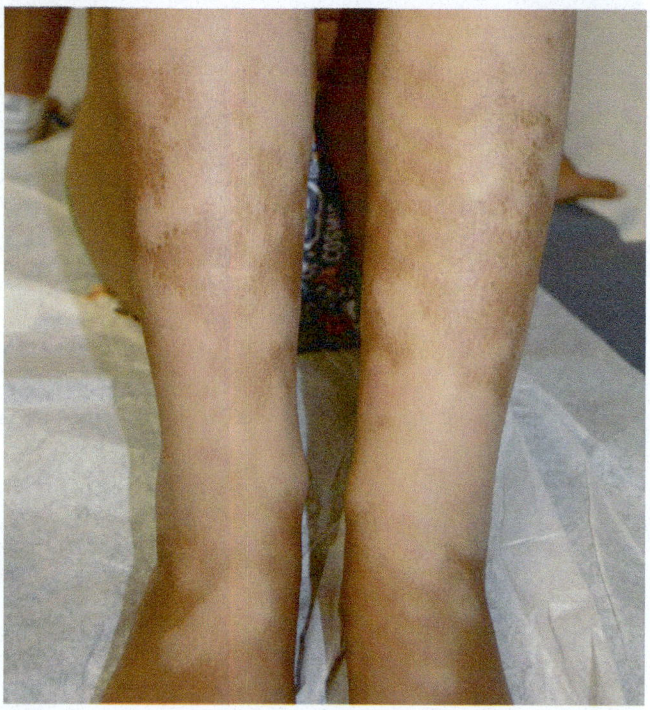

Fig. 9.13 Eczematous or ichthyosiform presentation of chronic GVHD

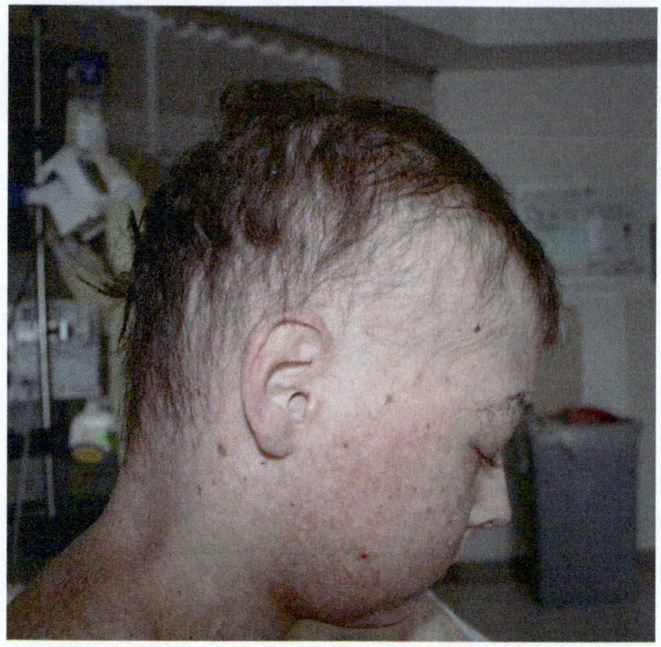

Fig. 9.14 Alopecia is common in children with chronic GVHD

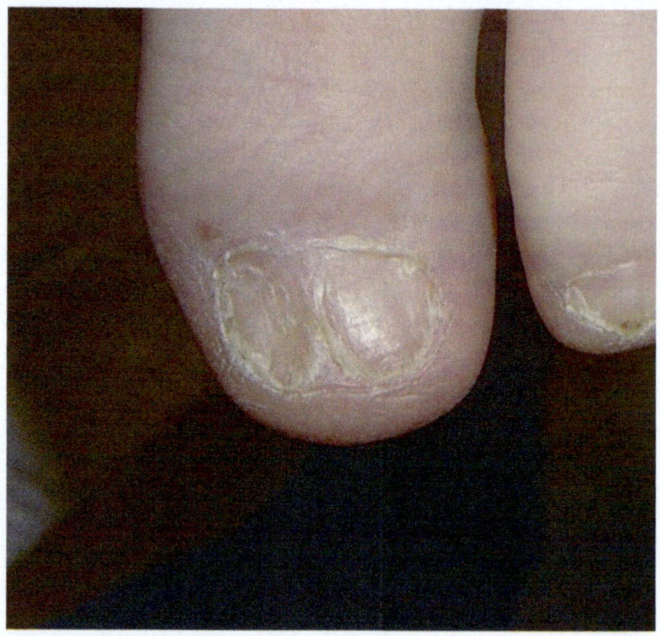

Fig. 9.15 Pterygium nail deformity may be a harbinger of severe lung involvement in children with chronic GVHD

Differential Diagnosis for Chronic GVHD

The differential diagnosis for sclerotic chronic GVHD includes lichen sclerosus, morphea, eosinophilic fasciitis, atrophoderma of Pasini and Pierini, and discoid lupus erythematosus. In patients with lichenoid lesions, lichenoid drug eruption, idiopathic lichen planus, and pityriasis lichenoides chronica should be considered. Voriconazole-induced phototoxicity may mimic chronic GVHD, but photodistribution of the rash should alert the clinician to this potential diagnosis (Fig. 9.16) [67].

Biopsy can help confirm the diagnoses of eczematoid, psoriasiform, or ichthyosiform chronic GVHD in children with a history of atopy or those who present with erythema, pruritus, scaling, xerosis, or follicular prominence.

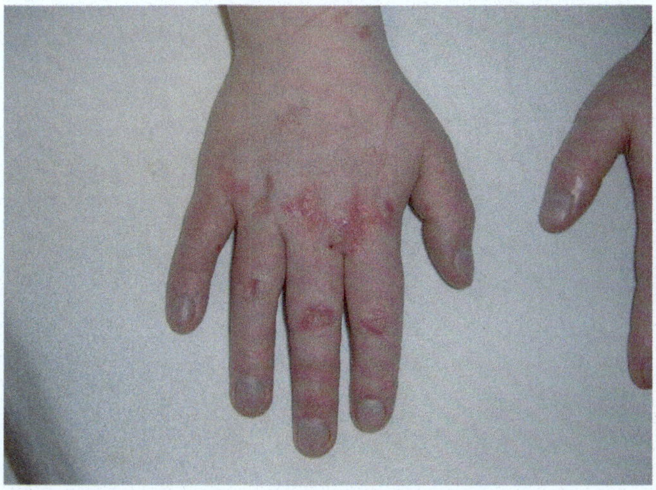

Fig. 9.16 Erythematous, scaly papules in photodistributed locations as a result of voriconazole phototoxicity

Histopathology and Laboratory Evaluation of Chronic GVHD

Histopathology of chronic GVHD is similar to adults and is required for diagnosis of chronic GVHD if features are distinctive but not diagnostic [16]. Peripheral eosinophilia has been noted in about half of children with chronic GVHD prior to disease onset [68]. Eosinophilia can be present in patients without chronic GHVD, however, particularly in association with eczema or infection [65].

Treatment of Chronic GVHD

First line therapy for chronic GVHD in children, based on data from adults, consists of topical immunosuppressive agents (steroids, calcineurin inhibitors) for limited cutaneous chronic GVHD and systemic steroids for extensive cutaneous (>20 % BSA or sclerotic features) or visceral involvement in children, which can be used in conjunction with other systemic immunosuppressants and/or topical calcineurin inhibitors [16, 69]. Photoprotection and topical moisturizers are also important aspects of care. Limited data is available on treatment practices, such as duration of therapy and frequency of first-line versus other agents, among pediatric patients. There is no consensus for treatment for steroid-refractory chronic GVHD. As demonstrated in Table 9.4, a wide range of therapies has been investigated for chronic GVHD in children with cutaneous features; unfortunately, the outcomes of these therapies are heterogeneous and inconclusive.

Challenges in treatment of children with chronic GVHD include lack of availability of newer agents such as IL-2 and basiliximab. Currently, extracorporeal photopheresis (ECP) units are designed for adult blood volumes, resulting in higher risk for fluid and electrolyte complications in children. Long-term central access and the long duration of ECP sessions can be difficult for small children [71].

Table 9.4 Treatment of chronic GVHD in pediatric patients

Agent(s)	Study design and reference	Study population	Patients with skin cGVHD, *n*	Global cGVHD assessment	Patients with cutaneous features or skin disease stage, *n*[a]	Median follow-up time, *months*	Outcomes (global or cutaneous assessment)
Narrow-band UVB phototherapy	Prospective case series [66]	cGVHD or overlap syndrome[a] refractory to steroids or cyclosporine with methotrexate	10	Severe	10 stage-3 skin disease: 5 lichenoid 5 lichen planus–like	24	5 cutaneous CR 2 cutaneous PR 3 lost-to-follow-up by 24 months but with cutaneous CR at 6 months
Extracorporeal photopheresis (ECP)	Retrospective case series [70]	Steroid-refractory acute *and* cGVHD or untreated cGVHD	4	Severe	3 stage-3 skin disease 1 stage-1 skin disease	15.5	2 globally quiescent 1 globally stable 1 global progression, deceased (GVHD)
	Retrospective case series [71]	Steroid-refractory or steroid-dependent cGVHD	8	Severe	5 stage-3 skin disease 3 stage-2 skin disease	9.5	2 global improvement 4 continuing on ECP 2 deceased (GVHD, disease relapse)
	Prospective case series [72]	Steroid-refractory cGVHD	12	11 extensive 1 limited	Not reported	39	5 cutaneous CR 5 cutaneous PR, 1 deceased (secondary neoplasm) 2 cutaneous progression, 1 deceased (GVHD)
	Multicenter retrospective case series [39]	Steroid-refractory GVHD at >100 days after transplant	36	Extensive in 38/44 with any cGVHD[b]	22 severe skin disease 9 moderate skin disease 5 mild skin disease 10 joint contractures 26 lichen planus	Not reported (likely >1 year)	20 cutaneous improvement 10 cutaneous NR 6 cutaneous progression
Imatinib	Case report [73]	Steroid-refractory cGVHD	2	Not reported	Modified Rodnan skin score of 17.5 and 11.1	24	Modified Rodnan skin score of 6 and 4
	Subset of open-label phase II trial [74]	Steroid-refractory sclerotic cGVHD	3	Severe	3 sclerotic disease affecting range of motion	6	Global cGVHD scores changed by −1, +2, and 0 with % change in body surface area −13 %, 0 %, and +2 %, respectively
Mycofenolate mofetil	Prospective case series [75]	Steroid and cyclosporine-refractory cGVHD	14	14 extensive disease	7 sclerotic 6 oral mucosa involvement	4	6 global CR (1 with sclerotic disease) 2 global PR 6 global NR (5 with sclerotic disease)

Pentostatin	Phase II multi-institution clinical trial [76]	Steroid-refractory cGVHD of any organ without severe lung or kidney involvement and Karnofsky score >40	51 with any cGVHD[b] (≥40 with skin cGVHD)	30/51 severe	40 lichenoid 27 sclerotic 30 oral involvement 7 fasciitis	33	In lichenoid and sclerotic lesions, respectively: 13/40, 11/27 CR 7/40, 5/27 PR 10/40, 6/27 stable 10/40, 5/27 worse
	Prospective case series [77]	Steroid-refractory cGVHD	5	Karnofsky score 60 % in 1, 70 % in 3, 80 % in 1	3 sclerotic with limited range of motion 5 dyspigmentation 3 lichenoid	18	1 cutaneous CR with Karnofsky score 90 % 4 cutaneous PR with Karnofsky score 80 %
Thalidomide	Prospective case series [78]	Steroid-refractory cGVHD plus one case of untreated cGVHD with thrombocytopenia	14	12 extensive 2 limited	Not reported	13.5	6 global CR 4 global PR, 1 deceased (thrombotic microangiopathy) 4 global NR, 3 deceased (GVHD)
	Retrospective case series and case reports from literature [79]	Steroid-refractory cGVHD also treated with azathioprine and/or cyclosporine	10	Severe extensive	Not fully described	17	2 global CR 6 global PR 1 globally stable 1 globally progressive, deceased (aspergillosis)
Hydroxy-chloroquine	Double-blind, placebo-controlled, randomized multi-center phase III trial [64]	Newly diagnosed cGVHD	27 with any cGVHD[b] (≥15 with skin cGVHD)	Moderate to severe	6 lichenoid 6 sclerotic 15 oral involvement 5 contractures	9	18/27 patients followed to 9 months, of whom: 5/18 global CR 2/18 global PR 11/18 global NR

cGVHD chronic graft-versus-host disease, *CR* complete response, *ECP* extracorporeal photopheresis, *NR* no response, *PR* partial response

[a]*Overlap syndrome* and *stage* refer to 2005 NIH consensus on cGVHD diagnosis and staging [17]

[b]Including noncutaneous cGVHD

Outcomes of Chronic GVHD

Symptoms of chronic GVHD resolve in as many as 70 % of children, with a median duration of 5 months with treatment [57]. Children with severe chronic GVHD tend to have a longer disease course, lower likelihood of responding to steroids, and lower chance of remission than patients with mild to moderate disease (20 % versus 65 % remission by 10–15 years after transplantation) [65, 80].

Chronic GVHD is a major cause of mortality in children, with an overall 5-year survival rate of 50–70 % [57, 81]. Children with severe chronic GVHD experience a 10-year nonrelapse mortality rate of about 35 %, compared with 4–5 % among children with mild to moderate chronic GVHD [80]. Causes of death in patients with chronic GVHD are most often transplant-related (typically infection), but they also include respiratory failure directly attributable to chronic GVHD and relapse [57]. Risk factors associated with higher mortality in children with chronic GVHD are similar to those in adults (*e.g.*, HLA mismatch, Karnofsky score <90 %) [81]. Chronic GVHD has also been shown to be protective against relapse, with the strongest protective effect observed in acute lymphoblastic leukemia [4, 57, 65, 80].

Chronic GVHD can cause numerous long-term sequelae, such as generalized sicca, mucositis, malabsorption, generalized wasting, and lower Karnofsky performance scores due to persisting skin, eye, and fascial involvement [60, 80]. Most children will have other co-existing long-term sequelae of HSCT, such as osteopenia, hypothyroidism, pulmonary compromise, cataracts, hypogonadism, growth hormone deficiency, chronic renal insufficiency, academic difficulty, and attention deficit hyperactivity disorder (ADHD) [82]. Long-term use of voriconazole in this population has been shown to cause accelerated photodamage, including lentigines, actinic keratoses, and nonmelanoma skin cancer (Fig. 9.17) [83]. Other long-term outcomes of treatment for chronic GVHD have not been well described.

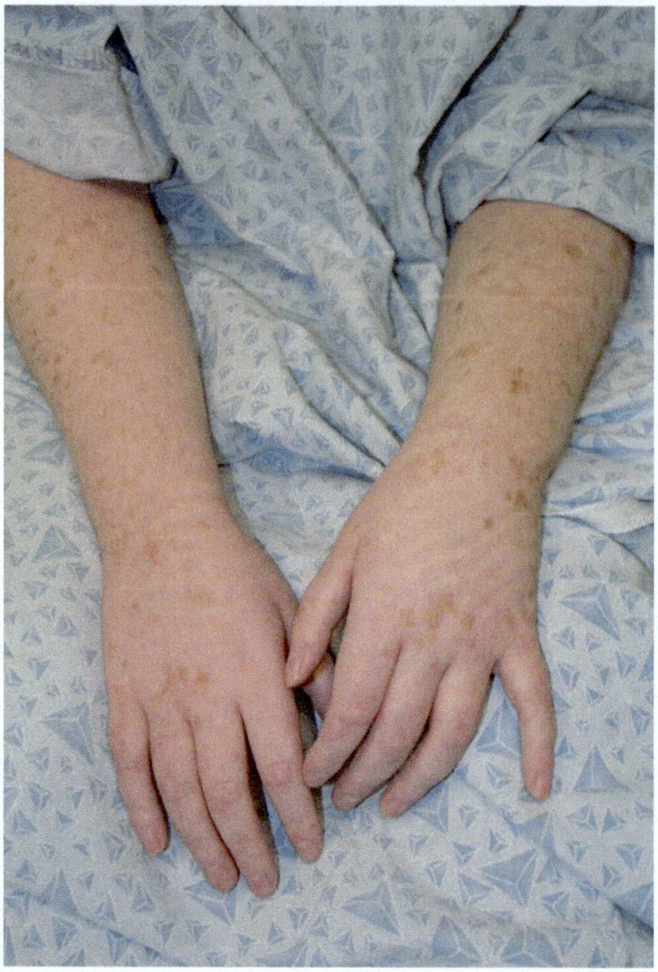

Fig. 9.17 Solar lentigos and actinic keratoses in a child after long-term use of voriconazole

Conclusion

Acute and chronic GVHD occur less commonly in children than in adults, but they remain major causes of morbidity and mortality. Clinicians should be aware of distinct differences in diagnosis and treatment when evaluating a child with possible GVHD. These differences include more frequent use of HSCT for nonmalignant conditions, higher likelihood of viral exanthema that may mimic or trigger GVHD, and hemodynamic considerations with use of ECP in small children. Currently, the management of children with acute and chronic GVHD of the skin is largely based on data from adults. The relatively low number of cases at each institution limits research on pediatric GVHD, so collaborative, multicenter studies are needed to better understand these conditions in children.

Acknowledgment Photographs are courtesy of Dr. Jennifer T. Huang.

References

1. Hymes SR, Alousi AM, Cowen EW. Graft-versus-host disease: part I. Pathogenesis and clinical manifestations of graft-versus-host disease. J Am Acad Dermatol. 2012;66:515.e1.
2. Jacobsohn DA. Acute graft-versus-host disease in children. Bone Marrow Transplant. 2008;41:215–21.
3. Center for International Blood and Marrow Transplant Research. Transplant activity report covering 2009–2013. US Department of Health and Human Services. 2015. Available from: http://bloodcell.transplant.hrsa.gov/research/transplant_data/transplant_activity_report/summary-tx_by_sex_disease_age_race_state_by_donor-type.pdf. Accessed 21 June 2016.
4. Eapen M, Horowitz MM, Klein JP, Champlin RE, FR Jr L, Ringden O, et al. Higher mortality after allogeneic peripheral-blood transplantation compared with bone marrow in children and adolescents: the Histocompatibility and Alternate Stem Cell Source Working Committee of the International Bone Marrow Transplant Registry. J Clin Oncol. 2004;22:4872–80.
5. Davies SM, Wang D, Wang T, Arora M, Ringden O, Anasetti C, et al. Recent decrease in acute graft-versus-host disease in children with leukemia receiving unrelated donor bone marrow transplants. Biol Blood Marrow Transplant. 2009;15:360–6.
6. Faraci M, Caviglia I, Biral E, Morreale G, Giardino S, Garbarino L, et al. Acute graft-versus-host disease in pediatric allogeneic hematopoietic stem cell transplantation. Single-center experience during 10 yr. Pediatr Transplant. 2012;16:887–93.
7. Giebel S, Giorgiani G, Martinetti M, Zecca M, Maccario R, Salvaneschi L, et al. Low incidence of severe acute graft-versus-host disease in children given haematopoietic stem cell transplantation from unrelated donors prospectively matched for HLA class I and II alleles with high-resolution molecular typing. Bone Marrow Transplant. 2003;31:987–93.
8. Rocha V, JE Jr W, Sobocinski KA, Klein JP, Zhang MJ, Horowitz MM, et al. Graft-versus-host disease in children who have received a cord-blood or bone marrow transplant from an HLA-identical sibling. Eurocord and International Bone Marrow Transplant Registry Working Committee on Alternative Donor and Stem Cell Sources. N Engl J Med. 2000;342:1846–54.
9. Wall DA, Carter SL, Kernan NA, Kapoor N, Kamani NR, Brochstein JA, et al. Busulfan/melphalan/antithymocyte globulin followed by unrelated donor cord blood transplantation for treatment of infant leukemia and leukemia in young children: the Cord Blood Transplantation study (COBLT) experience. Biol Blood Marrow Transplant. 2005;11:637–46.
10. Woolfrey AE, Anasetti C, Storer B, Doney K, Milner LA, Sievers EL, et al. Factors associated with outcome after unrelated marrow transplantation for treatment of acute lymphoblastic leukemia in children. Blood. 2002;99:2002–8.
11. Couriel DR, Saliba RM, Giralt S, Khouri I, Andersson B, de Lima M, et al. Acute and chronic graft-versus-host disease after ablative and nonmyeloablative conditioning for allogeneic hematopoietic transplantation. Biol Blood Marrow Transplant. 2004;10(3):178–85.
12. Harris AC, Ferrara JL, Levine JE. Advances in predicting acute GVHD. Br J Haematol. 2013;160:288–302.
13. Eisner MD, August CS. Impact of donor and recipient characteristics on the development of acute and chronic graft-versus-host disease following pediatric bone marrow transplantation. Bone Marrow Transplant. 1995;15:663–8.
14. Martin P, Bleyzac N, Souillet G, Galambrun C, Bertrand Y, Maire PH, et al. Clinical and pharmacological risk factors for acute graft-versus-host disease after paediatric bone marrow transplantation from matched-sibling or unrelated donors. Bone Marrow Transplant. 2003;32:881–7.
15. Ferrara JL, Levine JE, Reddy P, Holler E. Graft-versus-host disease. Lancet. 2009;373:1550–61.
16. Jagasia MH, Greinix HT, Arora M, Williams KM, Wolff D, Cowen EW, et al. National Institutes of Health consensus development project on criteria for clinical trials in chronic graft-versus-host disease: I. The 2014 diagnosis and staging working group report. Biol Blood Marrow Transplant. 2015;21:389–401.
17. Filipovich AH, Weisdorf D, Pavletic S, Socie G, Wingard JR, Lee SJ, et al. National Institutes of Health consensus development project on criteria for clinical trials in chronic graft-versus-host disease: I. Diagnosis and staging working group report. Biol Blood Marrow Transplant. 2005;11:945–56.
18. Exanthematous diseases of childhood. In: Paller A, Mancini AJ, editors. Hurwitz clinical pediatric dermatology: a textbook of skin disorders of childhood and adolescence. 4th ed. London: Elsevier; 2011. p. 370–89.
19. Spitzer TR. Engraftment syndrome following hematopoietic stem cell transplantation. Bone Marrow Transplant. 2001;27:893–8.
20. Bolognia JL, Cooper DL, Glusac EJ. Toxic erythema of chemotherapy: a useful clinical term. J Am Acad Dermatol. 2008;59:524–9.
21. Parker TL, Cooper DL, Seropian SE, Bolognia JL. Toxic erythema of chemotherapy following i.v. BU plus fludarabine for allogeneic PBSC transplant. Bone Marrow Transplant. 2013;48:646–50.
22. Graft-versus-host disease (GVHD). In: Brinster NK, Liu V, Diwan AH, McKee PH, editors Dermatopathology: high-yield pathology. Philadelphia: Elsevier; 2011. p. 42–e3.
23. Other non-neoplastic diseases. In: Rapini RP, editor. Practical dermatopathology. 2nd ed. Philadelphia: Elsevier; 2012. p. 239–5.
24. Byun HJ, Yang JI, Kim BK, Cho KH. Clinical differentiation of acute cutaneous graft-versus-host disease from drug hypersensitivity reactions. J Am Acad Dermatol. 2011;65:726–32.
25. Drijkoningen M, De Wolf-Peeters C, Tricot G, Degreef H, Desmet V. Drug-induced skin reactions and acute cutaneous graft-versus-host reaction: a comparative immunohistochemical study. Blut. 1988;56:69–73.
26. Firoz BF, Lee SJ, Nghiem P, Qureshi AA. Role of skin biopsy to confirm suspected acute graft-vs-host disease: results of decision analysis. Arch Dermatol. 2006;142:175–82.
27. Kohler S, Hendrickson MR, Chao NJ, Smoller BR. Value of skin biopsies in assessing prognosis and progression of acute graft-versus-host disease. Am J Surg Pathol. 1997;21:988–96.

28. Marra DE, McKee PH, Nghiem P. Tissue eosinophils and the perils of using skin biopsy specimens to distinguish between drug hypersensitivity and cutaneous graft-versus-host disease. J Am Acad Dermatol. 2004;51:543–6.
29. Zhou Y, Barnett MJ, Rivers JK. Clinical significance of skin biopsies in the diagnosis and management of graft-vs-host disease in early postallogeneic bone marrow transplantation. Arch Dermatol. 2000;136:717–21.
30. Przepiorka D, Weisdorf D, Martin P, HG K, Beatty P, Hows J, et al. 1994 consensus conference on acute GVHD grading. Bone Marrow Transplant. 1995;15:825–8.
31. Harris AC, Young R, Devine S, Hogan WJ, Ayuk F, Bunworasate U, et al. International, multicenter standardization of acute graft-versus-host disease clinical data collection: a report from the Mount Sinai Acute GVHD International Consortium. Biol Blood Marrow Transplant. 2016;22:4–10.
32. Ball LM, Bernardo ME, Roelofs H, van Tol MJ, Contoli B, Zwaginga JJ, et al. Multiple infusions of mesenchymal stromal cells induce sustained remission in children with steroid-refractory, grade III-IV acute graft-versus-host disease. Br J Haematol. 2013;163:501–9.
33. Dignan FL, Clark A, Amrolia P, Cornish J, Jackson G, Mahendra P, et al. Diagnosis and management of acute graft-versus-host disease. Br J Haematol. 2012;158:30–45.
34. Van Lint MT, Uderzo C, Locasciulli A, Majolino I, Scime R, Locatelli F, et al. Early treatment of acute graft-versus-host disease with high- or low-dose 6-methylprednisolone: a multicenter randomized trial from the Italian Group for Bone Marrow Transplantation. Blood. 1998;92:2288–93.
35. MacMillan ML, Weisdorf DJ, Wagner JE, DeFor TE, Burns LJ, Ramsay NK, et al. Response of 443 patients to steroids as primary therapy for acute graft-versus-host disease: comparison of grading systems. Biol Blood Marrow Transplant. 2002;8:387–94.
36. Cragg L, Blazar BR, Defor T, Kolatker N, Miller W, Kersey J, et al. A randomized trial comparing prednisone with antithymocyte globulin/prednisone as an initial systemic therapy for moderately severe acute graft-versus-host disease. Biol Blood Marrow Transplant. 2000;6:441–7.
37. Teachey DT, Bickert B, Bunin N. Daclizumab for children with corticosteroid refractory graft-versus-host disease. Bone Marrow Transplant. 2006;37:95–9.
38. Calore E, Marson P, Pillon M, Tumino M, Tison T, Mainardi C, et al. Treatment of acute graft-versus-host disease in childhood with extracorporeal photochemotherapy/photopheresis: the Padova experience. Biol Blood Marrow Transplant. 2015;21:1963–72.
39. Messina C, Locatelli F, Lanino E, Uderzo C, Zacchello G, Cesaro S, et al. Extracorporeal photochemotherapy for paediatric patients with graft-versus-host disease after haematopoietic stem cell transplantation. Br J Haematol. 2003;122:118–27.
40. Perotti C, Del Fante C, Tinelli C, Viarengo G, Scudeller L, Zecca M, et al. Extracorporeal photochemotherapy in graft-versus-host disease: a longitudinal study on factors influencing the response and survival in pediatric patients. Transfusion. 2010;50:1359–69.
41. Berger M, Pessolano R, Albiani R, Asaftei S, Barat V, Carraro F, et al. Extracorporeal photopheresis for steroid resistant graft versus host disease in pediatric patients: a pilot single institution report. J Pediatr Hematol Oncol. 2007;29:678–87.
42. Gonzalez Vicent M, Ramirez M, Sevilla J, Abad L, Diaz MA. Analysis of clinical outcome and survival in pediatric patients undergoing extracorporeal photopheresis for the treatment of steroid-refractory GVHD. J Pediatr Hematol Oncologia. 2010;32:589–93.
43. Levine JE, Paczesny S, Mineishi S, Braun T, Choi SW, Hutchinson RJ, et al. Etanercept plus methylprednisolone as initial therapy for acute graft-versus-host disease. Blood. 2008;111:2470–5.
44. Yang J, Cheuk DK, Ha SY, Chiang AK, Lee TL, Ho MH, et al. Infliximab for steroid refractory or dependent gastrointestinal acute graft-versus-host disease in children after allogeneic hematopoietic stem cell transplantation. Pediatr Transplant. 2012;16:771–8.
45. Sleight BS, Chan KW, Braun TM, Serrano A, Gilman AL. Infliximab for GVHD therapy in children. Bone Marrow Transplant. 2007;40:473–80.
46. Prasad VK, Lucas KG, Kleiner GI, Talano JA, Jacobsohn D, Broadwater G, et al. Efficacy and safety of ex vivo cultured adult human mesenchymal stem cells (Prochymal) in pediatric patients with severe refractory acute graft-versus-host disease in a compassionate use study. Biol Blood Marrow Transplant. 2011;17:534–41.
47. Kurtzberg J, Prockop S, Teira P, Bittencourt H, Lewis V, Chan KW, et al. Allogeneic human mesenchymal stem cell therapy (remestemcel-L, Prochymal) as a rescue agent for severe refractory acute graft-versus-host disease in pediatric patients. Biol Blood Marrow Transplant. 2014;20:229–35.
48. Inagaki J, Kodama Y, Fukano R, Noguchi M, Okamura J. Mycophenolate mofetil for treatment of steroid-refractory acute graft-versus-host disease after pediatric hematopoietic stem cell transplantation. Pediatr Transplant. 2015;19:652–8.
49. Inagaki J, Fukano R, Kodama Y, Nishimura M, Shimokawa M, Okamura J. Safety and efficacy of low-dose methotrexate for pediatric patients with steroid-refractory acute graft-versus-host disease after hematopoietic stem cell transplantation. Ann Hematol. 2014;93:645–51.
50. Inagaki J, Nagatoshi Y, Hatano M, Isomura N, Sakiyama M, Okamura J. Low-dose MTX for the treatment of acute and chronic graft-versus-host disease in children. Bone Marrow Transplant. 2008;41:571–7.
51. Bolanos-Meade J, Jacobsohn DA, Margolis J, Ogden A, Wientjes MG, Byrd JC, et al. Pentostatin in steroid-refractory acute graft-versus-host disease. J Clin Oncol. 2005;23:2661–8.
52. Kawahara Y, Morimoto A, Masuzawa A, Ikeda T, Hayase T, Kashii Y, et al. Successful treatment with pulse cyclophosphamide of a steroid-refractory hepatitic variant of liver acute graft-vs.-host disease in a child. Pediatr Transplant. 2012;16:E315–9.
53. Mehta P, Kedar A, Graham-Pole J, Skoda-Smith S, Wingard JR. Thalidomide in children undergoing bone marrow transplantation: series at a single institution and review of the literature. Pediatrics. 1999;103:e44.
54. Skin signs of other systemic diseases. In: Paller A, Mancini AJ, editors. Hurwitz clinical pediatric dermatology: a textbook of skin disorders of childhood and adolescence. 4th ed. London: Elsevier; 2011. p. 562–79.
55. Blazar BR, Murphy WJ, Abedi M. Advances in graft-versus-host disease biology and therapy. Nat Rev Immunol. 2012;12:443–58.
56. Center for International Blood and Marrow Transplant Research, a contractor for the C.W. Bill Young Cell Transplantation Program operated through the U.S. Department of Health and Human Services, Health Resources and Services Administration, Healthcare Systems Bureau. Transplant activity report covering 2009–2013. Available from http://bloodcell.transplant.hrsa.gov/research/transplant_data/transplant_activity_report/summary-tx_by_sex_disease_age_race_state_by_donortype.pdf. Last updated 18 May 2015. Accessed 5 July 2016.
57. Zecca M, Prete A, Rondelli R, Lanino E, Balduzzi A, Messina C, et al. Chronic graft-versus-host disease in children: incidence, risk factors, and impact on outcome. Blood. 2002;100:1192–200.
58. Wagner JE, Kernan NA, Steinbuch M, Broxmeyer HE, Gluckman E. Allogeneic sibling umbilical-cord-blood transplantation in children with malignant and non-malignant disease. Lancet. 1995;346:214–9.
59. Meisel R, Laws HJ, Balzer S, Bernbeck B, Kramm C, Schonberger S, et al. Comparable long-term survival after bone marrow versus peripheral blood progenitor cell transplantation from matched unrelated donors in children with hematologic malignancies. Biol Blood Marrow Transplant. 2007;13:1338–45.

60. Storb R, Prentice RL, Sullivan KM, Shulman HM, Deeg HJ, Doney KC, et al. Predictive factors in chronic graft-versus-host disease in patients with aplastic anemia treated by marrow transplantation from HLA-identical siblings. Ann Intern Med. 1983;98:461–6.
61. Atkinson K, Horowitz MM, Gale RP, van Bekkum DW, Gluckman E, Good RA, et al. Risk factors for chronic graft-versus-host disease after HLA-identical sibling bone marrow transplantation. Blood. 1990;75:2459–64.
62. Sullivan KM, Shulman HM, Storb R, Weiden PL, Witherspoon RP, McDonald GB, et al. Chronic graft-versus-host disease in 52 patients: adverse natural course and successful treatment with combination immunosuppression. Blood. 1981;57:267–76.
63. Treister NS, Woo SB, O'Holleran EW, Lehmann LE, Parsons SK, Guinan EC. Oral chronic graft-versus-host disease in pediatric patients after hematopoietic stem cell transplantation. Biol Blood Marrow Transplant. 2005;11:721–31.
64. Gilman AL, Schultz KR, Goldman FD, Sale GE, Krailo MD, Chen Z, et al. Randomized trial of hydroxychloroquine for newly diagnosed chronic graft-versus-host disease in children: a Children's Oncology Group study. Biol Blood Marrow Transplant. 2012;18:84–91.
65. Huang JT, Duncan CN, Boyer D, Khosravi H, Lehmann LE, Saavedra A. Nail dystrophy, edema, and eosinophilia: harbingers of severe chronic GVHD of the skin in children. Bone Marrow Transplant. 2014;49:1521–7.
66. Brazzelli V, Grasso V, Muzio F, Moggio E, Zecca M, Locatelli F, et al. Narrowband ultraviolet B phototherapy in the treatment of cutaneous graft-versus-host disease in oncohaematological paediatric patients. Br J Dermatol. 2010;162:404–9.
67. Patel AR, Turner ML, Baird K, Gea-Banacloche J, Mitchell S, Pavletic SZ, et al. Voriconazole-induced phototoxicity masquerading as chronic graft-versus-host disease of the skin in allogeneic hematopoietic cell transplant recipients. Biol Blood Marrow Transplant. 2009;15:370–6.
68. Jacobsohn DA, Schechter T, Seshadri R, Thormann K, Duerst R, Kletzel M. Eosinophilia correlates with the presence or development of chronic graft-versus-host disease in children. Transplantation. 2004;77:1096–100.
69. Baird K, Cooke K, Schultz KR. Chronic graft-versus-host disease (GVHD) in children. Pediatr Clin N Am. 2010;57:297–322.
70. Kapadia E, Wong E, Perez-Albuerne E, Jacobsohn D. Extracorporeal photopheresis performed on the CELLEX(R) compared with the UVAR-XTS(R) instrument is more efficient and better tolerated in children with steroid-refractory graft-versus-host disease. Pediatr Blood Cancer. 2015;62:1485–8.
71. Rangarajan HG, Punzalan RC, Camitta BM, Talano JA. The use of novel Therakos Cellex(R) for extracorporeal photopheresis in treatment of graft-versus-host disease in paediatric patients. Br J Haematol. 2013;163:357–64.
72. Salvaneschi L, Perotti C, Zecca M, Bernuzzi S, Viarengo G, Giorgiani G, et al. Extracorporeal photochemotherapy for treatment of acute and chronic GVHD in childhood. Transfusion. 2001;41:1299–305.
73. Kim H, Kim NH, Kang HJ, Lee JW, Kim MS, Park KD, et al. Successful long-term use of imatinib mesylate in pediatric patients with sclerodermatous chronic GVHD. Pediatr Transplant. 2012;16:910–2.
74. Baird K, Comis LE, Joe GO, Steinberg SM, Hakim FT, Rose JJ, et al. Imatinib mesylate for the treatment of steroid-refractory sclerotic-type cutaneous chronic graft-versus-host disease. Biol Blood Marrow Transplant. 2015;21:1083–90.
75. Busca A, Saroglia EM, Lanino E, Manfredini L, Uderzo C, Nicolini B, et al. Mycophenolate mofetil (MMF) as therapy for refractory chronic GVHD (cGVHD) in children receiving bone marrow transplantation. Bone Marrow Transplant. 2000;25:1067–71.
76. Jacobsohn DA, Gilman AL, Rademaker A, Browning B, Grimley M, Lehmann L, et al. Evaluation of pentostatin in corticosteroid-refractory chronic graft-versus-host disease in children: a Pediatric Blood and Marrow Transplant Consortium study. Blood. 2009;114:4354–60.
77. Goldberg JD, Jacobsohn DA, Margolis J, Chen AR, Anders V, Phelps M, et al. Pentostatin for the treatment of chronic graft-versus-host disease in children. J Pediatr Hematol Oncol. 2003;25:584–8.
78. Rovelli A, Arrigo C, Nesi F, Balduzzi A, Nicolini B, Locasciulli A, et al. The role of thalidomide in the treatment of refractory chronic graft-versus-host disease following bone marrow transplantation in children. Bone Marrow Transplant. 1998;21:577–81.
79. Cole CH, Rogers PC, Pritchard S, Phillips G, Chan KW. Thalidomide in the management of chronic graft-versus-host disease in children following bone marrow transplantation. Bone Marrow Transplant. 1994;14:937–42.
80. Inagaki J, Moritake H, Nishikawa T, Hyakuna N, Okada M, Suenobu S, et al. Long-term morbidity and mortality in children with chronic graft-versus-host disease classified by National Institutes of Health consensus criteria after allogeneic hematopoietic stem cell transplantation. Biol Blood Marrow Transplant. 2015;21:1973–80.
81. Jacobsohn DA, Arora M, Klein JP, Hassebroek A, Flowers ME, Cutler CS, et al. Risk factors associated with increased nonrelapse mortality and with poor overall survival in children with chronic graft-versus-host disease. Blood. 2011;118:4472–9.
82. El-Jawahri A, Pidala J, Inamoto Y, Chai X, Khera N, Wood WA, et al. Impact of age on quality of life, functional status, and survival in patients with chronic graft-versus-host disease. Biol Blood Marrow Transplant. 2014;20:1341–8.
83. Sheu J, Hawryluk EB, Guo D, London WB, Huang JT. Voriconazole phototoxicity in children: a retrospective review. J Am Acad Dermatol. 2015;72:314–20.

10 Diagnosis, Staging, and Treatment of Chronic Graft-Versus-Host Disease

Dominique C. Pichard and Edward W. Cowen

Chronic graft-versus-host disease (cGVHD) remains the primary cause of non–relapse-related morbidity and mortality after allogeneic hematopoietic stem cell transplantation (HSCT), and the incidence of cGVHD continues to rise [1]. Evolving transplantation practices, including the use of mobilized peripheral stem cells, transplantation of older recipients, and more frequent use of mismatched transplants, may explain the occurrence of this vexing problem.

Chronic GVHD is a multisystem disease, with the skin being the most common target organ. The clinical spectrum of cutaneous cGVHD includes "diagnostic" features (*e.g.*, sclerosis, poikiloderma), "distinctive" features (*e.g.*, dyspigmentation), and other manifestations that are neither diagnostic nor distinctive and which can also be present in acute GVHD (*e.g.*, pruritus). In 2005, the Diagnosis and Staging Working Group of the National Institutes of Health (NIH) Consensus Development Project on Criteria for Clinical Trials in cGVHD proposed diagnostic and staging criteria for cGVHD that are reviewed in this chapter [2]. The Diagnosis and Staging Working Group Report was updated in 2014, with clarification of the definition of the overlap cGVHD subcategory and the addition of numerous organ-specific refinements [3].

Treatment of cGVHD remains challenging. Fundamentally, effective evidence-based therapies are lacking. Corticosteroids are generally first-line therapy, but there is not sufficient evidence to support one second-line therapeutic option as superior. Many salvage therapies have been used with varying levels of success in cutaneous cGVHD. A multidisciplinary approach is recommended for treatment decisions, be it skin-directed, systemic, or a combination of both. Many factors are evaluated, including the type of skin involvement and its potential for long-term morbidity, other GVHD organ involvement, graft-versus-tumor effect, current comorbidities, and the toxicities of the treatments being considered.

D.C. Pichard • E.W. Cowen (✉)
Dermatology Branch, Center for Cancer Research,
National Cancer Institute, National Institutes of Health,
10 Center Drive, Bethesda, MD 20892, USA
e-mail: dominique.pichard@nih.gov; cowene@mail.nih.gov

J.A. Cotliar (ed.), *Atlas of Graft-versus-Host Disease*, DOI 10.1007/978-3-319-46952-2_10

Diagnosis and Staging

Chronic GVHD was historically defined as signs and symptoms of GVHD occurring after the first 100 days post-transplant. The 2005 NIH Consensus Project highlighted the arbitrary nature of the designation between acute and chronic GVHD. Chronic GVHD is now classified based on the clinical manifestations [2]. In addition, four categories of cGVHD clinical manifestations have been described for each organ system (Table 10.1, Figs. 10.1, 10.2, 10.3, 10.4, and 10.5):

- *Diagnostic* signs and symptoms that do not require additional diagnostic information to make the diagnosis of cGVHD
- *Distinctive* signs and symptoms, which are known characteristics of cGVHD but are not sufficient to make the diagnosis of cGVHD without additional testing
- *Nondiagnostic* features, which are controversial or rare
- Signs and symptoms that are *common* to both acute and chronic GVHD

Diagnosis of cutaneous cGVHD requires at least one clinical *diagnostic* feature or at least one *distinctive* clinical manifestation plus a skin biopsy demonstrating cGVHD. *Nondiagnostic* and *common* features of cutaneous cGVHD are not considered for the diagnosis of cGVHD, but they are included in the severity scoring, as discussed in the following section.

Classification of cGVHD severity is also guided by the Diagnosis and Staging Working Group report. Based on the 2014 report [3], two individual skin scores comprise the overall cGVHD severity (Table 10.2). The body surface area (BSA) involvement of five cutaneous findings (maculopapular rash/erythema, lichen planus–like features, sclerotic features, papulosquamous lesions or ichthyosis, and keratosis pilaris–like GVHD) is scored from 0 to 3 based on the percentage of body surface area involved. The second skin score is based on skin sclerosis. The presence of superficial sclerosis results in a score of 2 and presence of deep sclerosis, impaired mobility, or ulceration is given a score of 3. Six other features are listed on the screening document but do not contribute to the severity score. The highest of the two skin scores is used for the NIH Global Severity Score. The global score defines severity of cGVHD, with a skin score of 1 corresponding to mild cGVHD, 2 corresponding to moderate cGVHD, and three corresponding to severe cGVHD.

Table 10.1 NIH consensus project classification of signs and symptoms of cutaneous cGVHD

Site	Diagnostic	Distinctive	Other	Common
Skin	Poikiloderma Lichen planus–like Sclerotic features Morphea features Lichen sclerosus–like	Depigmentation Papulosquamous lesions	Sweat impairment Ichthyosis Keratosis pilaris Hypopigmentation Hyperpigmentation	Erythema Maculopapular rash Pruritus
Nails		Dystrophy Longitudinal ridging, splitting, or brittle features Onycholysis Pterygium unguis Nail loss		
Scalp and body hair		New-onset scarring or nonscarring alopecia Scaling	Thinning scalp hair Premature gray hair	

Adapted from Jagasia et al. [3]
NIH national institutes of health

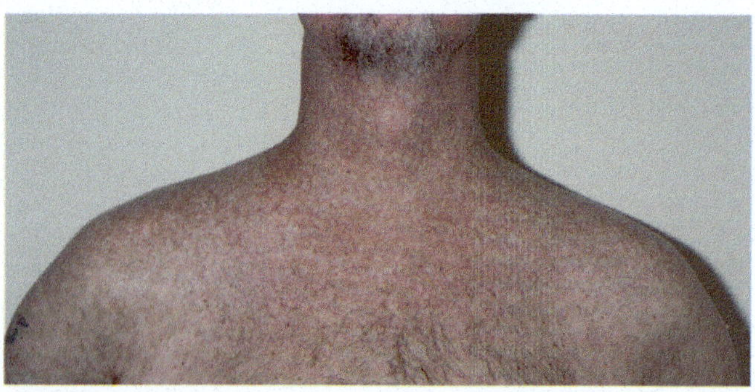

Fig. 10.1 Poikilodermic cGVHD on the neck and upper chest

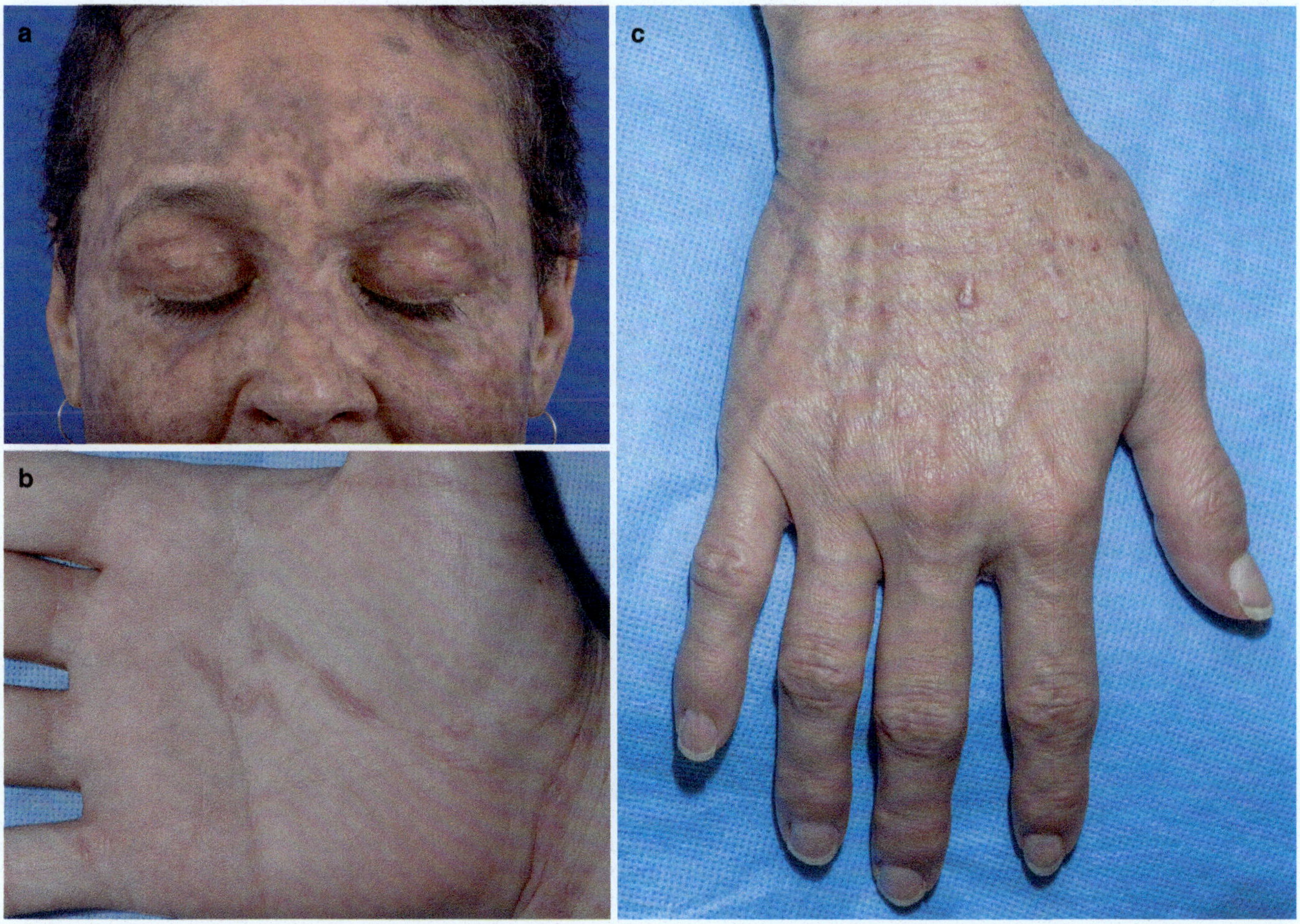

Fig. 10.2 Lichen planus–like chronic graft-versus-host disease (cGVHD). (**a**) Woman with lichen planus–like cGVHD on the face. (**b**) Man with lichen planus–like cGVHD on the palm and wrist. (**c**) Woman with lichen planus–like papules on the dorsal hand and wrist

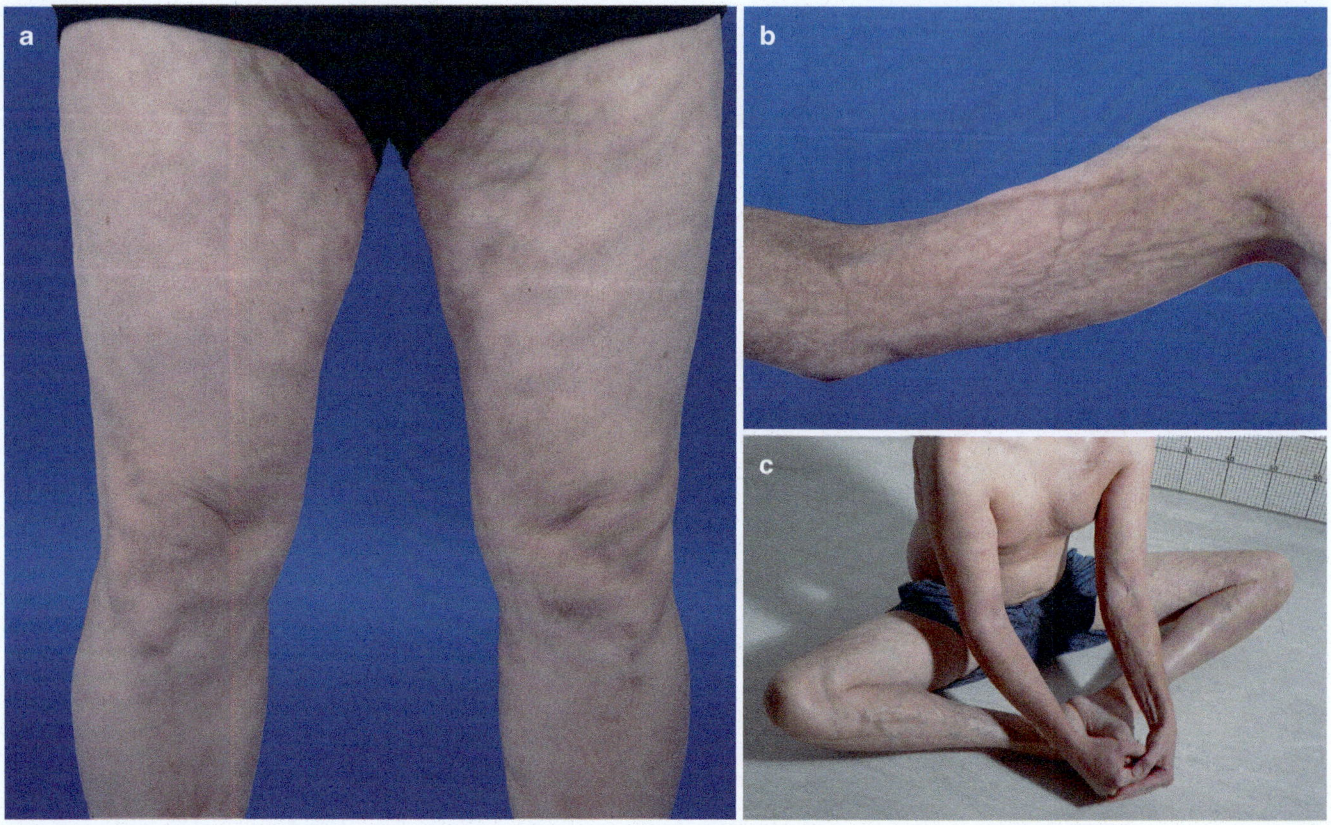

Fig. 10.3 Deep sclerosis. (**a**) Rippling of the subcutaneous tissue of the medial thighs from subcutaneous sclerosis. (**b**) Rippling and nodularity of the subcutaneous tissue of the upper extremity from subcutaneous sclerosis. (**c**) Rippling and nodularity of subcutaneous tissue of the upper and lower extremities accentuated by abduction and flexion of the hip

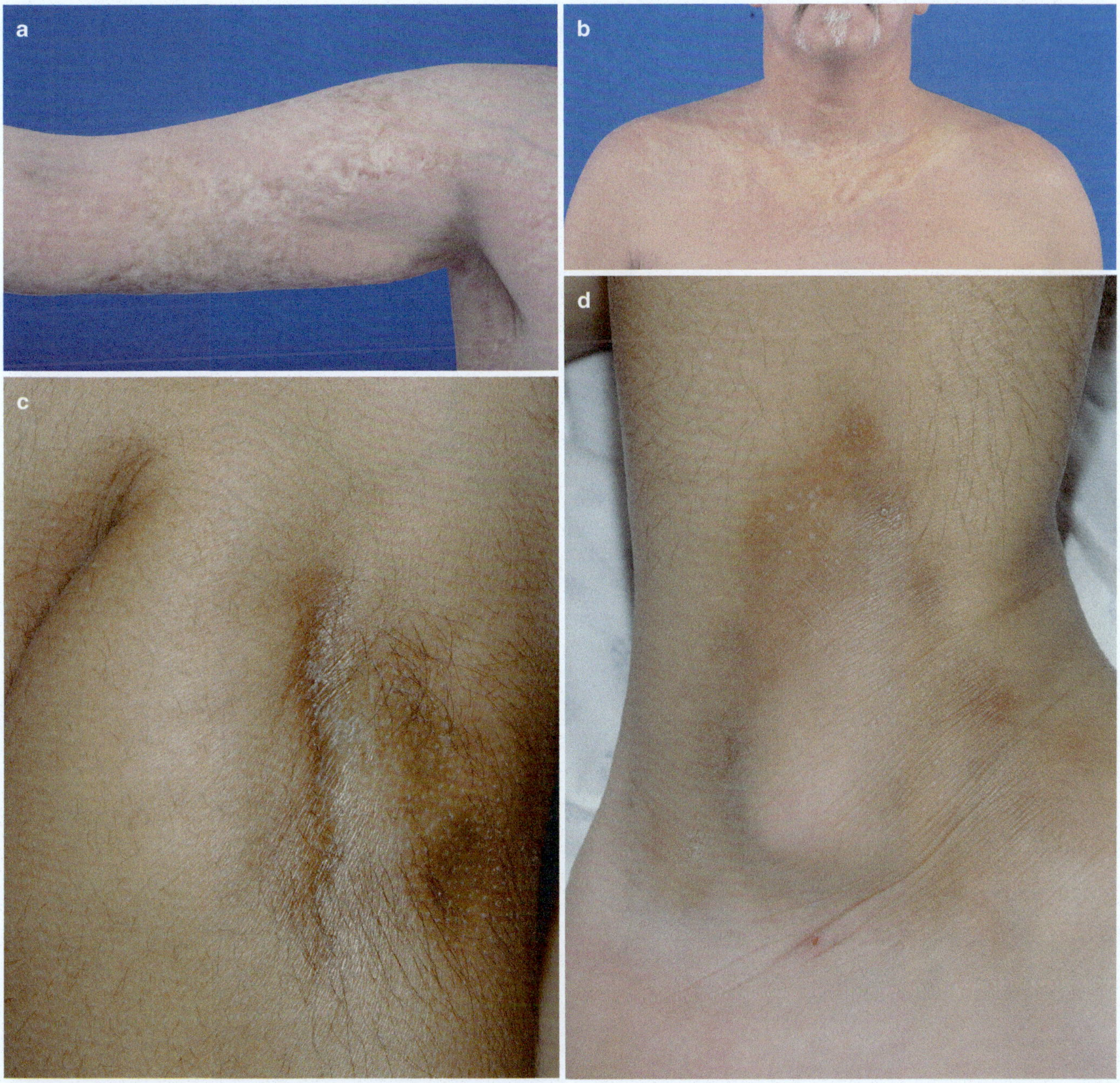

Fig. 10.4 Dermal sclerosis. (**a**) Thin, yellow morphea-like plaques and hyperpigmentation on the upper extremity. (**b**) Thin, yellow morphea-like plaques on the upper chest and anterior neck. (**c**) Bound down, hyperpigmented morphea-like plaque on the right leg. (**d**) Bound-down, hyperpigmented morphea-like plaque on right lower leg

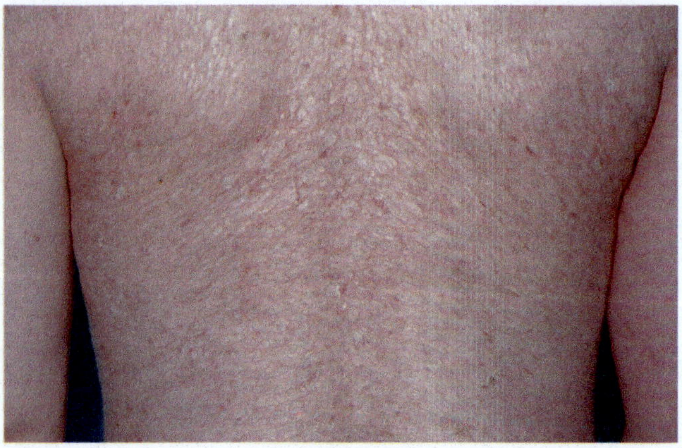

Fig. 10.5 Diffuse, thin, shiny lichen sclerosus–like plaques on the back

Table 10.2 NIH consensus project severity scoring of cutaneous cGVHD[a]

Cutaneous signs and symptoms	Score 0	Score 1	Score 2	Score 3	Highest score*
GVHD features to be scored by BSA: Maculopapular rash/erythema Lichen planus–like features Sclerotic features Papulosquamous lesions or ichthyosis Keratosis pilaris–like GVHD	No BSA	1–18% BSA	19–50% BSA	>50% BSA	
Sclerotic features	No sclerotic features		Superficial sclerotic features (able to pinch)	Deep sclerotic features Hidebound (unable to pinch) Impaired mobility Ulceration	
Other skin features not scored by BSA: Hyperpigmentation Hypopigmentation Poikiloderma Severe or generalized pruritus Hair involvement Nail involvement					

[a]Final scoring will be the highest of those marked
BSA **body surface area,** *GVHD* **graft-versus-host disease**

Treatment

It has been estimated that approximately 50 % of patients with cGVHD have resolution of symptoms within 7 years of initiation of systemic management, and approximately 10 % will require continued systemic treatment beyond 7 years. The remaining 40 % either die or have a relapse of malignancy within 7 years of initiating treatment for cGVHD [4]. Anticipating protracted systemic therapy, many factors must be considered when selecting therapies, including disease severity, preservation of the graft-versus-tumor effect, drug toxicity, other medical comorbidities, access to therapy, and drug interactions.

Treatment of Mild Cutaneous cGVHD

Symptomatic mild cutaneous cGVHD is generally treated locally with topical steroids or topical calcineurin inhibitors (CNIs) [5, 6]. Topical therapy minimizes systemic side effects and does not interfere with the graft-versus-tumor effect. Close monitoring for disease progression is important, as many patients will eventually require systemic therapy. In addition, active skin involvement should heighten surveillance for *de novo* development of cGVHD in other organs. Steroids of mid to high potency can be used for erythematous and scaling lesions [7]. The topical CNIs, tacrolimus and pimecrolimus, are recommended for treatment of mild cGVHD in areas where high potency steroids should be limited or avoided, including the face and intertriginous regions [8]. Pimecrolimus may be better tolerated at sites of non-intact skin, although it is not as potent as tacrolimus [5, 9].

Treatment of Moderate and Severe Cutaneous cGVHD

Systemic therapy is usually indicated for moderate or severe cGVHD (cutaneous disease with a skin severity score of at least 2). A skin severity score of 2 is given for the presence of skin sclerosis or at least 19 % BSA involvement with one of the specified features. Prednisone (typically 1 mg/kg per day) has been the primary first-line therapy since the 1980s [10]. Trials to determine the optimal duration and dose of corticosteroids are lacking, but based on consensus and expert opinion, it is recommended that 1 mg/kg per day be administered for 2 weeks, followed by a slow taper [4, 6]. Prednisone dosing should be changed to an alternate-day regimen of 1 mg/kg within 6–8 weeks and maintained at that level for 2–3 months to avoid a flare of cGVHD. One recommended taper schedule is to decrease the dose by 20–30 % every 2 weeks and to return to the penultimate dose for 2–4 weeks if there is a flare of cGVHD [4].

A recently published phase II study by Solomon et al. [11] suggests an alternative to corticosteroids as first-line therapy. In this study, 25 patients with new-onset cGVHD of any organ were treated with 375 mg/m^2 of rituximab once a week for 4 weeks, followed by infusions every 3 months for 1 year. Other noncorticosteroid immunosuppressive agents such as mycophenolate mofetil (MMF), tacrolimus, and sirolimus were permitted. Overall, 22 (88 %) of the patients responded to this corticosteroid-free treatment, with complete remission in 21 (95 %) of the 22 responders. Relapse of cGVHD occurred in 37 % within 24 months. This small prospective trial raises the possibility of a corticosteroid-free first-line regimen with fewer toxicities for new-onset cGVHD, but these results needs to be validated in a larger, controlled trial.

Combination first-line therapy of corticosteroids plus an additional agent has been evaluated in clinical trials using cyclosporine [12], azathioprine [13], thalidomide [14], MMF [15], and hydroxychloroquine [16]. No additional benefit was demonstrated in the treatment of cGVHD, but cyclosporine in combination with prednisone resulted in less osteonecrosis than prednisone alone [12]. Based on this study, CNIs are often given in combination with corticosteroids as first-line therapy for cGVHD, in an attempt to decrease toxicity associated with prolonged corticosteroid use.

Approximately 50 % of patients will respond to corticosteroids. The remaining patients with steroid-refractory cGVHD will require second-line treatment [17]. Three criteria are generally used to define steroid-refractory cGVHD:

- Progression despite 1 mg/kg per day of prednisone for 2 weeks
- Stable disease after 4–8 weeks of at least 0.5 mg/kg per day
- An inability to decrease the dosage of prednisone below 0.5 mg/kg per day

There is no standard second-line therapy, and limited evidence exists to guide salvage therapy. Selection of a second-line agent remains mostly trial-and-error, based on factors such as the organ systems involved, comorbidities, experience of the treating provider, and access to the treatment. The few randomized controlled trials of second-line agents in cGVHD often do not support the positive findings of case reports, case series, and small retrospective or prospective studies [15]. Therapies that have demonstrated particular benefit in cutaneous cGVHD include rituximab, extracorporeal photopheresis (ECP), phototherapy, imatinib mesylate, and mammalian target of rapamycin (mTOR) inhibitors, which are discussed in detail below. Additional salvage therapies are included in Table 10.3.

Table 10.3 Other systemic therapies reported for chronic GVHD

Drug	Results	Adverse events
Mycophenolate mofetil	There are no randomized trials. Response rates range from 40–75 % and steroid-sparing benefits have been reported	Diarrhea and GI discomfort, cytopenia [69, 70] and infection [70, 71] Increased risk of relapse when used as a third immunosuppressive agent [73]
Pentostatin	ORR in two prospective trials was 51 % [73] and 53 % [74]; skin was best-responding organ (ORR 69 %). Not recommended for pulmonary cGVHD	Nausea and infection
Methotrexate	Pooled ORR from eight studies was 77.6 %; cutaneous GVHD had best response (42–100 %) [75]	Cytopenia and hepatic toxicity
Hydroxychloroquine	Phase II study showed ORR of 53 % [76]. Phase III RCT did not confirm benefit [16].	Hypertension, GI toxicity, retinal toxicity
Clofazimine	Partial response in 55 % from one study; cutaneous GVHD had best response [77]	Skin discoloration, GI toxicity
Thalidomide	ORRs range from 20–59 %, with higher ORR in children [78–82]	Somnolence, constipation, neuropathy, neutropenia, venous thrombosis
Retinoids	ORR 74 % from one retrospective study of sclerotic GVHD [83]	Hyperlipidemia, transaminase elevation, teratogenicity, impaired wound healing
Alemtuzumab	One phase I study showed ORR of 70 % of evaluable patients; Cutaneous and fascial GVHD had best response [84]	Infection, cytopenia
Etanercept	Two prospective studies had ORRs of 52 % and 70 %, with the best response from GI and cutaneous GVHD [85, 86]	Infection
Mesenchymal stromal cells	ORRs from three prospective trials range from 0–87 % [87–89]	Infection; unclear impact on graft-versus-tumor effect
Azathioprine	In combination with prednisone, showed increased nonrelapse mortality and decreased overall survival [13]	Oral malignancy, infection

AE adverse event, *cGVHD* chronic graft-versus-host disease, *GI* gastrointestinal, *ORR* overall response rate, *RCT* randomized controlled trial

Rituximab

Rituximab is a chimeric monoclonal antibody reactive with CD20, found on the cell surface of B cells. Rituximab has been proposed as a treatment for cGVHD because of the suggested role of B cells and B cell–activating factor (BAFF) in cGVHD pathophysiology, the common finding of autoantibodies in patients with cGVHD, and the similarity between cGVHD manifestations and autoimmune conditions such as Sjögren's syndrome and systemic sclerosis [18, 19]. Prospective studies have reported overall response rates (ORR) of 63–88 % [11, 20–24]. A meta-analysis of six studies reported a pooled proportion ORR of 60 % for cutaneous cGVHD; the skin was the organ with the highest response rate to rituximab therapy [25]. Regimens can vary, but patients usually receive a minimum of four weekly rituximab infusions of 375 mg/m^2. Additional infusions at intervals of 1 to 3 months have also been given. Van Dorp et al. [22] studied the immunologic phenotype of 18 patients with steroid-refractory or steroid-dependent cGVHD who were treated with rituximab to evaluate predictors of response to therapy. The ORR of rituximab for skin cGVHD was greater than 75 % regardless of the type of cutaneous involvement. About three fourths of the patients were able to decrease or discontinue corticosteroids. No correlation was seen between BAFF levels and rituximab response, but an elevated B-cell number prior to treatment correlated with response to therapy with rituximab [22].

The most common adverse events (AEs) in rituximab cGVHD trials were infusion reactions and infections [21, 26]. In a phase II prospective trial, infections and recurrent malignancy accounted for most of the treatment failures [21].

Extracorporeal Photopheresis

Extracorporeal photopheresis (ECP) is an immunomodulatory therapy that was first reported as a treatment for GVHD in the 1980s. Since then, ECP has become a widely used therapeutic modality for cGVHD of the skin and other organs (Fig. 10.6) [27–29]. As with other interventions, published reports are primarily retrospective in nature. One multicenter, randomized controlled trial compared standard treatment plus ECP (weekly on two consecutive days) to standard treatment alone over 12 weeks, for treatment of cutaneous cGVHD. The primary endpoint, a lower total skin score (TSS), had a positive trend, but it did not reach statistical significance. However, there was a steroid-sparing effect in the group that received ECP. Patients in the ECP arm were more likely to achieve both a reduction in steroid dose greater than 50 % and a total daily dose of 10 mg or less. The difference in the reduction of the steroid dose became apparent after week 8, though improvement in the TSS was noted earlier [30]. A steroid-sparing benefit of ECP also has been demonstrated in other studies [31–33].

As with other salvage therapies for cGVHD, comparison of the published literature for ECP is limited because of the heterogeneity of the disease and organ-specific outcome measures, as well as the variability in the schedule of ECP administration. Nonetheless, the skin appears to be among the organs most responsive to this treatment modality. A meta-analysis of ECP for steroid-refractory cGVHD found that ECP has the greatest benefit in skin, oral, liver, and musculoskeletal disease, with pooled response rates of 74 %, 72 %, 68 %, and 64 % respectively. Response rates were lower for other organs [32]. Similarly, a systematic review of ECP for acute or chronic steroid-refractory or steroid-dependent GVHD found a pooled ORR of 71 % for cutaneous chronic GVHD, which was higher than for other target organs with cGVHD [31].

ECP is generally a safe therapeutic option for cGVHD. The most commonly reported AEs are nausea, headache, and fever. Serious infections, including line infection, are rare, and relapse of malignancy has not been reported [27, 33, 34]. Both the U.K. Photopheresis Expert Group [33] and the Ontario Stem Cell Transplant Steering Committee [35] have developed consensus statements that recommend ECP as second-line therapy for cGVHD. The U.K. consensus statement recommends delivery of ECP on two consecutive days every other week, tapering to every 4 weeks once a response is seen. At this time, there is no biologic marker of disease response, so clinical assessment is the standard outcome measure. The clinical response of cGVHD to ECP is slow; 4 months is the recommended timeframe for response assessment [33].

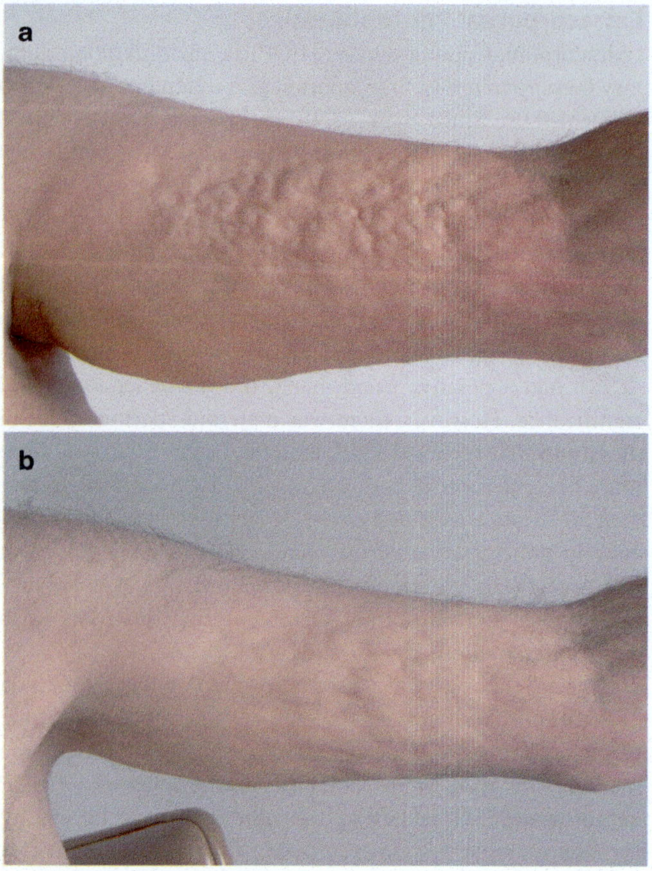

Fig. 10.6 Clinical improvement of sclerosis from extracorporeal photopheresis (ECP) therapy. (**a**) Localized rippling and nodularity from subcutaneous cGVHD on the left arm. (**b**) Decreased nodularity after 6 months of ECP

Phototherapy

Treatment of skin disease with ultraviolet (UV) radiation is commonly used for dermatologic conditions. As with many cGVHD therapies, high-quality trial data on the use of phototherapy is rare. In addition, different types of disease (*e.g.*, lichenoid *vs* sclerotic) would be expected to have different responses, given the therapeutic penetration of UV light. No prospective studies have been carried out to provide recommendations for the type, dose, or schedule of UV therapy. Psoralen plus ultraviolet A (PUVA) is the best-studied phototherapy in cGVHD. In a retrospective analysis of 40 patients with cGVHD, 77 % had a local response (cutaneous or oral), with 40 % experiencing a complete response [36]. However, all but one of the patients included had concomitant systemic therapy. UVA1, a subset of the UVA wavelength (340–400 nm), has been evaluated in three small studies [37–39]. Overall, 24 of 25 total patients in the three studies responded, including those with both lichenoid and sclerotic cGVHD. Calzavara Pinton et al. [37] reported that all patients with lichenoid cGVHD relapsed within a month and required maintenance phototherapy. Only two studies have evaluated UVB (280–320 nm) as a local therapy for cGVHD [40, 41]. Brazzelli et al. [41] administered narrow band UVB (311–312 nm) to 10 pediatric patients, 5 with cGVHD and 5 with overlap GVHD. Of the 10 patients, 8 had a complete response, which was sustained in 71 % of the responders at 2 years.

Phototherapy is generally well tolerated. Photosensitizing medications (*e.g.*, voriconazole, trimethoprim-sulfamethoxazole, and furosemide) should be discontinued prior to initiating phototherapy. Erythema is a common short-term AE. Oral psoralens may induce nausea, vomiting, dizziness, and hepatotoxicity, which can limit tolerability. Bath PUVA avoids the systemic side effects of psoralens, but is time-intensive. Strict sun protection (including eye protection) is required on the day psoralens are taken. Long-term phototherapy may cause accelerated photoaging and increase the risk of skin cancer, particularly with PUVA. Patients treated with PUVA develop squamous cell carcinoma more often than basal cell carcinoma or melanoma [42].

Imatinib Mesylate

Imatinib is a tyrosine kinase inhibitor (TKI) that targets the platelet-derived growth factor receptor (PDGFR) among other tyrosine kinases [43]. Stimulatory autoantibodies to the PDGFR were reported in patients with sclerotic cGVHD and in patients with systemic sclerosis, suggesting a potential pathway of skin fibrosis targetable by this drug [44, 45]. In addition, *in vitro* studies have demonstrated that treatment of fibroblasts with imatinib inhibited proliferation [46]. Clinical studies have reported an ORR in sclerotic GVHD ranging from 26 % to 63 % [47–52]. Comparisons between studies is challenging because of the heterogeneous disease manifestations and the range of end points used to determine efficacy. Even within studies, the benefit of this antifibrotic therapy was not consistent among patients with sclerotic GVHD.

Imatinib appears to be less well tolerated in the cGVHD setting than in chronic myeloid leukemia (CML) and other indications. AEs have been reported at doses as low as 100 mg in sclerotic GVHD patients, despite dosing of 400 to 800 mg in the CML setting [51]. Hematologic AEs include neutropenia, thrombocytopenia, leukopenia, and anemia. Nonhematologic AEs include fatigue, nausea, diarrhea, electrolyte abnormalities, fluid retention (peripheral and periorbital), and muscular cramps. Sclerotic cGVHD patients are particularly sensitive to discomfort from fluid retention and muscular cramps, as they often experience these symptoms as part of their primary disease.

Dasatinib, a second-generation TKI, has been evaluated as an alternative agent in patients with sclerotic cGVHD who are resistant or intolerant to imatinib. Three patients with sclerotic cGVHD who could not take imatinib were treated with dasatinib [53]. All three achieved a partial response and corticosteroids were decreased in all patients. In contrast to imatinib, the patients did not experience dose-limiting toxicities from dasatinib. There is overlap in the observed AEs between imatinib and dasatinib, but it appears that individual patients develop differing AEs to the two different drugs [54]. This limited experience in cGVHD suggests that dasatinib warrants further investigation as a better-tolerated treatment for some patients with sclerotic cGVHD.

Mammalian Target of Rapamycin (mTOR) Inhibitors

Sirolimus and its derivative everolimus are macrolide antibiotics that act through inhibition of the mTOR pathway. They act as immunosuppressive drugs and may also act via inhibition of proliferation of fibroblasts and smooth muscle cells. Additionally, they have a role in reconstitution of regulatory T cells in cGVHD [55]. mTOR inhibitors have been suggested as alternatives to CNIs for treatment of cGVHD because of the protective effect on skin cancer development that has been demonstrated in recipients of solid-organ transplants [56]. Data regarding the efficacy of mTOR inhibitors specifically for cutaneous cGVHD are scarce. One prospective study reported a response rate of 65 % in skin cGVHD, and one retrospective study of sclerotic cGVHD reported an ORR of 76 % [57, 58]. Additionally, mTOR inhibitors have demonstrated a steroid-sparing benefit.

The combination of CNIs and mTOR inhibitors is associated with increased risk of transplant-associated microangiopathy and renal toxicity [57]. Other toxicities seen with mTOR inhibitors include hyperlipidemia, infection, and cytopenias. mTOR inhibitors are substrates for cytochrome p450 3 A4, indicating that potential drug interactions may occur in GVHD patients, who often take multiple medications. Potential impairment of wound healing should also be considered for patients with skin breakdown or ulceration [59].

Low-Dose Interleukin (IL)-2

Regulatory T cells (Tregs), CD4+ T cells that play an important role in immune tolerance, are decreased in cGVHD. Tregs are stimulated by cytokines, including IL-2, which results in Treg expansion and survival [60]. Low-dose subcutaneous IL-2 has been evaluated in phase I and phase II prospective trials of patients with steroid-refractory cGVHD [61, 62]. IL-2 was given daily for 8–12 weeks. Although there were no complete responders in the trials, 94 % of patients experienced a partial response (32 of 56 patients) or stable disease (21 of 56 patients). In the phase II study of 33 evaluable patients, the best responses were seen in cGVHD of the liver (46 %) and skin (33 %) [62]. The spectrum of cutaneous disease that had a measurable response included papulosquamous, lichen planus-like, keratosis pilaris, poikiloderma, and superficial and deep sclerosis. This therapy allowed for reduction in dose of glucocorticoids for many patients. Adverse events from the trials included infection, injection site induration, constitutional symptoms, TMA, and renal dysfunction [61, 62]. Validation in randomized, controlled trials of subcutaneous low-dose IL-2 in cGVHD of the skin are needed.

Janus Kinase (JAK) Inhibitors

JAK inhibitors are a class of drugs that inhibit one or more of the Janus tyrosine kinases (JAK1, JAK2, JAK3, TYK2). Binding of interferons and other cytokines, such as IL-2, IL-4, IL-7, IL-9, IL-15, and IL-21, to their receptors results in activation of Janus kinases and the JAK-signal transducer and activator of transcription (STAT) pathway. Although there are no prospective studies of JAK inhibitors in cGVHD, retrospective studies and case reports are encouraging [63–65]. Khoury et al. [65] reported 16 patients with cGVHD treated with ruxolitinib, a JAK1/2 inhibitor. Patients with erythematous cGVHD had complete response and those with sclerotic cGVHD had subjective improvements. The majority (75 %) were able to taper or discontinue corticosteroids. Zeiser et al. [64] described a retrospective series of 41 patients with cGVHD from 19 institutions treated with ruxolitinib and found an ORR of 85.4 % (35 of 41 patents) for all sites of cGVHD involvement. Six patients had a complete response. Two patients had a relapse of cGVHD with a median follow-up of 22 weeks. The most common adverse events included cytopenia and CMV reactivation. One patient had a relapse of the primary malignancy. Larger, randomized, controlled studies are needed to validate the utility of JAK inhibitors in cutaneous cGVHD.

Prophylaxis

Patients who are exposed to long-term immunosuppressive medications, especially corticosteroids, require supportive therapy to minimize AEs from the treatment. Infection is the leading cause of death in patients with cGVHD. Prophylaxis against *Pneumocystis jirovecii* and encapsulated bacteria is recommended. Patients with GVHD are considered at high risk for fluconazole-resistant *Candida* species and molds. The recommended antifungal agent for prophylaxis in this population is posaconazole [65]. The use of voriconazole is considered a second-line alternative to posaconazole, but voriconazole is associated with phototoxicity, and long-term use of voriconazole in the GVHD setting has been associated with skin cancer, particularly squamous cell carcinoma [65–67].

References

1. Arai S, Arora M, Wang T, Spellman SR, He W, Couriel DR, et al. Increasing Incidence of chronic graft-versus-host disease in allogeneic transplantation: a report from the Center for International Blood and Marrow Transplant Research. Biol Blood Marrow Transplant. 2015;21:266–74.
2. Filipovich AH, Weisdorf D, Pavletic S, Socie G, Wingard JR, Lee SJ, et al. National Institutes of Health consensus development project on criteria for clinical trials in chronic graft-versus-host disease: I. Diagnosis and staging working group report. Biol Blood Marrow Transplant. 2005;11:945–56.
3. Jagasia MH, Greinix HT, Arora M, Williams KM, Wolff D, Cowen EW, et al. National Institutes of Health consensus development project on criteria for clinical trials in chronic graft-versus-host disease: I. The 2014 Diagnosis and Staging Working Group report. Biol Blood Marrow Transplant. 2015;21:389–401.
4. Flowers ME, Martin PJ. How we treat chronic graft-versus-host disease. Blood. 2015;125:606–15.
5. Marks C, Stadler M, Hausermann P, Wolff D, Buchholz S, Stary G, et al. German-Austrian-Swiss Consensus Conference on clinical practice in chronic graft-versus-host disease (GVHD): guidance for supportive therapy of chronic cutaneous and musculoskeletal GVHD. Br J Dermatol. 2011;165:18–29.
6. Wolff D, Gerbitz A, Ayuk F, Kiani A, Hildebrandt GC, Vogelsang GB, et al. Consensus conference on clinical practice in chronic graft-versus-host disease (GVHD): first-line and topical treatment of chronic GVHD. Biol Blood Marrow Transplant. 2010;16:1611–28.
7. Couriel D, Carpenter PA, Cutler C, Bolanos-Meade J, Treister NS, Gea-Banacloche J, et al. Ancillary therapy and supportive care of chronic graft-versus-host disease: National Institutes of Health consensus development project on criteria for clinical trials in chronic graft-versus-host disease: V. Ancillary Therapy and Supportive Care Working Group report. Biol Blood Marrow Transplant. 2006;12:375–96.
8. Choi CJ, Nghiem P. Tacrolimus ointment in the treatment of chronic cutaneous graft-vs-host disease: a case series of 18 patients. Arch Dermatol. 2001;137:1202–6.
9. Paller AS, Lebwohl M, Fleischer Jr AB, Antaya R, Langley RG, Kirsner RS, et al. Tacrolimus ointment is more effective than pimecrolimus cream with a similar safety profile in the treatment of atopic dermatitis: results from 3 randomized, comparative studies. J Am Acad Dermatol. 2005;52:810–22.
10. Sullivan KM, Shulman HM, Storb R, Weiden PL, Witherspoon RP, McDonald GB, et al. Chronic graft-versus-host disease in 52 patients: adverse natural course and successful treatment with combination immunosuppression. Blood. 1981;57:267–76.
11. Solomon SR, Sizemore CA, Ridgeway M, Zhang X, Smith J, Brown S, et al. Corticosteroid-free primary treatment of chronic extensive graft-versus-host disease incorporating rituximab. Biol Blood Marrow Transplant. 2015;21:1576–82.
12. Koc S, Leisenring W, Flowers ME, Anasetti C, Deeg HJ, Nash RA, et al. Therapy for chronic graft-versus-host disease: a randomized trial comparing cyclosporine plus prednisone versus prednisone alone. Blood. 2002;100:48–51.
13. Sullivan KM, Witherspoon RP, Storb R, Weiden P, Flournoy N, Dahlberg S, et al. Prednisone and azathioprine compared with prednisone and placebo for treatment of chronic graft-v-host disease: prognostic influence of prolonged thrombocytopenia after allogeneic marrow transplantation. Blood. 1988;72:546–54.
14. Flowers ME, Martin PJ. Evaluation of thalidomide for treatment or prevention of chronic graft-versus-host disease. Leuk Lymphoma. 2003;44:1141–6.
15. Martin PJ, Inamoto Y, Carpenter PA, Lee SJ, Flowers ME. Treatment of chronic graft-versus-host disease: Past, present and future. Korean J Hematol. 2011;46:153–63.
16. Gilman AL, Schultz KR, Goldman FD, Sale GE, Krailo MD, Chen Z, et al. Randomized trial of hydroxychloroquine for newly diagnosed chronic graft-versus-host disease in children: a Children's Oncology Group study. Biol Blood Marrow Transplant. 2012;18: 84–91.
17. Inamoto Y, Flowers ME, Sandmaier BM, Aki SZ, Carpenter PA, Lee SJ, et al. Failure-free survival after initial systemic treatment of chronic graft-versus-host disease. Blood. 2014;124:1363–71.
18. Sarantopoulos S, Ritz J, Aberrant B. Cell homeostasis in chronic GVHD. Blood. 2015;125:1703–7.
19. Kuzmina Z, Gounden V, Curtis L, Avila D, Rnp TT, Baruffaldi J, et al. Clinical significance of autoantibodies in a large cohort of patients with chronic graft-versus-host disease defined by NIH criteria. Am J Hematol. 2015;90:114–9.
20. Cutler C, Miklos D, Kim HT, Treister N, Woo SB, Bienfang D, et al. Rituximab for steroid-refractory chronic graft-versus-host disease. Blood. 2006;108:756–62.
21. Kim SJ, Lee JW, Jung CW, Min CK, Cho B, Shin HJ, et al. Weekly rituximab followed by monthly rituximab treatment for steroid-refractory chronic graft-versus-host disease: results from a prospective, multicenter, phase II study. Haematologica. 2010;95:1935–42.
22. van Dorp S, Resemann H, te Boome L, Pietersma F, van Baarle D, Gmelig-Meyling F, et al. The immunological phenotype of rituximab-sensitive chronic graft-versus-host disease: a phase II study. Haematologica. 2011;96:1380–4.
23. von Bonin M, Oelschlagel U, Radke J, Stewart M, Ehninger G, Bornhauser M, et al. Treatment of chronic steroid-refractory graft-versus-host disease with low-dose rituximab. Transplantation. 2008;86:875–9.
24. Canninga-van Dijk MR, van der Straaten HM, Fijnheer R, Sanders CJ, van den Tweel JG, Verdonck LF. Anti-CD20 monoclonal antibody treatment in 6 patients with therapy-refractory chronic graft-versus-host disease. Blood. 2004;104:2603–6.
25. Kharfan-Dabaja MA, Mhaskar AR, Djulbegovic B, Cutler C, Mohty M, Kumar A. Efficacy of rituximab in the setting of steroid-refractory chronic graft-versus-host disease: a systematic review and meta-analysis. Biol Blood Marrow Transplant. 2009;15: 1005–13.
26. Bates JS, Engemann AM, Hammond JM. Clinical utility of rituximab in chronic graft-versus-host disease. Ann Pharmacother. 2009;43:316–21.
27. Greinix HT, Volc-Platzer B, Rabitsch W, Gmeinhart B, Guevara-Pineda C, Kalhs P, et al. Successful use of extracorporeal photoche-

motherapy in the treatment of severe acute and chronic graft-versus-host disease. Blood. 1998;92:3098–104.
28. Seaton ED, Szydlo RM, Kanfer E, Apperley JF, Russell-Jones R. Influence of extracorporeal photopheresis on clinical and laboratory parameters in chronic graft-versus-host disease and analysis of predictors of response. Blood. 2003;102:1217–23.
29. Couriel DR, Hosing C, Saliba R, Shpall EJ, Anderlini P, Rhodes B, et al. Extracorporeal photochemotherapy for the treatment of steroid-resistant chronic GVHD. Blood. 2006;107:3074–80.
30. Flowers ME, Apperley JF, van Besien K, Elmaagacli A, Grigg A, Reddy V, et al. A multicenter prospective phase 2 randomized study of extracorporeal photopheresis for treatment of chronic graft-versus-host disease. Blood. 2008;112:2667–74.
31. Abu-Dalle I, Reljic T, Nishihori T, Antar A, Bazarbachi A, Djulbegovic B, et al. Extracorporeal photopheresis in steroid-refractory acute or chronic graft-versus-host disease: results of a systematic review of prospective studies. Biol Blood Marrow Transplant. 2014;20:1677–86.
32. Malik MI, Litzow M, Hogan W, Patnaik M, Murad MH, Prokop LJ, et al. Extracorporeal photopheresis for chronic graft-versus-host disease: a systematic review and meta-analysis. Blood Res. 2014;49:100–6.
33. Scarisbrick JJ, Taylor P, Holtick U, Makar Y, Douglas K, Berlin G, et al. U.K. consensus statement on the use of extracorporeal photopheresis for treatment of cutaneous T-cell lymphoma and chronic graft-versus-host disease. Br J Dermatol. 2008;158:659–78.
34. Kitko CL, Braun T, Couriel DR, Choi SW, Connelly J, Hoffmann S, et al. Combination therapy for graft-versus-host disease prophylaxis with etanercept and extracorporeal photopheresis: results of a phase II clinical trial. Biol Blood Marrow Transplant. 2016;22:862–8.
35. Bredeson C, Rumble RB, Varela NP, Kuruvilla J, Kouroukis CT. Stem Cell Transplant Steering Committee. Extracorporeal photopheresis in the management of graft-versus-host disease. Curr Oncol. 2014;21:e310–25.
36. Vogelsang GB, Wolff D, Altomonte V, Farmer E, Morison WL, Corio R, et al. Treatment of chronic graft-versus-host disease with ultraviolet irradiation and psoralen (PUVA). Bone Marrow Transplant. 1996;17:1061–7.
37. Calzavara Pinton P, Porta F, Izzi T, Venturini M, Capezzera R, Zane C, et al. Prospects for ultraviolet A1 phototherapy as a treatment for chronic cutaneous graft-versus-host disease. Haematologica. 2003;88:1169–75.
38. Wetzig T, Sticherling M, Simon JC, Hegenbart U, Niederwieser D, Al-Ali HK. Medium dose long-wavelength ultraviolet A (UVA1) phototherapy for the treatment of acute and chronic graft-versus-host disease of the skin. Bone Marrow Transplant. 2005;35:515–9.
39. Stander H, Schiller M, Schwarz T. UVA1 therapy for sclerodermic graft-versus-host disease of the skin. J Am Acad Dermatol. 2002;46:799–800.
40. Enk CD, Elad S, Vexler A, Kapelushnik J, Gorodetsky R, Kirschbaum M. Chronic graft-versus-host disease treated with UVB phototherapy. Bone Marrow Transplant. 1998;22:1179–83.
41. Brazzelli V, Grasso V, Muzio F, Moggio E, Zecca M, Locatelli F, et al. Narrowband ultraviolet B phototherapy in the treatment of cutaneous graft-versus-host disease in oncohaematological paediatric patients. Br J Dermatol. 2010;162:404–9.
42. Stern RS, Lange R. Non-melanoma skin cancer occurring in patients treated with PUVA five to ten years after first treatment. J Invest Dermatol. 1988;91:120–4.
43. Carroll M, Ohno-Jones S, Tamura S, Buchdunger E, Zimmermann J, Lydon NB, et al. CGP 57148, a tyrosine kinase inhibitor, inhibits the growth of cells expressing BCR-ABL, TEL-ABL, and TEL-PDGFR fusion proteins. Blood. 1997;90:4947–52.
44. Baroni SS, Santillo M, Bevilacqua F, Luchetti M, Spadoni T, Mancini M, et al. Stimulatory autoantibodies to the PDGF receptor in systemic sclerosis. N Engl J Med. 2006;354:2667–76.
45. Svegliati S, Olivieri A, Campelli N, Luchetti M, Poloni A, Trappolini S, et al. Stimulatory autoantibodies to PDGF receptor in patients with extensive chronic graft-versus-host disease. Blood. 2007;110:237–41.
46. Soria A, Cario-Andre M, Lepreux S, Rezvani HR, Pasquet JM, Pain C, et al. The effect of imatinib (Glivec) on scleroderma and normal dermal fibroblasts: a preclinical study. Dermatology. 2008;216:109–17.
47. Magro L, Mohty M, Catteau B, Coiteux V, Chevallier P, Terriou L, et al. Imatinib mesylate as salvage therapy for refractory sclerotic chronic graft-versus-host disease. Blood. 2009;114:719–22.
48. Olivieri A, Locatelli F, Zecca M, Sanna A, Cimminiello M, Raimondi R, et al. Imatinib for refractory chronic graft-versus-host disease with fibrotic features. Blood. 2009;114:709–18.
49. Chen GL, Arai S, Flowers ME, Otani JM, Qiu J, Cheng EC, et al. A phase 1 study of imatinib for corticosteroid-dependent/refractory chronic graft-versus-host disease: response does not correlate with anti-PDGFRA antibodies. Blood. 2011;118:4070–8.
50. Olivieri A, Cimminiello M, Corradini P, Mordini N, Fedele R, Selleri C, et al. Long-term outcome and prospective validation of NIH response criteria in 39 patients receiving imatinib for steroid-refractory chronic GVHD. Blood. 2013;122:4111–8.
51. Baird K, Comis LE, Joe GO, Steinberg SM, Hakim FT, Rose JJ, et al. Imatinib mesylate for the treatment of steroid-refractory sclerotic-type cutaneous chronic graft-versus-host disease. Biol Blood Marrow Transplant. 2015;21:1083–90.
52. Arai S, Pidala J, Pusic I, Chai X, Jaglowski S, Khera N, et al. A randomized phase II crossover study of imatinib or rituximab for cutaneous sclerosis after hematopoietic cell transplantation. Clin Cancer Res. 2015;22:319–27.
53. Sanchez-Ortega I, Servitje O, Arnan M, Orti G, Peralta T, Manresa F, et al. Dasatinib as salvage therapy for steroid refractory and imatinib resistant or intolerant sclerotic chronic graft-versus-host disease. Biol Blood Marrow Transplant. 2012;18:318–23.
54. Conchon M, Freitas CM, Rego MA, Braga Junior JW. Dasatinib – clinical trials and management of adverse events in imatinib resistant/intolerant chronic myeloid leukemia. Rev Bras Hematol Hemoter. 2011;33:131–9.
55. Sugiyama H, Maeda Y, Nishimori H, Yamasuji Y, Matsuoka K, Fujii N, et al. Mammalian target of rapamycin inhibitors permit regulatory T cell reconstitution and inhibit experimental chronic graft-versus-host disease. Biol Blood Marrow Transplant. 2014;20:183–91.
56. Euvrard S, Morelon E, Rostaing L, Goffin E, Brocard A, Tromme I, et al. Sirolimus and secondary skin-cancer prevention in kidney transplantation. N Engl J Med. 2012;367:329–39.
57. Couriel DR, Saliba R, Escalon MP, Hsu Y, Ghosh S, Ippoliti C, et al. Sirolimus in combination with tacrolimus and corticosteroids for the treatment of resistant chronic graft-versus-host disease. Br J Haematol. 2005;130:409–17.
58. Jedlickova Z, Burlakova I, Bug G, Baurmann H, Schwerdtfeger R, Schleuning M. Therapy of sclerodermatous chronic graft-versus-host disease with mammalian target of rapamycin inhibitors. Biol Blood Marrow Transplant. 2011;17:657–63.
59. Kuppahally S, Al-Khaldi A, Weisshaar D, Valantine HA, Oyer P, Robbins RC, et al. Wound healing complications with de novo sirolimus versus mycophenolate mofetil-based regimen in cardiac transplant recipients. Am J Transplant. 2006;6:986–92.
60. Zorn E, Nelson EA, Mohseni M, Porcheray F, Kim H, Litsa D, et al. IL-2 regulates FOXP3 expression in human CD4+CD25+ regulatory T cells through a STAT-dependent mechanism and induces the expansion of these cells in vivo. Blood. 2006;108(5):1571–9.
61. Koreth J, Matsuoka K, Kim HT, McDonough SM, Bindra B, Alyea EP 3rd, et al. Interleukin-2 and regulatory T cells in graft-versus-host disease. N Engl J Med 2011;365(22):2055–66.
62. Koreth J, Kim HT, Jones KT, Lange PB, Reynolds CG, Chammas MJ, et al. Efficacy, durability, and response predictors of low-dose

interleukin-2 therapy for chronic graft vs. host disease. Blood. 2016;128:130–7.
63. Spoerl S, Mathew NR, Bscheider M, Schmitt-Graeff A, Chen S, Mueller T, et al. Activity of therapeutic JAK 1/2 blockade in graft-versus-host disease. Blood. 2014;123(24):3832–42.
64. Zeiser R, Burchert A, Lengerke C, Verbeek M, Maas-Bauer K, Metzelder SK, et al. Ruxolitinib in corticosteroid-refractory graft-versus-host disease after allogeneic stem cell transplantation: a multicenter survey. Leukemia. 2015;29:2062–8.
65. Khoury HJ, Kota V, Arellano M, Bauer SL, Jillella AP, Langston A, et al. Ruxolitinib As Sparing Agent for Steroid-Dependent Chronic Graft-Versus-Host Disease (cGVHD). Blood. 2015;126(23):1938.
66. Tomblyn M, Chiller T, Einsele H, Gress R, Sepkowitz K, Storek J, et al. Guidelines for preventing infectious complications among hematopoietic cell transplantation recipients: a global perspective. Biol Blood Marrow Transplant. 2009;15:1143–238.
67. Sheu J, Hawryluk EB, Guo D, London WB, Huang JT. Voriconazole phototoxicity in children: a retrospective review. J Am Acad Dermatol. 2015;72:314–20.
68. Cowen EW, Nguyen JC, Miller DD, McShane D, Arron ST, Prose NS, et al. Chronic phototoxicity and aggressive squamous cell carcinoma of the skin in children and adults during treatment with voriconazole. J Am Acad Dermatol. 2010;62:31–7.
69. Furlong T, Martin P, Flowers ME, Carnevale-Schianca F, Yatscoff R, Chauncey T, et al. Therapy with mycophenolate mofetil for refractory acute and chronic GVHD. Bone Marrow Transplant. 2009;44:739–48.
70. Krejci M, Doubek M, Buchler T, Brychtova Y, Vorlicek J, Mayer J. Mycophenolate mofetil for the treatment of acute and chronic steroid-refractory graft-versus-host disease. Ann Hematol. 2005;84: 681–5.
71. Baudard M, Vincent A, Moreau P, Kergueris MF, Harousseau JL, Milpied N. Mycophenolate mofetil for the treatment of acute and chronic GVHD is effective and well tolerated but induces a high risk of infectious complications: a series of 21 BM or PBSC transplant patients. Bone Marrow Transplant. 2002;30:287–95.
72. Martin PJ, Storer BE, Rowley SD, Flowers ME, Lee SJ, Carpenter PA, et al. Evaluation of mycophenolate mofetil for initial treatment of chronic graft-versus-host disease. Blood. 2009;113:5074–82.
73. Jacobsohn DA, Chen AR, Zahurak M, Piantadosi S, Anders V, Bolanos-Meade J, et al. Phase II study of pentostatin in patients with corticosteroid-refractory chronic graft-versus-host disease. J Clin Oncol. 2007;25
74. Jacobsohn DA, Gilman AL, Rademaker A, Browning B, Grimley M, Lehmann L, et al. Evaluation of pentostatin in corticosteroid-refractory chronic graft-versus-host disease in children: a Pediatric Blood and Marrow Transplant Consortium study. Blood. 2009;114: 4354–60.
75. Nassar A, Elgohary G, Elhassan T, Nurgat Z, Mohamed SY, Aljurf M. Methotrexate for the treatment of graft-versus-host disease after allogeneic hematopoietic stem cell transplantation. J Transplant. 2014;2014:980301.
76. Gilman AL, Chan KW, Mogul A, Morris C, Goldman FD, Boyer M, et al. Hydroxychloroquine for the treatment of chronic graft-versus-host disease. Biol Blood Marrow Transplant. 2000;6: 327–34.
77. Lee SJ, Wegner SA, McGarigle CJ, Bierer BE, Antin JH. Treatment of chronic graft-versus-host disease with clofazimine. Blood. 1997;89:2298–302.
78. Vogelsang GB, Farmer ER, Hess AD, Altamonte V, Beschorner WE, Jabs DA, et al. Thalidomide for the treatment of chronic graft-versus-host disease. N Engl J Med. 1992;326:1055–8.
79. Parker PM, Chao N, Nademanee A, O'Donnell MR, Schmidt GM, Snyder DS, et al. Thalidomide as salvage therapy for chronic graft-versus-host disease. Blood. 1995;86:3604–9.
80. Rovelli A, Arrigo C, Nesi F, Balduzzi A, Nicolini B, Locasciulli A, et al. The role of thalidomide in the treatment of refractory chronic graft-versus-host disease following bone marrow transplantation in children. Bone Marrow Transplant. 1998;21:577–81.
81. Browne PV, Weisdorf DJ, DeFor T, Miller WJ, Davies SM, Filipovich A, et al. Response to thalidomide therapy in refractory chronic graft-versus-host disease. Bone Marrow Transplant. 2000;26:865–9.
82. Kulkarni S, Powles R, Sirohi B, Treleaven J, Saso R, Horton C, et al. Thalidomide after allogeneic haematopoietic stem cell transplantation: activity in chronic but not in acute graft-versus-host disease. Bone Marrow Transplant. 2003;32:165–70.
83. Marcellus DC, Altomonte VL, Farmer ER, Horn TD, Freemer CS, Grant J, et al. Etretinate therapy for refractory sclerodermatous chronic graft-versus-host disease. Blood. 1999;93:66–70.
84. Nikiforow S, Kim HT, Bindra B, McDonough S, Glotzbecker B, Armand P, et al. Phase I study of alemtuzumab for therapy of steroid-refractory chronic graft-versus-host disease. Biol Blood Marrow Transplant. 2013;19:804–11.
85. Busca A, Locatelli F, Marmont F, Ceretto C, Falda M. Recombinant human soluble tumor necrosis factor receptor fusion protein as treatment for steroid refractory graft-versus-host disease following allogeneic hematopoietic stem cell transplantation. Am J Hematol. 2007;82:45–52.
86. Chiang KY, Abhyankar S, Bridges K, Godder K, Henslee-Downey JP. Recombinant human tumor necrosis factor receptor fusion protein as complementary treatment for chronic graft-versus-host disease. Transplantation. 2002;73:665–7.
87. Peng Y, Chen X, Liu Q, Zhang X, Huang K, Liu L, et al. Mesenchymal stromal cells infusions improve refractory chronic graft versus host disease through an increase of CD5+ regulatory B cells producing interleukin 10. Leukemia. 2015;29:636–46.
88. Introna M, Lucchini G, Dander E, Galimberti S, Rovelli A, Balduzzi A, et al. Treatment of graft versus host disease with mesenchymal stromal cells: a phase I study on 40 adult and pediatric patients. Biol Blood Marrow Transplant. 2014;20:375–81.
89. Weng JY, Du X, Geng SX, Peng YW, Wang Z, ZS L, et al. Mesenchymal stem cell as salvage treatment for refractory chronic GVHD. Bone Marrow Transplant. 2010;45:1732–40.

11 Wound Care in the Management of Chronic Graft-Versus-Host Disease

Jae Y. Jung and Timothy H. Almazan

Chronic graft-versus-host disease (cGVHD) affects a substantial proportion of long-term survivors of hematopoietic stem cell transplantation (HSCT). cGVHD of the skin has a varied presentation, ranging from mild, local sclerosis to extensive complex wounds and/or ulcerations. Treatment of cGVHD affecting the skin requires knowledge of local and systemic immunosuppressive therapy, along with basic wound care knowledge Multiple modalities of therapy are often needed.

Introduction

Graft-versus-host disease (GVHD) is a frequent complication of HSCT, and is a major cause of morbidity and mortality. Both acute and chronic graft-versus-host diseases are multisystem disorders that commonly affect the skin. Severe sclerotic features result in tight, fragile skin prone to poor wound healing, inadequate lymphatic drainage, and skin ulcer formation [1]. Adequate skin and wound care are essential in providing optimal treatment for patients with cutaneous manifestations.

The incidence of cGVHD following HSCT ranges from 60 to 80 %. The syndrome may occur with or without a history of acute GVHD, and presents with lichen planus-like or sclerotic skin manifestations. Lichen planus-like GVHD is characterized by erythematous to violaceous papules or plaques, often at the dorsal hands, feet, forearms and trunk. Sclerotic manifestations may be morphea-like (firm, hyper or hypopigmented plaques), or lichen-sclerosus-like (epidermal atrophy, dermal fibrosis, and the presence of white or gray thin plaques). Subcutaneous fibrosis and rippled appearance of the skin, a hallmark of deep sclerosis, may also be present. Other cutaneous findings of chronic GVHD include poikiloderma, depigmentation, and both hypo and hyperpigmented areas of skin. In the most severe cases, chronic ulceration may develop. Chronic GVHD-related ulcers are prone to bacterial infection and may result in frequent hospitalization for infected wounds.

Pathogenically, cGVHD appears to be the result of autoreactive T cells derived from donor hematopoetic cells. Some host-reactive T cells escape from the elimination mechanisms in the thymus, resulting in persistent alloreactive and autoreactive T cell clones [2].

The treatment for cutaneous GVHD requires multiple dimensions of therapy, employing both systemic treatment and localized wound care. Additionally, such patients must receive regular preventive skin care, including skin cancer surveillance, management of pruritus, monitoring for adverse effects of corticosteroids, infection control measures, and wound care. Topical therapy is critical in the treatment of GVHD. Although there are no randomized control studies on the effect of skin-care protocols in the evolution of the disease, ancedotal data suggest that adequate skin care improves prognosis [2]. This chapter reviews the basic principles of wound care in patients with chronic GVHD affecting the skin. There is a paucity of published data on this topic and we have included illustrative cases to provide practical management strategies for these complex patients.

Cleaning and Compression

Skin care in chronic graft-versus-host disease employs the basic principles of wound management. To ensure proper healing, therapy is directed toward promoting vascularization, maintaining skin moisture, and preventing infection. While all wounds are colonized with microbes, not all wounds are necessarily infected [3].

J.Y. Jung (✉) • T.H. Almazan
Division of Dermatology, City of Hope Comprehensive Cancer Center, 1500 East Duarte Road, Duarte, CA 91010, USA
e-mail: jjung@coh.org; talmazan@coh.org

J.A. Cotliar (ed.), *Atlas of Graft-versus-Host Disease*, DOI 10.1007/978-3-319-46952-2_11

Cleaning

Wounds that have devitalized tissue require debridement. The accumulation of devitalized tissue, decreased angiogenesis, hyperkeratosis, exudate, and biofilm formation prevent healing. Irrigation is important for decreasing bacterial load and is a recommended part of routine wound management [4, 5]. Warm, isotonic saline is often used; however, no significant differences in rates of infection have been seen when using tap water rather than saline for wound cleansing [6]. Regular use of soap and warm water should be encouraged in most patients who do not have profound immunosuppression. Adding iodine or other antiseptic solutions such as chlorhexidine or hydrogen peroxide is generally unnecessary, as these solutions have minimal action against bacteria and may prevent wound healing through toxic effects on normal tissue. Dilute hypochlorite is preferred in cases where wounds are heavily colonized with resistant bacteria.

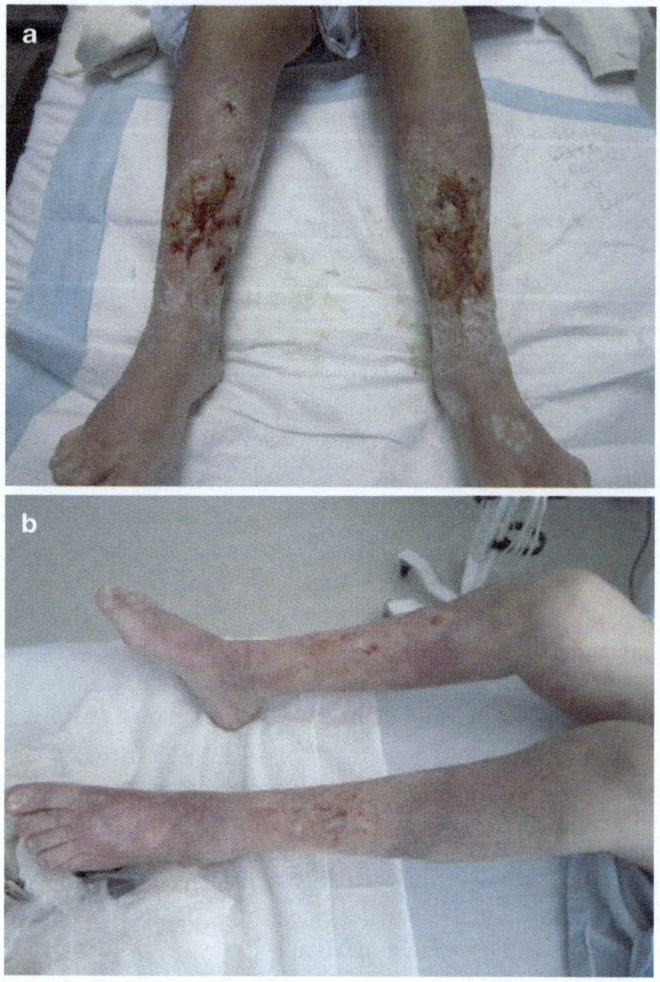

Fig. 11.1 Cleansing daily with soap and warm water should be encouraged for patients with sclerotic chronic GVHD. Before (**a**) and after (**b**); 2 days of soap and water cleansing followed by application of good emollient (100 % petrolatum)

Case 1 Many patients are not given any skin or wound care instructions and are repeatedly admitted to the hospital with suspected cellulitis (Fig. 11.1). This patient was admitted to the hospital three times in the prior 6 months with cellulitis. She was afraid of showering and did not receive any skin or wound care instructions after discharge. On presentation, she had nearly confluent sclerotic plaques on her lower extremities with retention hyperkeratosis and foul-smelling purulent drainage without frank ulceration (Fig. 11.1a). She demonstrated dramatic improvement after 2 days of soap and water cleansing and application of 100 % petrolatum (Fig. 11.1b). The emollient is helpful to loosen the retained scale and to facilitate cleansing. Reassurance and education can have pivotal roles in the management of these complex patients. Although her sclerotic plaques did not significantly improve, this patient was not readmitted for cellulitis in over 2 years of follow-up.

Excisional debridement is a form of wound cleaning that uses a scalpel or curette to remove non-viable tissue and adherent biofilm. The procedure also stimulates contraction and wound re-epithelialization [7]. Serial surgical debridement in a clinical setting may be associated with an increased likelihood of healing [8], but for patients with cGVHD, repeated aggressive surgical debridement often results in progressively larger ulcers.

Compression

Compression bandages and compression hosiery are forms of static compression therapy. Compression produces beneficial effects in wounds through multifactorial mechanisms. Traditionally, compression therapy has been most applied to the treatment of lower extremity venous stasis ulcerations, though similar principles may be useful in the treatment of GVHD wounds. Compression increases deep venous blood flow velocity and improves lymphatic flow and the local microcirculation. Compression therapy may also decrease the expression of pro-inflammatory matrix metalloproteinases, resulting in a wound milieu that favors ulcer healing [9]. Compression therapy is contraindicated in patients with peripheral artery disease, cellulitis, and acute deep vein thrombosis.

Compression bandages are generally divided into rigid (inelastic) and elastic types. The most common example of inelastic compression therapy is the Unna boot. Inelastic compression provides a high working pressure with muscle contraction during ambulation, but does not provide resting pressure. Elastic compression can be applied using elastic compression stockings, cotton/elastic wraps, short stretch bandages, or specialized multi-layered systems. Elastic compression bandaging systems conform to changes in leg size and sustain compression during activity and rest. Compression bandages should be applied by trained personnel and changed once or twice a week, depending on the degree of wound drainage [10].

Traditional compression stockings are often difficult for patients with sclerotic GVHD because of their restricted range of motion, neuropathic pain, skin fragility, and ulcer drainage. GVHD patients may respond better to multilayered wraps or combination therapy using specialized dressings directly placed on the ulcer bed that are then wrapped with compressive bandages.

Case 2 This patient, with extensive sclerotic chronic GVHD, was treated at a local wound center with serial debridement. At presentation, his legs demonstrated confluent sclerotic plaques with superficial and extensive erosions (Fig. 11.2a). He had poorly palpable pulses and pitting edema bilaterally. After starting a combination therapy including oral doxycycline, topical clindamycin and topical clobetasol ointment, he had significant improvement after 2 weeks (Fig. 11.2b). Although he had been given compression stockings by his hematologist and wound care physician, he could not apply them himself (due to his inability to bend at the hip or knees), and when placed by a caregiver the stockings would tear his fragile skin, worsening the erosions and causing additional pain. We recommended using cotton/elastic bandage wraps, which can be easily applied without causing additional trauma and can be adjusted to modify the amount of compression. Once his legs improved, we transitioned him to full length (foot, leg, and thigh) wraps secured with Velcro® straps that were much easier to apply and remove.

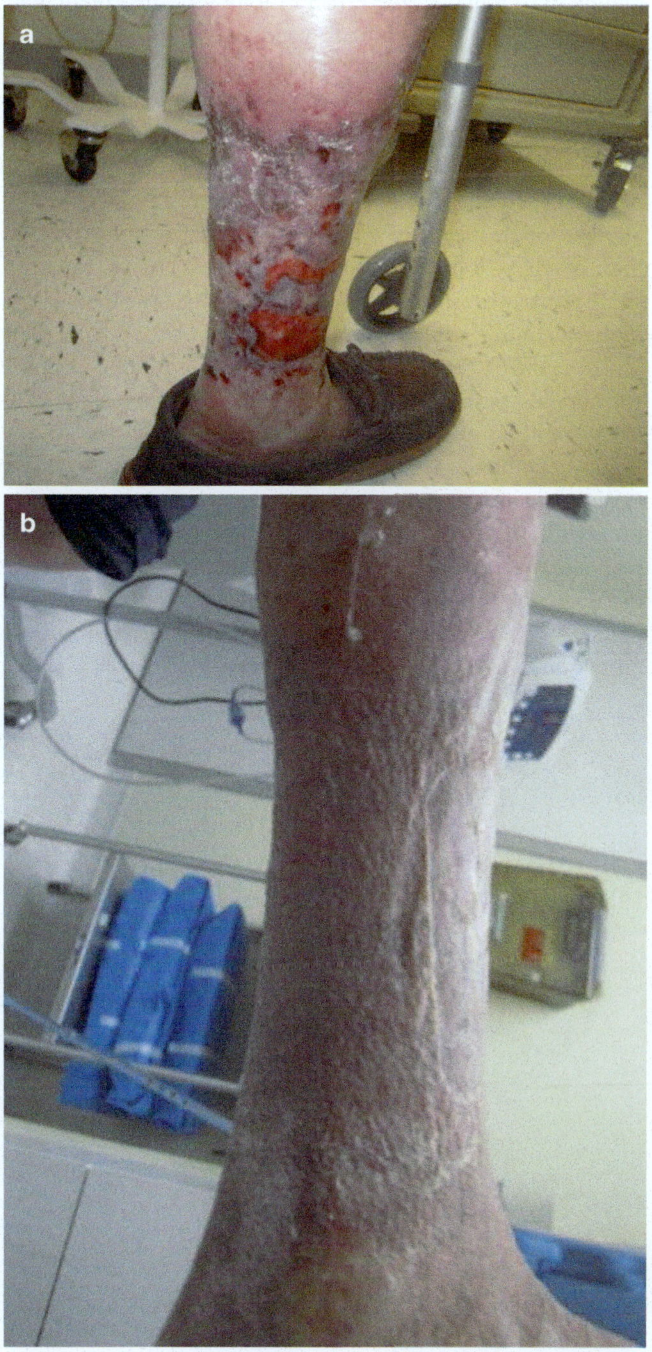

Fig. 11.2 (**a, b**) Surgical debridement is common in wound care centers but can lead to worsening chronic GVHD ulcers due to poor healing. A combination of topical steroid and compression was used for this patient, who demonstrated significant and lasting improvement

Topical and Intralesional Steroids

Topical Steroids

Topical corticosteroids are an appropriate first-line therapy for patients with mild cutaneous disease. As skin atrophy is known to be a major side-effect of long-term treatment, care should be taken in prolonged use, particularly for the face and intertriginous areas of the body. However, for many of these patients, the benefit of decreasing systemic immunosuppression far outweighs the risk of epidermal atrophy. Systemic absorption of topical steroids may be a concern in pediatric patients, but in these patients benefits also generally outweigh these risks [11]. Treatment should start with high-potency topical steroids. In unresponsive patients, short-term occlusion with damp dressings increases skin hydration and steroid penetration.

Topical treatment of mild GVHD is important especially for patients with a high risk of relapse, as increasing systemic immunosuppression may interfere with the desired graft-versus-malignancy effect [11]. In moderate-to-severe GVHD, topical immunosuppression may be used in conjunction with systemic immunosuppression to increase local response rates. Furthermore, topical immunosuppressive therapies for cGVHD are associated with less toxicity compared with systemic treatment, and may allow for dose reduction of systemic immunosuppression [11].

Intralesional Steroids

Intralesional steroids may be helpful for localized cutaneous GHVD refractory to high-dose topical steroid therapy. Mid-potency steroids such as triamcinolone 1 mg/kg is often used, and often requires multiple treatments. While effective in clinical practice, its use is often limited by a lack of consensus guidelines and patient discomfort associated with the procedure. However, in patients who have refractory localized disease, intralesional injections can resolve their lesions and allow them to discontinue systemic immunosuppression.

Case 3 A 10-year-old male patient had extensive sclerotic cGVHD affecting 60–70 % BSA. He developed chronic ulcerations of his scalp that were resistant to systemic immunosuppression. At presentation, he had numerous crusted erosions localized to the scalp (Fig. 11.3, left panel). Numerous topical therapies were attempted without significant improvement, including antibiotics, steroids, and calcineurin inhibitors. After extensive discussion of the risks and benefits, we elected for a trial of intralesional steroids. The patient required sedation for the procedure and a total of 1 mg/kg was injected into four trial areas. After significant improvement was noted in these lesions, the patient underwent three additional treatments using 1–2 mg/kg of intralesional triamcinolone at each treatment. He had complete resolution of his lesions (Fig. 11.3, right panel) and was weaned completely off systemic immunosuppression. Of note, he also exhibited partial reversal of his alopecia.

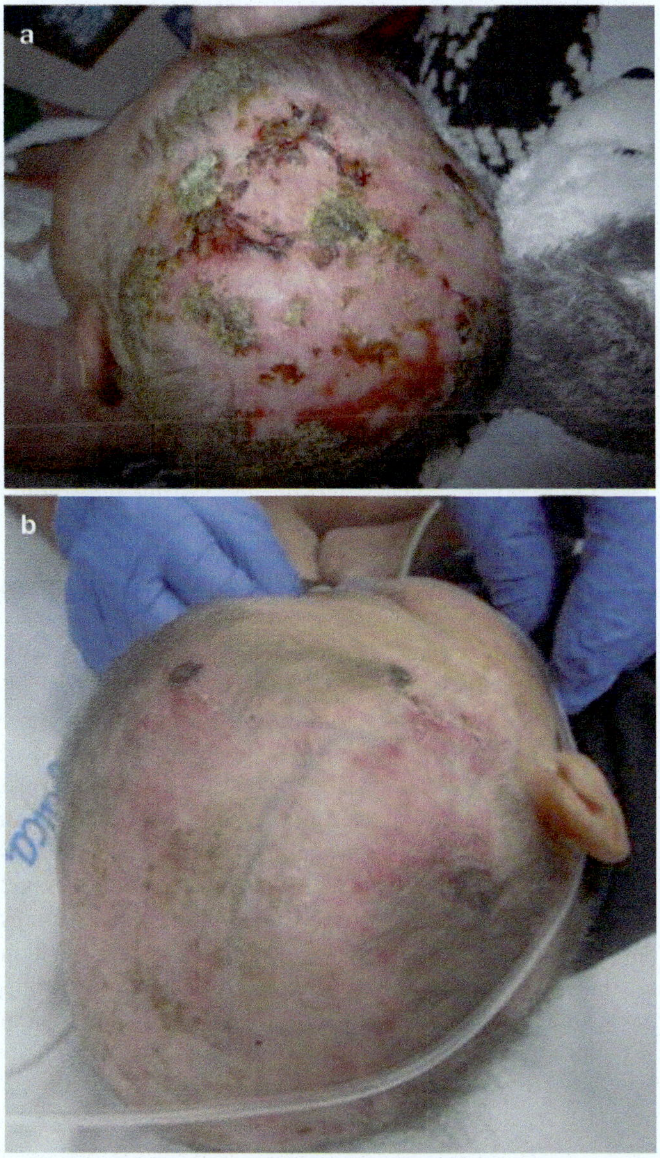

Fig. 11.3 (**a**, **b**) When ulcers are localized, intralesional steroids can be used to heal chronic ulcers and decrease systemic immunosuppression

Topical Calcineurin Inhibitors

For patients who fail topical or intralesional therapy, topical calcineurin inhibitors (CNIs) may be considered. Topical CNIs (e.g., tacrolimus and pimecrolimus) are useful localized steroid-sparing medications. However, most patients who initially respond to topical calcineurin inhibitors eventually require additional treatment. Topical CNIs may be of particular benefit for sites at high risk of skin atrophy (lips, eyelids, and intertriginous surfaces). CNIs are generally poorly tolerated at areas of very active skin involvement with erosions [12].

Complex Wounds

Complex, chronic wounds, such as those associated with cGVHD, contain a persistently high amount of inflammatory exudate, an environment that impedes the proliferation of fibroblasts [13]. Local therapy plays an important role in diminishing skin inflammation and promoting wound healing. Ideal dressings are those that control exudate, prevent bacterial proliferation, and absorb excessive wound drainage while preventing drying.

Collagen Gel and Matrix

Collagen is a primary component of the extracellular matrix and plays a vital role in connective tissue support within the skin. Collagen (applied to a wound as either a gel or matrix) supplies the wound with intact bovine or porcine collagen. The collagen is thought to serve as a sacrificial substrate for matrix metalloproteinases—enzymes associated with chronic wound inflammation and poor healing. Additionally, collagen may possess chemotactic properties resulting in fibroblast and keratinocyte recruitment.

Case 4 The patient developed chronic ulcerations localized to his back. He was started on systemic immunosuppression and extracorporeal photophoresis, with little improvement of the lesions. A series of topical treatments and dressings were applied, including silver sponge dressings and collagen gel (Fig. 11.4). His ulcers healed after 3 months of twice weekly dressing changes.

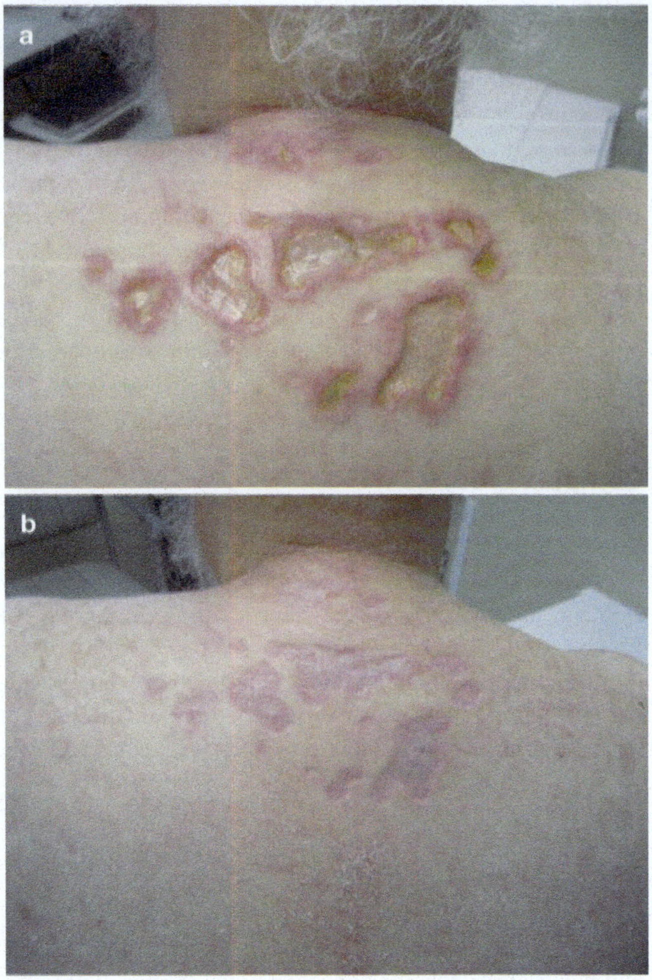

Fig. 11.4 Many collagen wound care products are available. (**a**, **b**) In this patient, a combination of collagen gel and silver alginate dressings led to significant resolution of the ulcers

Silver Dressings

Addition of a silver-containing collagen scaffold dressing may assist in replenishing some of the structure, components, and signaling mechanisms needed for wound healing [14]. Silver dressings are used by many clinicians to decrease heavy bacterial burden within wounds. Silver-impregnated foam dressings are absorbent and have broad-spectrum antimicrobial activity. They are slightly adherent on one side, facilitating application and allowing the dressing to be left on wounds for up to 7 days. The dressing consists of a silicone-based wound contact layer, an absorbent polyurethane foam pad comprised of silver sulfate and activate carbon, and a vapor-permeable waterproof film. Silver ions target thiol groups on bacterial enzymes causing unraveling; the ions also inhibit bacterial growth, damage the cell wall, and cause structural abnormalities in bacterial nucleic acids. The bactericidal properties of silver have led to its common use in burn patients.

Case 5 The patient presented with sclerotic cGVHD affecting primarily the lower extremities. She had an ulcer on her right lower extremity that slowly enlarged over a period of 10 months. She was a poorly controlled diabetic and had multiple hospitalizations for lower extremity cellulitis with bacteremia. She underwent surgical debridement, intravenous antibiotics, and 4 weeks of negative pressure-wound therapy followed split-thickness skin graft. Five months later, the ulcer recurred (Fig. 11.5a). We used a combination of collagen matrix and silver sponge dressings with compression (Fig. 11.5b). The ulcer resolved completely within 3 months and did not recur (Fig. 11.5c).

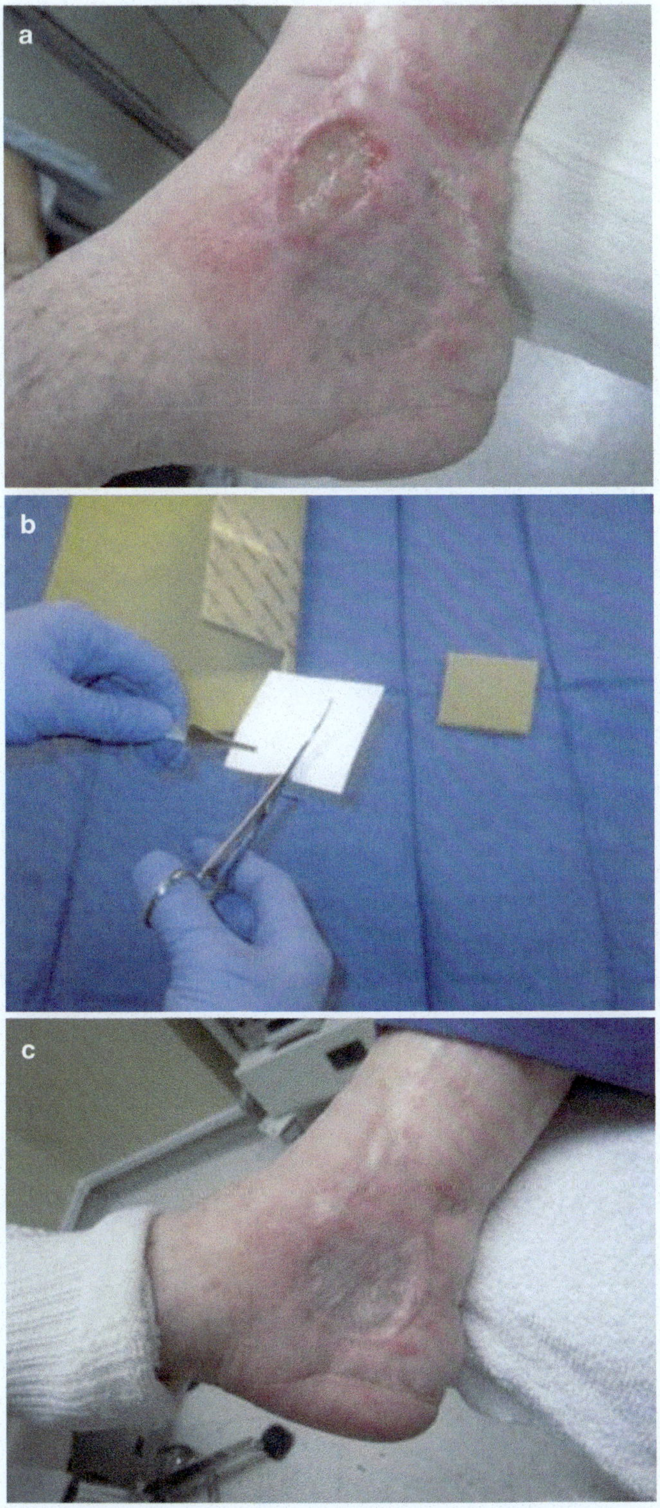

Fig. 11.5 (**a–c**) This patient responded rapidly to a combination of collagen silver matrix dressings (*white*) and silver sponge dressings (*gray*) with compression

Maggot Debridement Therapy

An effective method of wound debridement utilizes larvae of the Australian sheep blow fly (*Lucilia cuprina*) or green bottle fly (*Lucilia sericata*). Maggot therapy is often used for debridement of chronic wounds when surgical debridement is not available or cannot be performed. Maggot therapy may also decrease the duration of antibiotic use in certain patients, though this has not been well studied in the setting of GVHD [15]. Larvae secrete proteolytic enzymes that degrade necrotic tissue, which the maggots then ingest; healthy tissue is preferentially left intact. Maggot therapy has also shown benefit through antimicrobial action and stimulation of wound healing [16]. Maggot therapy has been classically used in the treatment of pressure ulcers, chronic venous stasis ulcers, diabetic ulcers, and other chronic wounds including GVHD-related ulcers. However, no consistent reductions have been demonstrated in the time elapsed to wound healing compared to standard wound therapy [17].

Case 6 The patient presented with extensive sclerotic cGVHD primarily involving the lower extremities. He developed bilateral dorsal feet ulcers recalcitrant to systemic therapies including steroids, photophoresis, tacrolimus, sirolimus, and mycophenolate mofetil. Topically, we also tried liquid collagen, collagen matrix, silver alginate, silver sponge, collagenase, and cadexomer iodine with minimal improvement. After more than 1 year of worsening ulcers (Fig. 11.6a), we discussed maggot debridement therapy. Maggots are placed directly onto the ulcer bed with a mesh "cage" constructed around the ulcer (Fig. 11.6b). He completed two treatment cycles (2–3 days) and the ulcer bed was clean with healthy granulation tissue following each debridement (Fig. 11.6c). He had significant improvement after 3 months (Fig. 11.6d) and near complete resolution after 6 months (Fig. 11.6e).

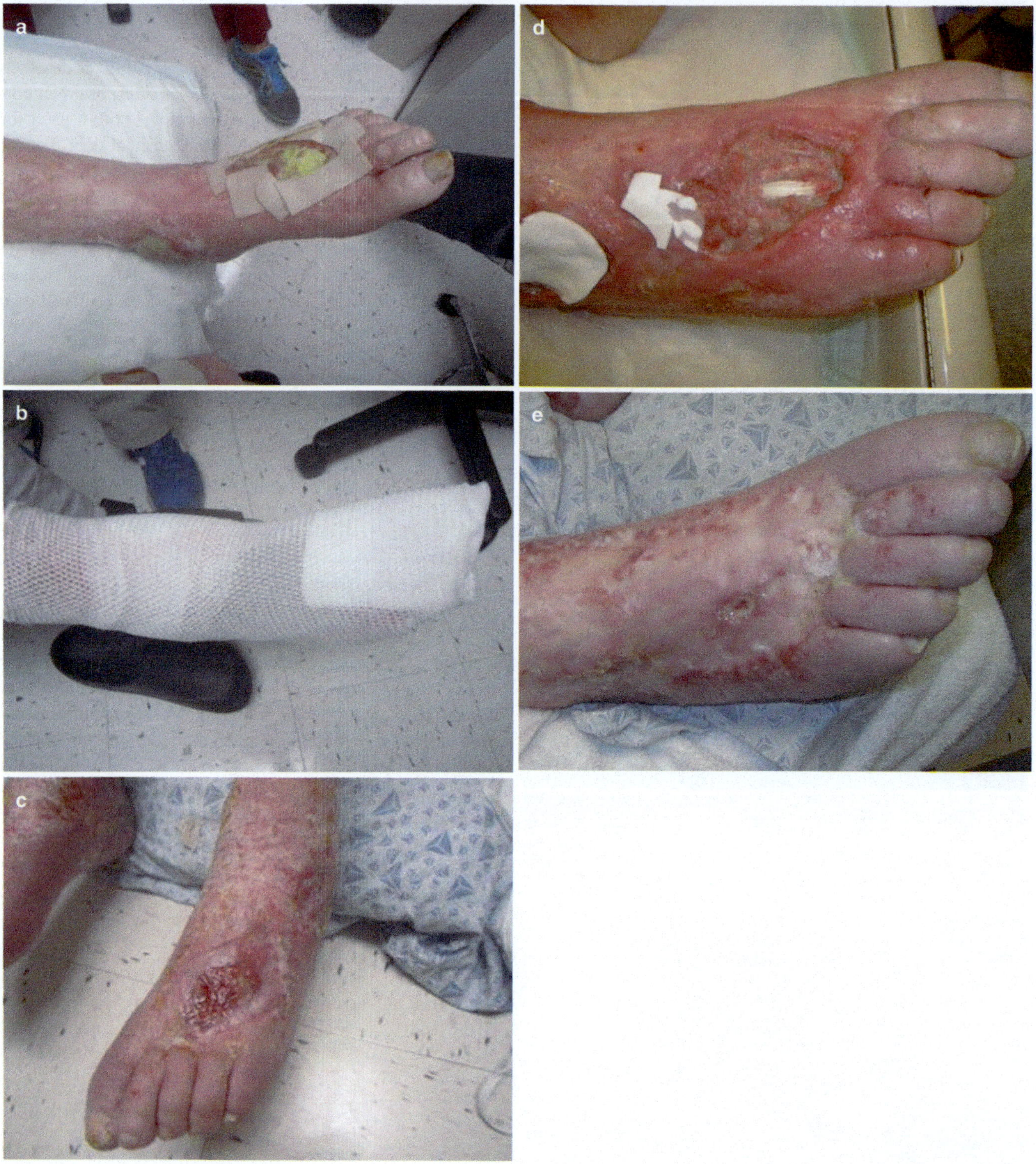

Fig. 11.6 (**a–e**) Maggot debridement therapy is an effective and rapid method of non-surgical debridement that facilitates ulcer improvement and resolution

Summary

The skin is the most commonly affected organ in graft-versus-host disease. Cutaneous cGVHD has a varied clinical presentation ranging from mild, localized sclerosis to poorly healing wounds with large areas of ulceration. Multiple treatment options for cutaneous cGVHD exist, though lack of standardized treatment algorithms makes clinical decisions challenging. A multifaceted approach to treatment, employing both systemic immunosuppression and aggressive localized wound care, is often the most effective course of action.

References

1. Jachiet M, de Masson A, Peffault de Latour R, Rybojad M, Robin M, Bourhis JH, et al. Skin ulcers related to chronic graft-versus-host disease: clinical findings and associated morbidity. Br J Dermatol. 2014;171:63–8.
2. Peñas PF, Fernández-herrera J, García-diez A. Dermatologic treatment of cutaneous graft versus host disease. Am J Clin Dermatol. 2004;5(6):403–16.
3. Bowler PG, Duerden BI, Armstrong DG. Wound microbiology and associated approaches to wound management. Clin Microbiol Rev. 2001;14(2):244–69.
4. Atiyeh BS, Ioannovich J, Al-amm CA, El-musa KA. Management of acute and chronic open wounds: the importance of moist environment in optimal wound healing. Curr Pharm Biotechnol. 2002;3(3):179–95.
5. Stevenson TR, Thacker JG, Rodeheaver GT, Bacchetta C, Edgerton MT, Edlich RF. Cleansing the traumatic wound by high pressure syringe irrigation. JACEP. 1976;5(1):17–21.
6. Fernandez R, Griffiths R. Water for wound cleansing. Cochrane Database Syst Rev. 2012;(2):CD003861.
7. Brem H, Stojadinovic O, Diegelmann RF, Entero H, Lee B, Pastar I, et al. Molecular markers in patients with chronic wounds to guide surgical debridement. Mol Med. 2007;13(1–2):30–9.
8. Wilcox JR, Carter MJ, Covington S. Frequency of debridements and time to heal: a retrospective cohort study of 312 744 wounds. JAMA Dermatol. 2013;149(9):1050–8.
9. Beidler SK, Douillet CD, Berndt DF, Keagy BA, Rich PB, Marston WA. Multiplexed analysis of matrix metalloproteinases in leg ulcer tissue of patients with chronic venous insufficiency before and after compression therapy. Wound Repair Regen. 2008;16(5):642–8.
10. Keller A, Müller ML, Calow T, Kern IK, Schumann H. Bandage pressure measurement and training: simple interventions to improve efficacy in compression bandaging. Int Wound J. 2009;6(5):324–30.
11. Marks C, Stadler M, Häusermann P, Wolff D, Buchholz S, Stary G, et al. German-Austrian-Swiss Consensus Conference on clinical practice in chronic graft-versus-host disease (GVHD): guidance for supportive therapy of chronic cutaneous and musculoskeletal GVHD. Br J Dermatol. 2011;165(1):18–29.
12. Hymes SR, Alousi AM, Cowen EW. Graft-versus-host disease: part II. Management of cutaneous graft-versus-host disease. J Am Acad Dermatol. 2012;66(4):535.e1–16.
13. Bucalo B, Eaglstein WH, Falanga V. Inhibition of cell proliferation by chronic wound fluid. Wound Repair Regen. 1993;1(3):181–6.
14. Iorio ML, Shuck J, Attinger CE. Wound healing in the upper and lower extremities: a systematic review on the use of acellular dermal matrices. Plast Reconstr Surg. 2012;130(5 Suppl 2):232S–41S.
15. Armstrong DG, Salas P, Short B, Martin BR, Kimbriel HR, Nixon BP, et al. Maggot therapy in "lower-extremity hospice" wound care: fewer amputations and more antibiotic-free days. J Am Podiatr Med Assoc. 2005;95(3):254–7.
16. Margolin L, Gialanella P. Assessment of the antimicrobial properties of maggots. Int Wound J. 2010;7(3):202–4.
17. Dumville JC, Worthy G, Soares MO, Bland JM, Cullum N, Dowson C, et al. VenUS II: a randomised controlled trial of larval therapy in the management of leg ulcers. Health Technol Assess 2009;13(55):1–182, iii–iv.

12 Atypical Manifestations of Graft-Versus-Host Disease

Christine M. Cornejo and Robert G. Micheletti

The cutaneous manifestations of graft-versus-host disease (GVHD) are protean and often diagnostically challenging. Acute GVHD (aGVHD) of the skin most often presents with a morbilliform exanthem, which may progress to generalized erythema and bullae in severe cases, bearing striking resemblance to toxic epidermal necrolysis. The manifestations of chronic GVHD (cGVHD) are more diverse and often resemble other dermatologic conditions. For example, diagnostic signs of cGVHD, based on the NIH Consensus Criteria, include poikiloderma, lichen planus-like features, sclerotic features, morphea-like features, and lichen sclerosus-like features [1]. More atypical presentations of cutaneous GVHD also often mimic other disorders, in which case histologic findings supportive of GVHD can help establish the diagnosis. This chapter highlights the many atypical and under-recognized manifestations of both acute and chronic cutaneous GVHD (Table 12.1).

C.M. Cornejo
Department of Dermatology, Perelman School of Medicine, University of Pennsylvania, 3600 Spruce Street, 2 Maloney Building, Philadelphia, PA 19104, USA
e-mail: christine.cornejo@uphs.upenn.edu

R.G. Micheletti (✉)
Department of Dermatology and Medicine, Perelman School of Medicine, University of Pennsylvania, 3600 Spruce Street, 2 Maloney Building, Philadelphia, PA 19104, USA
e-mail: robert.micheletti@uphs.upenn.edu

J.A. Cotliar (ed.), *Atlas of Graft-versus-Host Disease*, DOI 10.1007/978-3-319-46952-2_12

Table 12.1 Signs and symptoms of acute and chronic cutaneous GVHD

Common manifestations		Atypical manifestations	
aGVHD	cGVHD[a]	aGVHD	cGVHD
Maculopapular rash	**Poikiloderma**	Eczematous eruptions (contact dermatitis [2], eczema craquele [3])	Eczematous eruptions [4, 5] (atopic dermatitis [6], eczema craquele [7], and eczematoid [8])
Generalized erythroderma	**Lichen planus-like features**	Psoriasiform [9, 10]	Psoriasiform [1, 4, 5, 11, 12]
Bullae	**Sclerotic features**	Type II PRP [13]	PR [14] and inverse PR [3]
	Morphea-like features	Acquired ichythosis [15, 16]	Reactive erythema (EM [12, 17] and EAC [4])
	Lichen sclerosis-like features	Extensive follicular eruption [18–20]	Erythroderma and exfoliative dermatitis [4, 8, 12, 21]
	Papulosquamous lesions	Total body leukoderma [22]	Extensive follicular or comedonal eruption [3, 23–26]
	Depigmentation	Wolf isotopic pattern [27]	Acral keratosis [2, 28]
	Alopecia		Angiomatous papules [29–33]
	Hypo- and hyper-pigmentation		LE [4, 34, 35] and hypertrophic LE [34]
	Sweat impairment		Dermatomyositis [36]
	Ichthyosis		Blaschko-linear [37–44]
	Keratosis pilaris		Dermatomal (Wolf isotopic pattern) [12, 35, 39, 45–56]
	Erythema		Wolf isotopic pattern (non-dermatomal) [46, 47, 54, 57, 58]
	Maculopapular rash		Koebner isomorphic pattern [5, 46, 52, 54, 59–62]
	Pruritus		Isoradiotopic pattern [46, 63–66]
			Total body leukoderma [67, 68]
			Calcinosis cutis universalis [69]
			Bullae [70]
			Ulceration [71–79]

EAC erythema annulare centrifugum, *EM* erythema multiforme, *LE* lupus erythematosus, *PR* pityriasis rosea, *PRP* pityriasis rubra pilaris
[a]Based on National Institutes of Health (NIH) Consensus Criteria [1]. Diagnostic features of cGVHD based on NIH Consensus Criteria are shown in *bold*

Eczematous Eruptions

Chronic cutaneous GVHD may present with eczematous eruptions [4, 5] and variants such as atopic dermatitis-like [6] and eczematoid GVHD [8]. This manifestation is not associated with a history of atopy in patients or donors. It is characterized by pronounced pruritus and either widespread or limited areas of dry skin, erythema, papules, and perifollicular accentuation. Peripheral eosinophilia and elevated IgE levels are common in cases of atopic dermatitis-like GVHD [6]. Histology demonstrates findings consistent with GVHD in addition to features of eczematous dermatitis in most cases. Atopic dermatitis-like chronic GVHD is associated with a favorable outcome, with a good response to topical therapies such as emollients, topical corticosteroids, and topical tacrolimus, as well as to ultraviolet phototherapy and prednisone, with or without immunosuppressant agents for GVHD [6]. Conversely, eczematoid GVHD, which has been described as a more aggressive variant that often progresses to erythroderma, can be difficult to manage and is associated with a poor prognosis [8]. It is important to note that some have suggested that eczematoid GVHD may be more accurately classified as a variant of late-onset acute GVHD based on precipitating factors and histopathologic findings [80].

There have also been reports of GVHD presenting as eczema craquele in both acute [3] and chronic GVHD [7], with diffuse or localized areas of reticulated erythema on exam (Fig. 12.1), and findings of GVHD and eczema on histology.

Acute cutaneous GVHD presenting as a contact dermatitis has been reported in one case of an infant who developed a hyperemic belt-shaped eruption in the diaper region following allogeneic stem cell transplant [2]. The clinical presentation in this case was progressive and fatal.

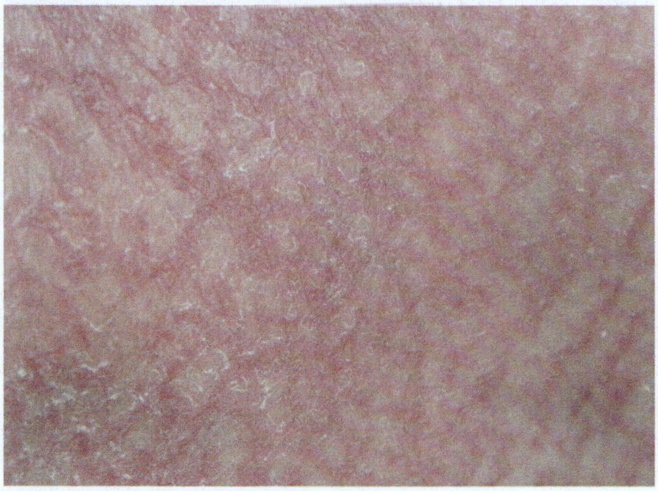

Fig. 12.1 Chronic GVHD presenting as reticulated erythema with fine scale mimicking eczema craquelé

Papulosquamous Eruptions

Psoriasiform eruptions have been described in both acute [9, 10] and chronic [1, 4, 5, 11, 12] cutaneous GVHD. Typical skin findings include discrete guttate, annular, or confluent erythematous scaly patches and plaques with micaceous scale that may involve any part of the body, including the scalp, face, hands, and feet [1, 4, 5, 10, 11]. Histology demonstrates features of GVHD as well as psoriasis in most cases. This manifestation is not associated with a history of psoriasis in either donors or patients.

An eruption resembling type II (atypical adult) pityriasis rubra pilaris (PRP) has been described as a very rare variant of acute GVHD, with only one reported case [13]. Clinically, this variant reveals a pattern of PRP with erythematous follicular hyperkeratotic papules coalescing to form diffuse red-orange plaques with islands of unaffected skin, palmoplantar keratoderma, and marked ichthyosiform scaling. Histology shows typical changes of acute GVHD, such as basal vacuolar degeneration, scattered apoptotic keratinocytes at the dermoepidermal junction, and lymphocyte satellitosis adjacent to dyskeratotic keratinocytes, as well as some characteristics of PRP, including psoriasiform hyperplasia, parakeratosis, and follicular plugging. The patient in this report achieved a partial response with treatment [13].

Few cases of pityriasis rosea (PR)-like [14] and inverse PR-like [3] chronic GVHD have been reported (Fig. 12.2). A herald patch preceded the development of a more diffuse eruption in half of the reported PR-like cases [14]. Histopathology in these cases demonstrated features of both PR and GVHD.

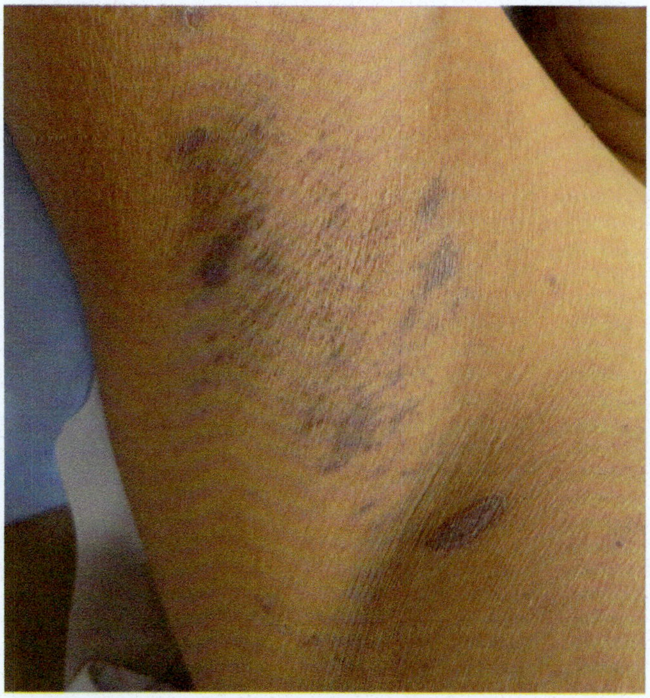

Fig. 12.2 A case of chronic cutaneous GVHD mimicking inverse pityriasis rosea

Reactive Erythema

Reactive erythemas such as erythema multiforme [12, 17] and erythema annulare centrifugum [4] have been reported as unusual variants of chronic GVHD.

Erythroderma and Exfoliative Dermatitis

Erythroderma and exfoliative dermatitis have been reported as a variant of chronic GVHD [4, 8, 12, 21]. This is often preceded by papulosquamous, morbilliform, or annular eruptions [4]. While exfoliative dermatitis can be seen in progressive acute GVHD, this manifestation does not necessarily reflect a progression of disease in chronic GVHD.

Ichthyosiform GVHD

Ichthyosis is an acknowledged feature of chronic cutaneous GVHD [1]. Acquired ichthyosis has also been reported as a manifestation of acute GVHD and is typically preceded by or associated with other signs of cutaneous and extracutaneous GVHD [15, 16]. A personal or family history of ichthyosis is not felt to be a relevant factor in this presentation.

Extensive Follicular Eruptions in GVHD

Follicular erythema and follicular keratosis or keratosis pilaris-like lesions can be early manifestations of acute and chronic GVHD, respectively. However, a follicular eruption as a major clinical manifestation of acute or chronic GVHD is uncommon (Fig. 12.3). In acute follicular GVHD, diffuse eruptions of erythematous, follicular papules develop early in the course of disease and precede or are simultaneous with the classic morbilliform rash. In some reported cases, the eruption was progressive and persistent, and the patients died shortly after the diagnosis was made; however, because of the small number of reports, it is unknown if acute follicular GVHD indicates a more severe course than other types of acute GVHD [18–20]. In contrast, chronic follicular GVHD develops late in the course of disease and is considered a clinical variant with more favorable prognosis [3, 23–25]. Another variant of chronic follicular GVHD that resembles open and closed acne-like comedones, termed comedonal-GVHD, has been reported in a few patients (Fig. 12.4). Like other forms of chronic follicular GVHD, this variant has been associated with a good clinical outcome [26].

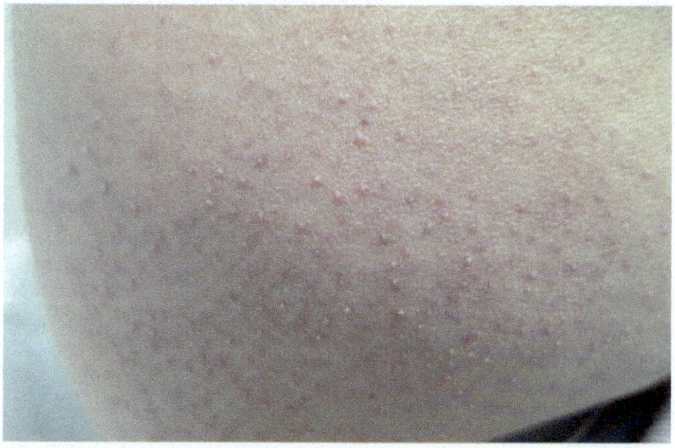

Fig. 12.3 Chronic GVHD manifesting as follicular hyperkeratosis on the flank

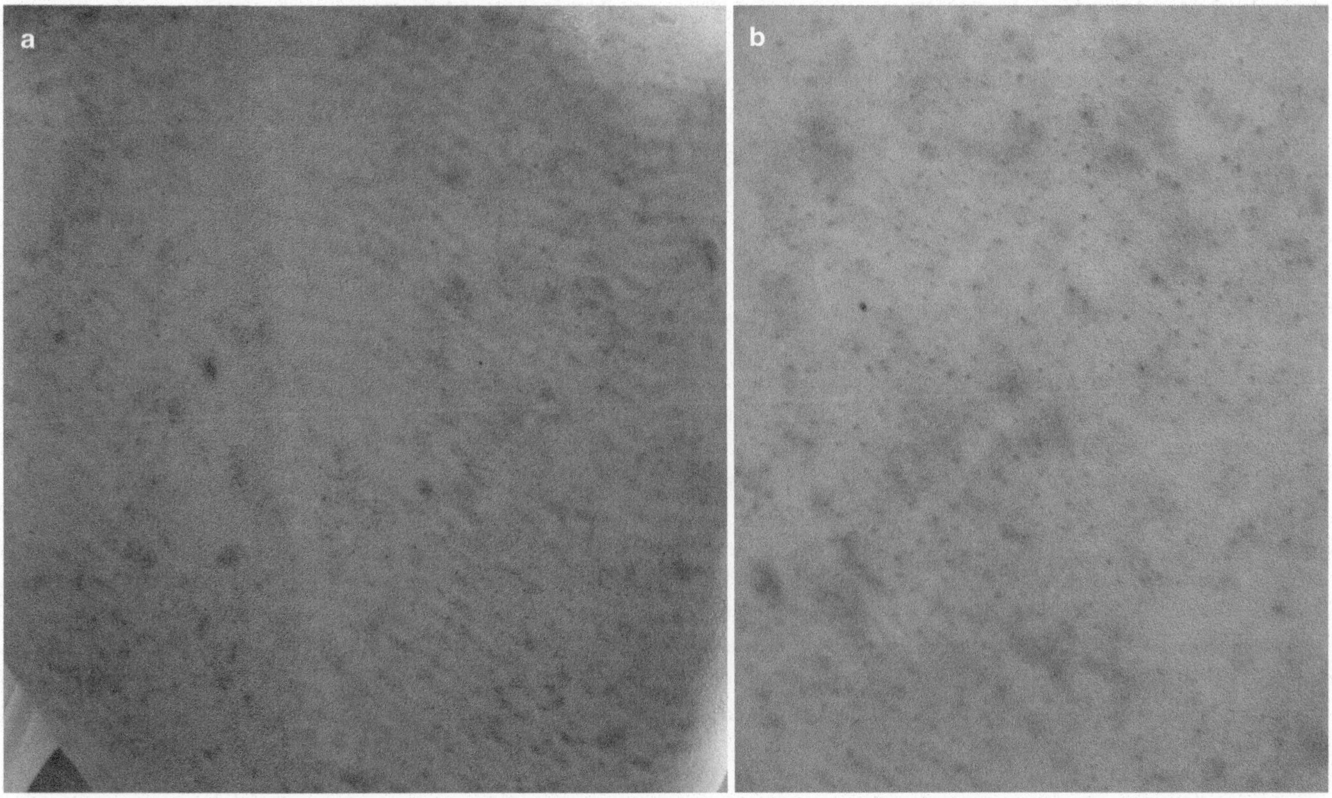

Fig. 12.4 (**a**, **b**) Chronic GVHD presenting with comedone-like lesions on the back

Atypical Acral Lesions in GVHD

While acral involvement in general is not uncommon in GVHD, lesions can be variable. These include less common presentations such as vesicles and scales resembling eczema [12, 81]; acral keratoses resembling warts [2, 28]; and targetoid lesions resembling erythema multiforme [17].

GVHD-Associated Angiomatosis

Eruptive angiomas are an uncommon and poorly understood manifestation of cGVHD [29–33]. The term "GVHD–associated angiomatosis" (GVHD-AA) has been proposed to describe this entity, which is believed to fall within the spectrum of reactive angiomatosis [30]. In GVHD-associated angiomatosis, patients with sclerotic cGVHD develop vascular plaques and nodules within areas of skin fibrosis [30]. Histologically, these lesions display hemorrhagic crust, irregular epidermal acanthosis, or atrophy overlying vague lobular architecture with endothelial proliferation and fibroblast-rich stroma, without atypia [30]. The pathogenesis of these lesions is not clearly understood but may involve increased lymphatic pressure, elevated angiogenic cytokines, and aberrant endothelial damage and repair in the setting of tissue chimerism [30]. These lesions have been associated with a poor prognosis, primarily because of their association with active GVHD and their recalcitrant nature. Data on the management of GVHD-AA are limited, and modalities such as shave, excision, cryotherapy, radiotherapy, thalidomide, and electrocautery have been largely unsuccessful [29–33]. Some success has been demonstrated with combination sirolimus and propranolol [30].

GVHD-Mimicking Connective Tissue Diseases

Chronic cutaneous GVHD may present with an eruption resembling cutaneous lupus erythematosus (LE) [4, 34, 35]. Skin exam may demonstrate a variety of clinical features similar to LE, including a malar rash [4, 35], lesions resembling hypertrophic LE [34], and annular plaques resembling subacute cutaneous lupus erythematosus (SCLE) (Fig. 12.5). Skin biopsy demonstrates features of lichenoid cGVHD, but may also show characteristics seen in LE [34, 35]. This clinical presentation can be associated with a poor prognosis, with either development of sclerotic GVHD or a relapse of hematological disease, as seen in one case series of five patients who presented with malar rash [35]. While autoantibodies such as antinuclear antibody, anti-Ro, and anti-La are variably positive in chronic GVHD, their significance is unknown. This presentation is not associated with the development of systemic LE symptoms.

Chronic cutaneous GVHD resembling dermatomyositis has been described in a patient who developed a heliotrope rash, edema of the eyelids, erythema of the knuckles, and weakness of proximal muscles with myalgias. Muscle biopsy was characteristic of dermatomyositis, and skin biopsy had features of both GVHD and dermatomyositis [36]. Similarly, chronic cutaneous GVHD can also rarely present with overlapping features of both dermatomyositis and LE [82].

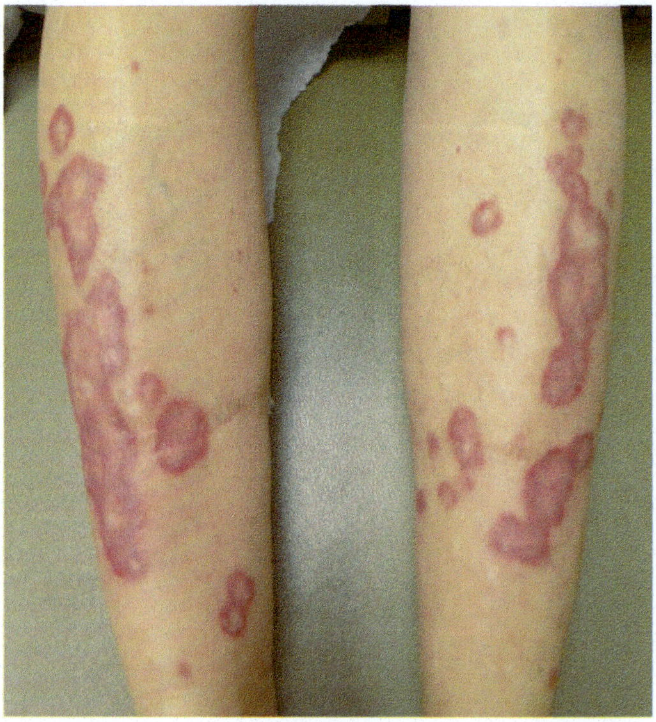

Fig. 12.5 Chronic GVHD mimicking the annular lesions of subacute cutaneous lupus

Unusual Distributions of GVHD

There have been numerous cases of chronic lichen planus-like GVHD presenting along Blaschko's lines (Fig. 12.6) [37–44]. One hypothesis explaining the linear and whorled distribution of these lesions is an unmasking of genetic mosaicism by the donor's lymphocytes recognizing altered cell surface antigens which were previously tolerated by the patient's own lymphocytes [43].

Chronic sclerotic-type and lichen planus-like GVHD may rarely occur in a dermatomal distribution [12, 35, 39, 45–56], often, but not always, at the site of antecedent zoster eruption. It has been hypothesized that viral proteins could play a role by altering the surface antigenicity of keratinocytes, which then serve as targets for the donor effector cells [38, 49, 50, 63, 83]. Interestingly, there has been one reported case of extensive chronic GVHD sparing dermatomes previously affected by herpes zoster, demonstrating a Renbök or inverse Koebner isomorphic phenomenon [84].

Chronic GVHD, typically sclerotic-type, has also demonstrated other isotopic and isomorphic responses, with lesions developing at sites of skin friction (waistband, brassiere) [5, 46, 59, 60], previous central venous catheter placement, with [46] or without [60] cellulitis, repeated needle sticks [46], suction blisters [54], Bacillus Calmette Guerin vaccination [54], influenza vaccination [52], subcutaneous interferon alpha injections [61], healed lesions of aGVHD [47, 54], previous measles exanthem [57], striae distensae [62], external beam radiotherapy [46, 63–65], sun or ultraviolet exposure [66], and other sites of prior trauma or scar (Fig. 12.7). There has been one reported case of sclerotic-type cGVHD presenting as annular plaques in a patient with prior similar annular morphology of his cutaneous lymphoma [58]. Whether this represents a true isotopic response is unclear. These responses are not necessarily limited to chronic GVHD. There has been one reported case of acute GVHD affecting only the lesional skin of a patient with piebaldism [27]. Overall, these isomorphic, isotopic, and isoradiotopic responses may be unified by the concept of the cutaneous immunocompromised district [85]. The cutaneous immunocompromised district, as described by Ruocco et al., is an area of skin where the local effective immunity has been altered, permitting the development of infection, tumor, or a dysimmune reaction, such as GVHD [85]. Though the exact mechanism of GVHD development at these sites remains unknown, this concept may provide some insight into the pathophysiology of cGVHD.

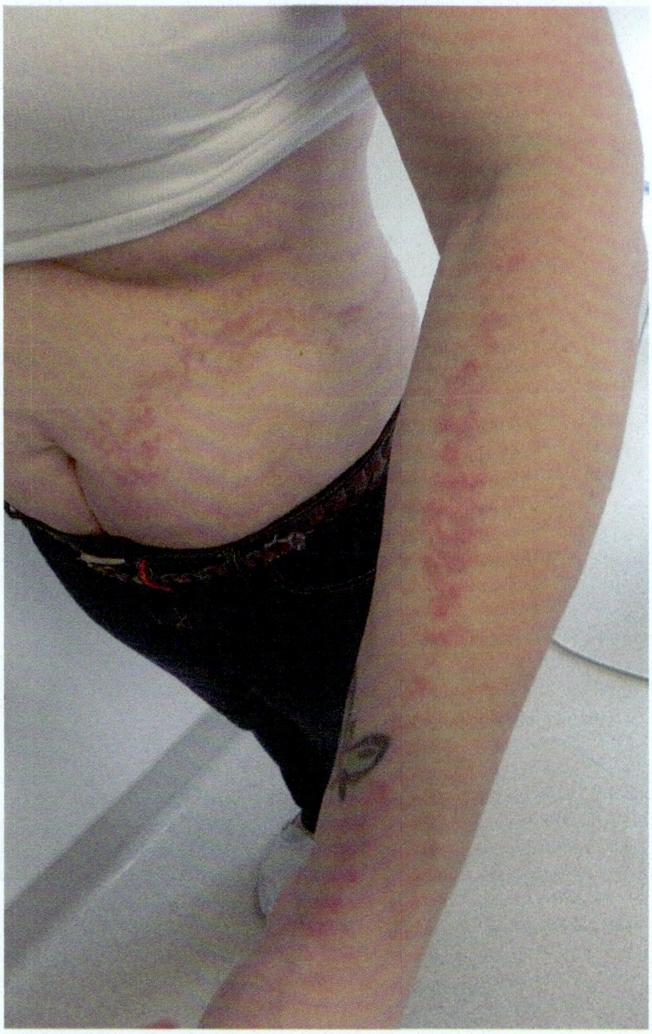

Fig. 12.6 Chronic lichen planus-like GVHD occurring along Blaschko's lines

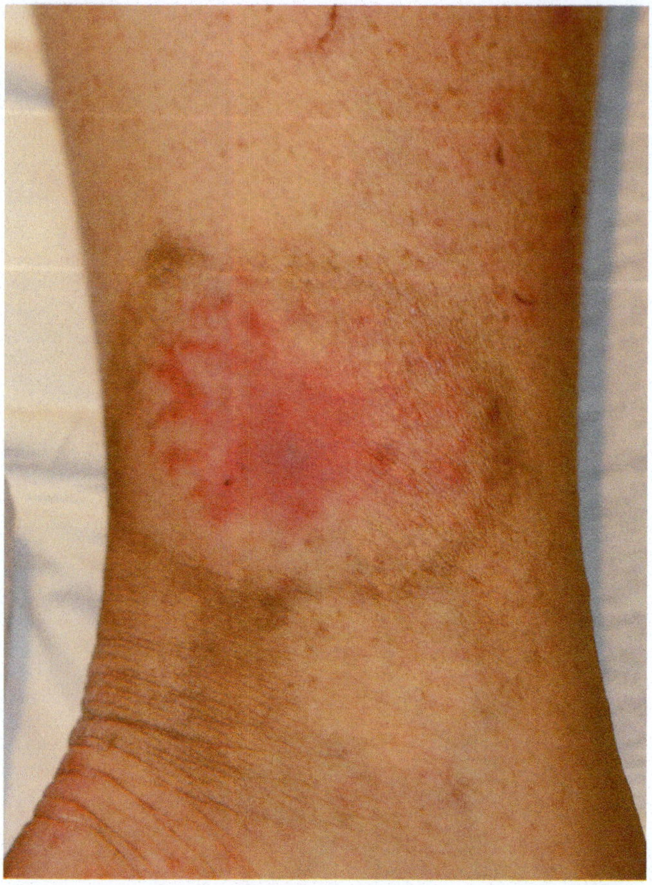

Fig. 12.7 Cutaneous GVHD presenting at the site of a scar from prior skin graft

Atypical Oral Manifestations

Under-recognized oral manifestations of GVHD include black hairy tongue and thick-appearing white tongue. Black hairy tongue (BHT), or lingua villosa, is an unusual condition in adults characterized by marked accumulation of keratin on the dorsum of the tongue, resulting in a hair-like appearance that has been reported as an unusual manifestation of GVHD [86]. BHT-like GVHD presents with pronounced black-brownish pigment of the dorsal tongue, with the appearance of elongated filiform papillae. Histopathology of tongue biopsy specimens reveals acanthosis and hyperkeratosis with evident filiform projections in the epidermis, consistent with BHT, as well as basal cell hydropic degeneration, lymphocyte satellitosis, and scattered apoptotic keratinocytes in the basal part of the epithelium and lamina propria, consistent with GVHD. In the reported cases, BHT was generally accompanied by other manifestations of cutaneous GVHD or preceded its onset. Cornejo et al. reported development of an entirely white and thick-appearing tongue as a striking end-complication of oral lichen planus-like cGVHD that has been seen in the context of extensive cutaneous GVHD (Fig. 12.8) [3].

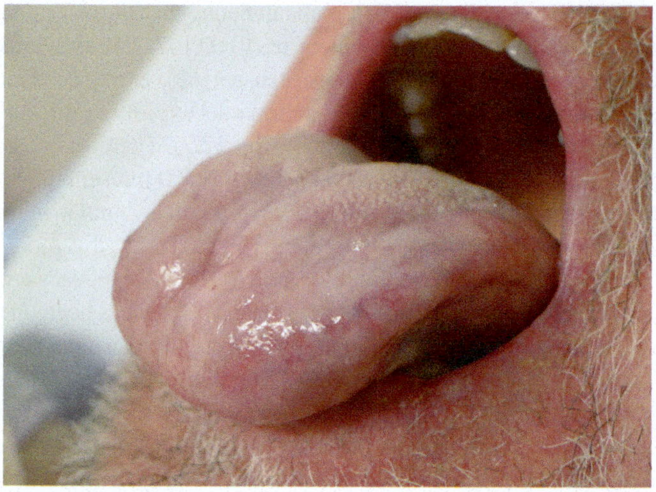

Fig. 12.8 Thick-appearing white tongue as a manifestation of oral lichen planus-like GVHD

Unusual Sequelae of Cutaneous GVHD

While partial depigmentation or vitiligo is considered a distinctive feature of chronic GVHD, total body leukoderma with leukotrichia is extremely unusual, with only three reported cases [22, 67, 68]. Onset of depigmentation can occur after or alongside other manifestations of active GVHD and can progress to total depigmentation within weeks [68] to months [67]. Histopathology in these cases reveals a total absence of melanocytes in the skin [22, 68, 69], as well as features consistent with GVHD [67]. The presence of cytotoxic anti-melanocyte antibodies in the blood has been reported [67]. It has been hypothesized that total leukoderma occurs as a selective immune response against melanocytes in the skin and hair, as in vitiligo [67]. The clinical presentation in these cases is associated with an otherwise benign course, though total leukoderma is persistent. No successful treatments for reversal of post-transplant total leukoderma have been reported in the literature to date. However, Jacobsohn et al. suggested one could consider treating these patients with therapies approved for vitiligo, given the histological similarities between the two conditions [68]. As in vitiligo and other depigmenting conditions, it is important for these patients to follow adequate sun protective measures and have close follow-up for cutaneous malignancies.

Dystrophic calcinosis cutis caused by chronic skin inflammation in the setting of sclerotic cGVHD is another important complication to recognize [69]. Calcinosis cutis can cause significant pain and may lead to skin breakdown and infection, restrictions in joint mobility, and overall reduced quality of life. Treatment of this condition is difficult and highlights the importance of prevention with aggressive, early treatment of GVHD.

Bullae formation and subsequent breakdown of the skin into ulcers is an additional, potentially serious complication of scleroderma-like cGVHD. While these lesions can occur anywhere on the trunk or extremities, they typically involve the lower limbs, where there is concomitant edema (Fig. 12.9) [70]. These ulcers are often painful and slow to heal and can serve as nidi for infection, severely affecting the patient's quality of life and prognosis. Sclerosis and ulceration can be particularly extensive in some cases (Fig. 12.10). There are no standardized approaches for the treatment of GVHD-associated bullae or ulcers. Though ulcers are often unresponsive to traditional therapy, wound care and local therapy play a major role. Split-thickness skin transplantation from an HLA-matched donor can be a successful permanent option [71].

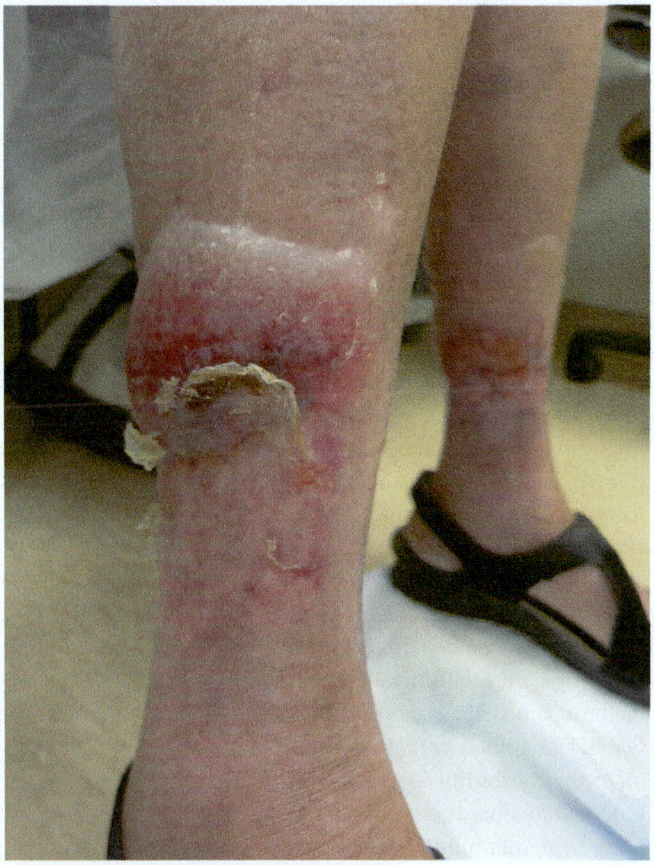

Fig. 12.9 Tense bullae superimposed on scleroderma-like changes of chronic GVHD

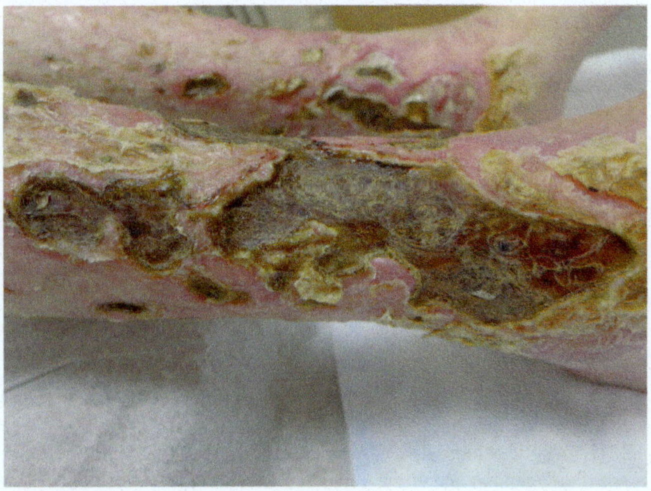

Fig. 12.10 Severe, end-stage ulcerations in a patient with scleroderma-like GVHD

Summary

Reports describing atypical presentations of GVHD generally describe small numbers of patients, limiting our understanding of the pathogenesis of these presentations and their significance with respect to disease course and prognosis. Some subjectivity also exists in regard to classifying these manifestations, and in cases that mimic other disorders, there is an assumption that a single disease process exists. However, it is possible that two separate diseases, one of which is GVHD, co-exist at the same location, altering the clinical appearance. Or, one disease may develop and then induce GVHD at the same site. Complex mechanisms, including not only the Koebner phenomenon, but also the role of viral infections, such as in zosteriform or pityriasis rosea-like GVHD, and epidermal mosaicism, as in Blaschkoid GVHD, may play a role.

Recognizing the many protean manifestations of GVHD presents a diagnostic challenge. Although histologic findings of GVHD can be nonspecific, skin biopsy with close clinicopathologic correlation may enable diagnosis of likely GVHD in these unusual cases. Early recognition and diagnosis of GVHD facilitates initiation of proper management to minimize the morbidity associated with severe or long-standing mucocutaneous disease. This chapter illustrates the importance of maintaining a high index of suspicion when evaluating typical and atypical-appearing rashes in patients with a history of stem cell transplantation.

References

1. Jagasia MH, Greinix HT, Arora M, Williams KM, Wolff D, Cowen EW, et al. National Institutes of Health Consensus Development Project on Criteria for Clinical Trials in Chronic Graft-versus-Host Disease: I. The 2014 Diagnosis and Staging Working Group report. Biol Blood Marrow Transplant. 2015;21(3):389–401.e1.
2. Kuskonmaz B, Gucer S, Boztepe G, Cetin M, Uckan D. Atypical skin graft-vs.-host disease following bone marrow transplantation in an infant. Pediatr Transplant. 2007;11(2):214–6.
3. Cornejo CM, Kim EJ, Rosenbach M, Micheletti RG. Atypical manifestations of graft-versus-host disease. J Am Acad Dermatol. 2015;72(4):690–5.
4. Hymes SR, Turner ML, Champlin RE, Couriel DR. Cutaneous manifestations of chronic graft-versus-host disease. Biol Blood Marrow Transplant. 2006;12(11):1101–13.
5. Hymes SR, Alousi AM, Cowen EW. Graft-versus-host disease: part I. Pathogenesis and clinical manifestations of graft-versus-host disease. J Am Acad Dermatol. 2012;66(4):515.e1–515.e18.
6. Wei J, Zhang Y, Xu H, Jin J, Zhang J. Atopic dermatitis-like presentation of graft-versus-host disease: a novel form of chronic cutaneous graft-versus-host disease. J Am Acad Dermatol. 2013;69(1):34–9.
7. Cohen EW. Graft-versus-host disease. In: Bolognia JL, Jorizzo JL, Scaffer JV, editors. Dermatology. 3rd ed. New York: Elsevier; 2012. p. 755.
8. Creamer D, Martyn-Simmons CL, Osborne G, Kenyon M, Salisbury JR, Devereux S, et al. Eczematoid graft-vs-host disease: a novel form of chronic cutaneous graft-vs-host disease and its response to psoralen UV-A therapy. Arch Dermatol. 2007;143(9):1157–62.
9. Taguchi S, Kawachi Y, Fujisawa Y, Nakamura Y, Furuta J, Otsuka F. Psoriasiform eruption associated with graft-versus-host disease. Cutis. 2013;92(3):151–3.
10. Matsushita T, Hasegawa M, Shirasaki F, Fujimoto M, Yamazaki H, Sato S, et al. A case of acute cutaneous graft-versus-host disease mimicking psoriasis vulgaris. Dermatology. 2008;216(1):64–7.
11. Kawakami Y, Oyama N, Nakamura K, Kaneko F, Kikuta A, Suzuki H. Psoriasiform eruption associated with graft-versus-host disease. Acta Derm Venereol. 2007;87(5):436–8.
12. Kim SJ, Choi JM, Kim JE, Cho BK, Kim DW, Park HJ. Clinicopathologic characteristics of cutaneous chronic graft-versus-host diseases: a retrospective study in Korean patients. Int J Dermatol. 2010;49(12):1386–92.
13. Surjana D, Robertson I, Kennedy G, James D, Weedon D. Acute cutaneous graft-versus-host disease resembling type II (atypical adult) pityriasis rubra pilaris. Australas J Dermatol. 2013;56(1):e21–3.
14. Spelman LJ, Robertson IM, Strutton GM, Weedon D. Pityriasis rosea-like eruption after bone marrow transplantation. J Am Acad Dermatol. 1994;31(2 Pt 2):348–51.
15. Chao SC, Tsao CJ, Liu CL, Lee JY. Acute cutaneous graft-versus-host disease with ichthyosiform features. Br J Dermatol. 1998;139(3):553–5.
16. Huang J, Pol-Rodriguez M, Silvers D, Garzon MC. Acquired ichthyosis as a manifestation of acute cutaneous graft-versus-host disease. Pediatr Dermatol. 2007;24(1):49–52.
17. Doherty C, Ulitsky O, Petronic-Rosic V. Erythema multiforme-like presentation of chronic graft versus host disease. J Am Acad Dermatol. 2008;59(5 Suppl):S127–8.
18. Friedman KJ, LeBoit PE, Farmer ER. Acute follicular graft-vs-host reaction. A distinct clinicopathologic presentation. Arch Dermatol. 1988;124(5):688–91.
19. Lycka BA, Kaye VN. Acute follicular graft-vs-host disease. Arch Dermatol. 1988;124(9):1442.
20. Tani M, Adachi A. Acute follicular graft-versus-host disease. Dermatology. 1992;185(4):281–3.
21. Ahn HS, Park HJ, Lee JY, Cho BK. A case of chronic cutaneous graft versus host disease with the clinical features of exfoliative dermatitis. Ann Dermatol. 2009;21(3):319–22.
22. Nambudiri VE, Tsiaras WG, Schmidt BA, Huang JT. Total leukoderma and leukotrichia in a child after hematopoietic SCT: report of a case and review of the literature. Bone Marrow Transplant. 2014;49(3):460–2.
23. Marti N, Martin JM, Monteagudo C, Lopez V, Jorda E. Follicular graft-versus-host disease: a rare manifestation of chronic cutaneous graft-versus-host disease. Am J Dermatopathol. 2008;30(6):620–1.
24. Valks R, Vargas E, Fraga J, Penas PF, Fernandez-Herrera J. A follicular lichenoid eruption as manifestation of chronic graft-vs-host disease. Acta Derm Venereol. 1998;78(5):386.
25. Miyazaki K, Higaki S, Maruyama T, Takahashi S, Morohashi M, Ito K. Chronic graft-versus-host disease with follicular involvement. J Dermatol. 1993;20(4):242–6.
26. Llamas-Velasco M, Solano-López Morel GE, Gruber-Wackernagel A, Concha-Garzón MJ, Requena L, Cerroni L. Comedonal graft-vs-host disease: a distinct clinical expression of a lichenoid follicular GVHD. J Cutan Pathol. 2014;41(11):853–8.
27. Chow RKP, Steward WD, Ho VC. Graft-versus-host reaction affecting lesional skin but not normal skin in a patient with piebaldism. Br J Dermatol. 1996;134(1):134–7.
28. Kossard S, Ma DD. Acral keratotic graft versus host disease simulating warts. Australas J Dermatol. 1999;40(3):161–3.
29. Adamski H, Le Gall F, Cartron L, Dauriac C, Lancien G, Wechsler J, et al. Eruptive angiomatous lesions associated with graft-versus-host disease. Br J Dermatol. 2003;149(3):667–8.

30. Kaffenberger BH, Zuo RC, Gru A, Plotner AN, Sweeney SA, Devine SM, et al. Graft-versus-host disease-associated angiomatosis: a clinicopathologically distinct entity. J Am Acad Dermatol. 2014;71(4):745–53.
31. Garnis S, Billick RC, Srolovitz H. Eruptive vascular tumors associated with chronic graft-versus-host disease. J Am Acad Dermatol. 1984;10(5 Pt 2):918–21.
32. Barnadas MA, Brunet S, Sureda A, López R, Curell R, Sierra J, et al. Exuberant granulation tissue associated with chronic graft-versus-host disease after transplantation of peripheral blood progenitor cells. J Am Acad Dermatol. 1999;41(5 Suppl):876–9.
33. Soo JK, Mortimer PS. Eruptive angiomas associated with graft-versus-host disease. Br J Dermatol. 2006;154(2):376–8.
34. Hu SW, Myskowski PL, Papadopoulos EB, Busam KJ. Chronic cutaneous graft-versus-host disease simulating hypertrophic lupus erythematosus-a case report of a new morphologic variant of graft-versus-host disease. Am J Dermatopathol. 2012;34(6):e81–3.
35. Goiriz R, Penas PF, Delgado-Jimenez Y, Fernandez-Herrera J, Aragues-Montanes M, Fraga J, et al. Cutaneous lichenoid graft-versus-host disease mimicking lupus erythematosus. Lupus. 2008;17(6):591–5.
36. Ollivier I, Wolkenstein P, Gherardi R, Wechsler J, Kuentz M, Cosnes A, et al. Dermatomyositis-like graft-versus-host disease. Br J Dermatol. 1998;138(3):558–9.
37. Vassallo C, Derlino F, Ripamonti F, Borroni G. Lichenoid cutaneous chronic GVHD following Blaschko lines. Int J Dermatol. 2014;53(4):473–5.
38. Beers B, Kalish RS, Kaye VN, Dahl MV. Unilateral linear lichenoid eruption after bone marrow transplantation: an unmasking of tolerance to an abnormal keratinocyte clone? J Am Acad Dermatol. 1993;28(5 Pt 2):888–92.
39. Cohen PR, Hymes SR. Linear and dermatomal cutaneous graft-versus-host disease. South Med J. 1994;87(7):758–61.
40. Freemer CS, Farmer ER, Corio RL, Altomonte VL, Wagner JE, Vogelsang GB, et al. Lichenoid chronic graft-vs-host disease occurring in a dermatomal distribution. Arch Dermatol. 1994; 130(1):70–2.
41. Lee SW, Kim YC, Lee E, Kang HY. Linear lichenoid graft versus host disease: an unsual configuration following Blaschko's lines. J Dermatol. 2006;33(8):583–4.
42. Kennedy FE, Hilari H, Ferrer B, Garcia-Patos V. Lichenoid chronic graft-vs-host disease following Blaschko lines. Actas Dermosifiliogr. 2014;105(1):89–92.
43. Kikuchi A, Okamoto S, Takahashi S, Asano S, Nishikawa T. Linear chronic cutaneous graft-versus-host disease. J Am Acad Dermatol. 1997;37(6):1004–6.
44. Wilson BB, Lockman DW. Linear lichenoid graft-vs-host disease. Arch Dermatol. 1994;130(9):1206–8.
45. Anli H, Anadolu R, Arat M, Ekmekci P, Birol A, Erdem C, et al. Dermatomal lichenoid graft-versus-host disease within herpes zoster scars. Int J Dermatol. 2003;42(7):562–4.
46. Martires KJ, Baird K, Citrin DE, Hakim FT, Pavletic SZ, Cowen EW. Localization of sclerotic-type chronic graft-vs-host disease to sites of skin injury: potential insight into the mechanism of isomorphic and isotopic responses. Arch Dermatol. 2011;147(9):1081–6.
47. White JML, Creamer D, Du Vivier AWP, Pagliuca A, Ho AY, Devereux S, et al. Sclerodermatous graft-versus-host disease: clinical spectrum and therapeutic challenges. Br J Dermatol. 2007; 156(5):1032–8.
48. Baselga E, Drolet BA, Segura AD, Leonardi CL, Esterly NB. Dermatomal lichenoid chronic graft-vs-host disease following varicella-zoster infection despite absence of viral genome. J Cutan Pathol. 1996;23(6):576–81.
49. Lacour JP, Sirvent N, Monpoux F, Perrin C, Castanet J, Michel G, et al. Dermatotmal chronic cutaneous graft-versus-host disease at the site of prior herpes zoster. Br J Dermatol. 1999;141(3):587–9.
50. Cordoba S, Fraga J, Bartolome B, Garcia-Diez A, Fernandez-Herrera J. Giant cell lichenoid dermatitis within herpes zoster scars in a bone marrow recipient. J Cutan Pathol. 2000;27(5):255–7.
51. Hymes SR, Hood AF, Farmer ER. Graft-versus-host disease. In: Jordan RE, editor. East Norwalk: Appleton & Lange; 1991. p. 509–23.
52. Palacios-Alvarez I, Santos-Briz A, Jorge-Finnigan C, Cañueto J, Fernandez-López E, Roman-Curto C. Chronic cutaneous lichenoid graft-versus-host disease at the area of herpes zoster infection and at a vaccination site. Br J Dermatol. 2015;173(4):1050–3.
53. Reisfeld PL. Lichenoid chronic graft-vs-host disease. Arch Dermatol. 1994;130(9):1207.
54. Chosidow O, Bagot M, Vernant JP, Roujeau JC, Cordonnier C, Kuentz M, et al. Sclerodermatous chronic graft-versus-host disease. Analysis of seven cases. J Am Acad Dermatol. 1992;26(1):49–55.
55. Mehra T, Metzler G, Bauer J, Koberle M, Garbe C. Isotopic response of graft versus host disease following herpes zoster infection: case report and review of the literature. Acta Derm Venereol. 2012;92(4):383–4.
56. Raymond AK, Singletary HL, Nelson K, Sidhu-Malik NK. Dermatomal sclerodermoid graft-vs-host disease following varicella-zoster virus infection. Arch Dermatol. 2011;147(9):1122–3.
57. Fenyk JRJ, Smith CM, Warkentin PI, Krivit W, Goltz RW, Neely JE, et al. Sclerodermatous graft-versus-host disease limited to an area of measles exanthem. Lancet. 1978;1(8062):472–3.
58. Alexander LJ, Paravar T, Duvic M, Prieto V, Hymes SR. Annular plaques: an unusual manifestation of graft-versus-host disease. Dermatol Online J. 2012;18(6):4.
59. Patel AR, Pavletic SZ, Turner ML, Cowen EW. The isomorphic response in morphealike chronic graft-vs-host disease. Arch Dermatol. 2008;144(9):1229–31.
60. Schaffer JV, McNiff JM, Seropian S, Cooper DL, Bolognia JL. Lichen sclerosus and eosinophilic fasciitis as manifestations of chronic graft-versus-host disease: expanding the sclerodermoid spectrum. J Am Acad Dermatol. 2005;53(4):591–601.
61. White JML, Devereux S, Pagliuca A, Salisbury JR, Du Vivier AWP, Creamer D. Koebnerizing sclerodermatous graft-versus-host disease caused by donor lymphocyte infusion and interferon? Br J Dermatol. 2006;155(3):621–3.
62. Girault PY, Waton J, Barbaud A, Bordigoni P, Schmutz JL. Isomorphic disposition of chronic graft-versus-host disease in striae distensae. J Eur Acad Dermatol Venereol. 2009;23(5):574–5.
63. Okamoto S, Takahashi S, Inoue T, Tojo A, Tani K, Kikuchi A, et al. Cutaneous chronic graft-versus-host disease localized to the field of total lymphoid irradiation. Bone Marrow Transplant. 1996;17(1):111–3.
64. Socie G, Gluckman E, Cosset JM, Devergie A, Girinski T, Esperou H, et al. Unusual localization of cutaneous chronic graft-versus-host disease in the radiation fields in four cases. Bone Marrow Transplant. 1989;4(1):133–5.
65. Zwaan FE, Jansen J, Noordijk EM. Graft-versus-host disease limited to an area of irradiated skin. Lancet. 1980;315(8177):1081–2.
66. Vassallo C, Brazzelli V, Zecca M, Locatelli F, Alessandrino P, Borroni G. Isomorphic cutaneous graft-versus-host disease reaction after ultraviolet exposure: clinical, histological and direct immunofluorescence studies of four allo-transplanted patients. J Eur Acad Dermatol Venereol. 2009;23(8):913–8.
67. Nagler A, Goldenhersh MA, Levi-Schaffer F, Bystryn JC, Klaus SN. Total leucoderma: a rare manifestation of cutaneous chronic graft-versus-host disease. Br J Dermatol. 1996;134(4):780–3.
68. Jacobsohn DA, Ruble K, Moresi JM, Vogelsang GB. Rapid-onset leucoderma associated with graft-versus-host disease. Bone Marrow Transplant. 2002;30(10):705–6.
69. Man J, Kalisiak M, Birchall IW, Salopek TG. Chronic cutaneous graft-versus-host disease manifesting as calcinosis cutis universalis on a background of widespread sclerodermatoid changes. J Cutan Med Surg. 2010;14(5):249–53.

70. Hymes S, Farmer ER, Burns WH, Morison WL, Tutschka PJ, Walters LL, et al. Bullous sclerodermalike changes in chronic graft-vs-host disease. Arch Dermatol. 1985;121:1189–92.
71. Jachiet M, de Masson A, Peffault de Latour R, Rybojad M, Robin M, Bourhis J, et al. Skin ulcers related to chronic graft-versus-host disease: clinical findings and associated morbidity. Br J Dermatol. 2014;171(1):63–8.
72. Ammer J, Prantl L, Holler B, Landfried K, Wolff D, Karrer S, et al. Successful treatment of a refractory skin ulcer in chronic cutaneous GvHD after allogeneic HSCT with split-thickness skin allografting from the stem cell donor. Bone Marrow Transplant. 2012; 47(10):1368–9.
73. Knobler HY, Sagher U, Peled IJ, Wexler MR, Steiner D, Rubinstein N, et al. Tolerance to donor-type skin in the recipient of a bone marrow allograft. Treatment of skin ulcers in chronic graft-versus-host disease with skin grafts from the bone marrow donor. Transplantation. 1985;40(2):223–5.
74. Kondo S, Tamura K, Makino S, Takamatsu Y. Allogeneic skin grafting for extensive skin chronic graft-versus-host disease. Int J Hematol. 1994;60(2):151–5.
75. Kamei Y, Torii S, Hasegawa M, Toriyama K, Kodera Y. Simultaneous allografting and autografting of skin for ulcers in a bone marrow transplant patient. Transplantation. 1993;56(6):1530–1.
76. Berg JO, Vindelov L, Schmidt G, Drzewiecki KT. Allogeneic split-skin grafting in stem cell transplanted patients. J Plast Reconstr Aesthet Surg. 2008;61(12):1512–5.
77. Caffee HH, Miller TA. Skin rejection in graft-versus-host disease. Plast Reconstr Surg. 1978;61(5):753–5.
78. Crocchiolo R, Nicolini FE, Sobh M, Ducastelle-Lepretre S, Labussiere H, Dubois V, et al. Treatment of a severe extensive cutaneous chronic GVHD after allo-HSCT using glycerolyzed skin allografts and cultured epidermis from the same donor. Bone Marrow Transplant. 2011;46(8):1153–5.
79. Storb R, Thomas ED, Buckner CD, Clift RA, Fefer A, Fernando LP, et al. Allogeneic marrow grafting for treatment of aplastic anemia: a follow-up on long-term survivors. Blood. 1976;48(4): 485–90.
80. Cook-Norris RHWR. Eczematoid graft-vs-host disease. Arch Dermatol. 2008;144(8):1066.
81. Schauder CS, Hymes SR, Rapini RP, Zipf TF. Vesicular graft-versus-host disease. Int J Dermatol. 1992;31(7):509–10.
82. Arin MJ, Scheid C, Hübel K, Krieg T, Groth W, Haerrmann G. Chronic graft-versus-host disease with skin signs suggestive of dermatomyositis. Clin Exp Dermatol. 2006;31(1):141–3.
83. Kawano N, Gondo H, Kamimura T, Aoki K, Iino T, Ishikawa F, et al. Chronic graft-versus-host disease following varicella-zoster virus infection in allogeneic stem cell transplant recipients. Int J Hematol. 2003;78(4):370–3.
84. Korth J, Tischer J, Samtleben W, Weiss C, Ruzicka T, Wollenberg A. Isotopic response, Köbner phenomenon and Renbök phenomenon following herpes zoster. J Dermatol. 2011;38(11): 1058–61.
85. Ruocco V, Brunetti G, Puca R, Ruocco E. The immunocompromised district: a unifying concept for lymphoedematous, herpes-infected and otherwise damaged sites. J Eur Acad Dermatol Venereol. 2009;23(12):1364–73.
86. Akay BN, Sanli H, Topcuoglu P, Zincircioglu G, Gurgan C, Heper AO. Black hairy tongue after allogeneic stem cell transplantation: an unrecognized cutaneous presentation of graft-versus-host disease. Transplant Proc. 2010;42(10):4603–7.

Index

J.A. Cotliar (ed.), *Atlas of Graft-versus-Host Disease*, DOI 10.1007/978-3-319-46952-2

D

E

F

G

The manufacturer's authorised representative in the EU is Springer
Nature Customer Service Centre GmbH, Europaplatz 3, 69115 Heidelberg,
Germany. If you have any concerns regarding our products, please
contact ProductSafety@springernature.com

Printed and bound by CPI Group (UK) Ltd, Croydon, CR0 4YY
26/09/2026
02222871-0006